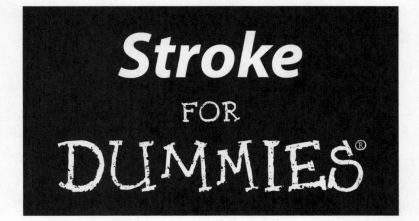

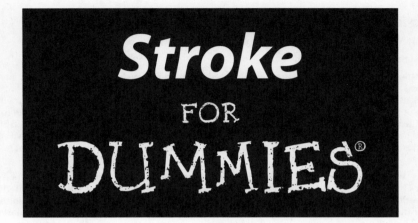

Stroke FOR DUMMIES®

by John R. Marler, MD

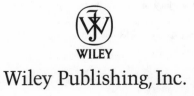

WILEY

Wiley Publishing, Inc.

Stroke For Dummies®

Published by
Wiley Publishing, Inc.
111 River St.
Hoboken, NJ 07030-5774
www.wiley.com

WILEY

About the Author

John R. Marler, MD (Bethesda, Maryland), a board-certified neurologist and stroke researcher, is Associate Director for Clinical Trials at the National Institute of Neurological Disorders and Stroke. He is a fellow of the American Stroke Association and recipient of the association's Feinberg Award for Excellence in Clinical Research. He has been administering clinical research in stroke since 1984. He completed his neurology residency training at Mayo Clinic in Rochester, Minnesota and graduated from West Virginia University Medical School in Morgantown, West Virginia.

Dedication

This book is dedicated to participants in clinical research who are leading the way toward new opportunities to treat stroke.

Author's Acknowledgments

This book could not have been produced without the help of Corbin Collins, editor, and Betsy Sheldon, writer, who took me step by step from rough draft to finished product. I thank them for their insights and suggestions. Likewise, Kathryn Born's illustrations are remarkable for their clarity and precision. I couldn't respect any stroke clinician any more than I do the technical editor, J. Donald Easton, MD. His comments have added greatly to this book. I want to thank Sandra Sewell, RN, at Suburban Hospital in Bethesda, Maryland, who helped me understand many of the difficulties faced by stroke patients and their families after hospitalization. Mary Dombovy, MD, MHSA, Unity Health System in Rochester, New York, took the time to talk with me about the basic approach to stroke recovery and rehabilitation. Jeffrey Saver, MD, at the UCLA Stroke Center, along with his colleagues David S. Liebeskind, MD and Reza Jahan, MD, provided the CT and MR images for the figures in the book. And last but far from least, there is Kathy Cox at Wiley whose dare got me to start this project in the first place and whose patience and encouragement motivated me to finish. Thank you all.

Publisher's Acknowledgments

We're proud of this book; please send us your comments through our Dummies online registration form located at www.dummies.com/register/.

Some of the people who helped bring this book to market include the following:

Acquisitions, Editorial, and Media Development

Editor: Corbin Collins

Acquisitions Editor: Kathy Cox

Technical Editor: J. Donald Easton, MD

Editorial Manager: Michelle Hacker

Editorial Supervisor and Reprint Editor: Carmen Krikorian

Editorial Assistants: Hanna Scott, Melissa Bennett

Cover Photos: Barros & Barros/Getty Images/ The Image Bank

Cartoons: Rich Tennant (www.the5thwave.com)

Composition Services

Project Coordinator: Maridee Ennis

Layout and Graphics: Carl Byers, Andrea Dahl, Kelly Emkow, Lauren Goddard, Joyce Haughey, Stephanie D. Jumper

Special Art: Kathryn Born

Proofreaders: Leeann Harney, Joe Niesen, Carl William Pierce, TECHBOOKS Production Services

Indexer: TECHBOOKS Production Services

Special Help: Betsy Sheldon, Patricia Harrington

Publishing and Editorial for Consumer Dummies

Diane Graves Steele, Vice President and Publisher, Consumer Dummies

Joyce Pepple, Acquisitions Director, Consumer Dummies

Kristin A. Cocks, Product Development Director, Consumer Dummies

Michael Spring, Vice President and Publisher, Travel

Kelly Regan, Editorial Director, Travel

Publishing for Technology Dummies

Andy Cummings, Vice President and Publisher, Dummies Technology/General User

Composition Services

Gerry Fahey, Vice President of Production Services

Debbie Stailey, Director of Composition Services

Contents at a Glance

Table of Contents

Introduction

*W*elcome to *Stroke For Dummies*.

In a nutshell: *Stroke* is the often severely damaging result of a sudden interruption of blood to part of the brain, whether due to a blockage or bleeding.
Stroke's impact on the brain can be catastrophic, causing paralysis, loss of
speech, loss of memory, and, of course, death in as many as 30 percent of
those who experience stroke.

Stroke is serious stuff. If you have one, you want to get to the emergency
room as fast as possible and begin treatment. If you survive one, you want to
recover as fully as possible and do everything in your power to *never* have
one again. Helping you achieve these things is what this book is about.

About This Book

This book is full of useful information to help you understand the who-what-
where-when-why-and-how of stroke. Information is critical in helping you get
the most out of stroke treatment, recovery, and adjustment to life after stroke.
And, most importantly, information is essential in helping you prevent future
stroke. But it's worthless if it's so technical you can't understand it. That's
why I wrote this book.

Stroke For Dummies explains stroke in a simple, straightforward manner,
guiding you through a complex field of knowledge with a minimum of technical vocabulary and a maximum of fundamental facts needed to understand
this medical condition and take action. The difficult issues are presented
unflinchingly — I don't soft-pedal the cold, hard facts. Stroke is scary. The
better you understand that, the more fervently you'll pursue a focused and
effective course of prevention.

Stroke For Dummies offers well-tested, clinically proven courses of action for
treatment and prevention of stroke. I spend my life trying to find out which
treatments for stroke and other brain diseases really work. You can count on
the fact that every treatment mentioned in this book is proven, unless I state
otherwise.

Still, every treatment plan poses risks, and doctors don't agree on everything. Your doctor may not agree that certain treatments described in this

book will work for you. This is to be expected and doesn't mean that either one of us is wrong. The point here is to gather as much good information as possible to help you make the best choices for you.

Stroke For Dummies is not a do-it-yourself book — I do not recommend any specific treatment plan but, instead, offer general information for you to discuss with your physician. Each individual is unique and must develop a customized approach to stroke in partnership with an experienced doctor. This book gives you the basic knowledge you need to be an effective partner in that relationship.

Conventions Used in This Book

The following conventions are used throughout the text to make things consistent and easy to understand:

- New terms appear in *italics* and are closely followed by an easy-to-understand definition.
- **Bold** is used to highlight the action parts of numbered steps or keywords in bulleted lists.
- Sidebars, which are enclosed in a shaded gray box, include information that may intrigue you but isn't critical to your understanding of stroke.
- Case studies, set off like sidebars but with a "Case Study" icon, present summarized accounts of fairly typical stroke victims.

What You're Not to Read

You can safely skip the case studies in this book and still understand the topic at hand. The case studies are merely meant to illustrate and dramatize some aspect of stroke or stroke prevention or care. Some may find them helpful, but they are not essential to understanding the basics of stroke as discussed here.

Likewise, if you came to this book to understand a particular type of stroke that you or a loved one has had, don't waste time boning up on the other kinds of stroke described in Part II. Many aspects of stroke and its accompanying events and treatments are time sensitive. This book is designed to make it as easy as possible to get in and get out with as much specific and easy-to-digest information as you need depending on your particular circumstances.

Finally, the "Jargon Alert" icon may warn you of impending Latin tongue-twisters, but in many cases you will have to grit your teeth and read the material in the indicated paragraphs in order to get a full understanding of the discussion. Due to the nature of the topic of stroke, some technical terms are unavoidable, and if stroke has touched your life or that of a loved one, you will be glad to have absorbed a few of these when it comes time to discuss the stroke and possible treatments.

Foolish Assumptions

It's unlikely that someone would pick up a book like this at random. Here is what I assume about you — that you fall into one of three categories:

- ✔ You've recently suffered a stroke and are now on the road to recovery. Perhaps you're re-learning to walk. Or talk. Or button your shirt. You seek an easy-to-understand resource that can shed light on your new circumstances.

- ✔ You are a spouse or family member of a stroke survivor who wants to learn as much as possible so you can be a better caregiver.

- ✔ You returned recently from a visit to your doctor and learned that your high blood pressure, high LDL blood cholesterol, and extra weight put you on a path toward something called stroke and you want to learn more about it.

Or maybe you picked up this book by mistake because you thought it had something to do with golf. In that case, I can't help you.

In any event, now that I have your attention, I hope to persuade you to continue reading. *Stroke is the number three cause of death in the United States.* This book could very well save your life — or the life of a loved one. At the very least, *Stroke For Dummies* can enlighten you about the recovery and treatment process and help you avoid future strokes.

How This Book Is Organized

Stroke For Dummies is organized into six parts. The chapters within each part cover specific topic areas in detail. Because I've structured the book this way, you can easily find the topic you're looking for. Check out the Table of Contents or the Index for your general area of interest and then find the chapter that concerns your particular needs.

Part I: The Brain and Stroke

I begin with some rudimentary background on stroke and how and why it happens. The basic principles of stroke are quite simple, but often get obscured by the terminology used by doctors to describe it. I've tried to simplify the explanations so that you can understand what you are told by or what you may overhear from your medical team. I begin in Chapter 1 by describing exactly what happens when you have a stroke. In Chapter 2, I offer a basic biology lesson in the workings of your brain and what happens when things go wrong.

Part II: Types of Stroke

For simplicity, I break stroke down into five types, stemming from two major causes. The most common cause of stroke is a blood clot blocking an artery to or inside the brain — I call these white strokes because they involve a *lack* of blood. The other cause is bleeding inside the skull, either inside or outside of the brain — I call these red strokes.

Chapters 3, 4, and 7 cover different types of white strokes, and Chapters 5 and 6 deal with the two kinds of red strokes. It's important to know which type of stroke one is dealing with, because treatment is different for each. For each type, I present the causes, what actually occurs during it, symptoms, risks, how to treat — and how to prevent.

Bear in mind that my "red" and "white" distinction is my own invention. I believe it helps to visualize what is happening in the brain. Of course, I also give you all types of technical terms for each type of stroke and explain them as clearly as I can.

Part III: Preventing Stroke

Three chapters are devoted to ways of reducing risk of stroke in the future — whether you've already suffered a stroke or want to maintain your stroke-free record.

Chapter 8 in this part deals with blood pressure, the major risk factor for stroke. I explain how high blood pressure beats down the blood vessels, leading the way for damage and blood clots. Even more importantly, I give you steps you can take to lower your blood pressure.

Chapter 9 addresses another key risk factor for both stroke and heart disease: cholesterol. I discuss the differences between *bad* cholesterol and *good* cholesterol — and how you can change your diet and take action to control your blood cholesterol levels and reduce stroke risk.

Finally, Chapter 10 rounds up other prevention steps that you can take to reduce your chances of having a stroke — or *another* stroke.

Part IV: Treating Stroke

This part focuses on the critical steps required for treating stroke. Chapter 11 is perhaps the most essential — responding *fast* when stroke occurs. Call 911: Stroke is an emergency! The faster you get to the hospital, the more brain you can save. I walk you through the emergency response process, including which actions and procedures are likely to be done. I also offer important advice to the stroke victim and family members — that will help ensure the best care. Chapter 12 deals with the hospital stay and what to expect in terms of care and follow-up testing. And Chapter 13 addresses the rehabilitation process, giving you a sense of what to expect as you make your way along the path toward recovery.

Part V: Living with Stroke

Life after stroke can be daunting for the stroke survivor and family members. It's a culture shock of sorts that involves learning a "language" of adjustment to new limitations and challenges. You will likely have to make changes to familiar routines and, perhaps, compromises to future plans.

Chapters 14 through 17 help you face the changes brought on by stroke, including returning home from the hospital, considering residential placement, confronting the cost implications, wrestling with family dynamics, returning to normal life, and confronting end-of-life issues.

You'll pick up on a recurring theme in this section: the importance of asking for help — whether you are the stroke survivor who must give up driving or a caregiver spouse who needs a support group. Asking for help is often difficult, but failing to do so causes a lot of unnecessary pain and impedes recovery.

Part VI: The Part of Tens

In these short and sweet chapters, I offer helpful information that I hope will enhance your understanding of the consequences of stroke and motivate you to do your part to take care of yourself — and others.

Chapter 18 offers ideas for helping your community manage stroke. I especially like Chapter 19, about the notable personalities who've contributed to the world — despite their history of stroke. From presidents to beauty queens, from authors to actors, stroke survivors have proven that productive life isn't over with the onset of stroke. Chapter 20 lists concrete steps you can take to improve your personal stroke care and prevent stroke. The last chapter is a glossary of terms — anytime you feel confused or unsure about a technical term, check the glossary for a quick definition.

Icons Used in This Book

Icons are handy little graphic images meant to point out particularly important information about stroke. You'll find the following icons in this book, conveniently located along the left margins.

This icon points out stroke stories that illustrate a point and help you recognize stroke issues in yourself and others. They are technically fictional and don't identify any single patient, but they are based on typical stroke events. They are similar to stories doctors hear over and over as they see the hundreds of stroke patients that come to their hospitals every year.

This icon alerts you to a paragraph that contains new medical terms in case you're severely allergic to them. The terms will be defined, so don't get too stressed out about it.

Remember these important points of information, if nothing else. In fact, if you've had a stroke, or even if you haven't, it's probably a good idea to write them down to put them on the refrigerator or bathroom mirror.

This icon directs you to helpful hints or practical advice for taking care of or preventing stroke.

Everything you do to treat, prevent, or recover from stroke may have side effects or complications. Stroke is a very serious disease and surgery and powerful drugs are warranted in many situations. You need to be aware that there can be problems.

Where to Go from Here

Where you go from here depends on why you are reading the book. You can read it cover to cover or look up specific topics of interest in the Table of Contents or Index.

Part I is written for everyone — stroke victims, family members, and any individual committed to protecting good health. It offers a basic understanding of stroke.

In Part II, you may only want to read about the particular type of stroke that is of most immediate concern or interest to you.

Part III is for the whole world. Preventing stroke isn't that hard, especially considering the payoff. And preventing *another* stroke may be absolutely paramount.

If you or a loved one is in the hospital or rehabilitation unit, Part IV is for you.

Part V is for patients, caretakers, and family members struggling with the realities of life after stroke.

Part VI also has something for everyone — particularly the Glossary, which you may find yourself flipping to repeatedly.

If you are a stroke survivor, it is my hope that you will be inspired to maximize your rehabilitation efforts and make the most of your life after stroke. If you are a caregiver, I hope you will increase your understanding of stroke and do what you can to partner in your loved one's adjustment. If you are an individual concerned with preventing stroke, I hope you will make lifestyle changes to reduce your chances of stroke.

And for all readers, I hope that, armed with knowledge bound in this book, you will move forward with a greater appreciation for your brain — its power and its delicacy — and do everything within your capacity to protect it.

Part I
The Brain and Stroke

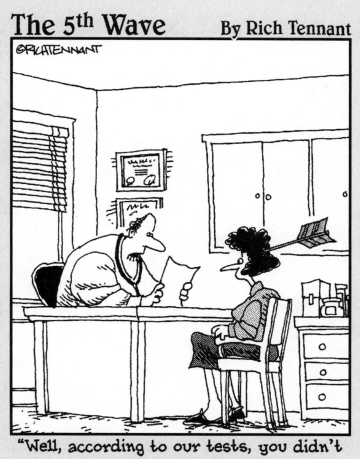

The 5th Wave   By Rich Tennant

"Well, according to our tests, you didn't have a stroke at all."

In this part . . .

*W*hat is stroke, what does it do to the brain — and how and why does it do this? These are a few of the questions I tackle in this part. I begin in Chapter 1 by describing the process and mechanisms of the different kinds of stroke. Chapter 2 covers the basics of how the brain does what it does and how stroke disrupts its natural workings.

Chapter 1

A Brain Attack

*L*et me hit you with the bad news first: Stroke kills, stroke destroys, stroke debilitates. Stroke is the third most common cause of death in the United States, and the number-one cause of serious disability. One year after the most common kind of stroke, approximately 30 percent of those afflicted will have died, and another 30 percent will have a moderate to severe disability.

Now for some good news: Of those who experience the most common type of stroke, approximately 40 percent are left with only a mild or no disability one year later. And each year more people survive and recover from stroke as medical research continues to advance effective treatment. Today, recovery with improvement is the rule rather than the exception.

Stroke is sometimes called a brain attack. I wish this label would catch on, because I think that people might then understand that stroke is an emergency — like a heart attack — and call 911 right away! A heart attack threatens your heart; a stroke threatens your brain. In truth, most stroke *is* like a heart attack: It's a problem with blood vessels, and time is really important. However, heart attack is a little easier to recognize. First of all, the pain tells you something is wrong — and it is usually near your heart. Most strokes are painless, and the symptoms, a paralyzed arm or leg for instance, are not obviously related to the brain.

Clearly, the more you know about stroke — its symptoms, causes, risks, treatment, and prevention — the better your chances of living a full and productive life with or, better yet, without stroke. And the first lesson is to learn what stroke is and how and why stroke occurs.

Real-life examples

A 57-year-old man arrives early at work to prepare for an important presentation he has to make at 10 a.m. At about 9:15 he notices a headache. He thinks this is unusual, because he doesn't have many headaches. He remembers that he did forget his blood pressure medication. He continues to work for a few minutes and then notices his right hand is not working and he can't concentrate. He calls for his assistant who finds him looking very unusual. His mouth is twisted. He starts to talk but his speech is difficult to understand. She asks if he is okay. He says no. He starts to get up but his right arm gives way and he almost falls. His assistant calls 911.

A 68-year-old woman is preparing breakfast for herself and her husband. He has made the coffee and is reading the newspaper. He hears her drop a plate and looks up to see her standing and looking at her left hand. He asks her what's wrong. She says she doesn't know. Her face — particularly the way she is holding her mouth — looks unusual. She keeps looking at her hand. "My hand is numb," she says. He asks her to sit down. She seems confused as he leads her to a chair. He asks if it hurts. She says no. "I think you're having a stroke," he says. He dials 911.

A 38-year-old lawyer is out jogging on a canal towpath. She starts to feel pain in her head that gets worse and worse. She stops, puts her hand to her head, and falls to the ground. A man walking ahead of her sees her fall. He runs to her but she is unconscious. He pulls out his cellphone and dials 911.

If you've already had a stroke, there are many opportunities to reduce the disability that stroke causes and prevent another stroke attack. A serious stroke will affect your entire family. You can fight back together.

Attacking Out of the Blue

Stroke is nothing if not *fast*. Each year, as many as 750,000 people in the United States suffer a sudden and unexpected attack of the brain. When part of the brain is deprived of oxygen — which is what is happening when stroke hits — it doesn't take long for the catastrophe to make itself evident. A minute or less.

Whether it's a sudden inability to speak, the crash of a dish from a hand that can no longer grasp, or loss of consciousness, a brain attack strikes its victims quickly and powerfully and without warning.

Or does it? Although your stroke may occur in a lightning flash, it has most likely been years in the making, with conditions such as high blood pressure, high cholesterol, obesity, and diabetes possibly serving as warning signs that the brain is in danger. Basically, as these conditions cause wear and tear on your blood vessels, your risks increase of suffering either a blockage or rupture of a brain artery. And — suddenly — you're in stroke mode.

So how does it happen? It starts with the brain.

Going to the source: Stroke is in the brain

Because of a number of possible causes — which I explain in detail in this book — part of your brain may be deprived of blood. When that happens, it doesn't take long for your brain to suffer. In a nutshell, the glucose and oxygen transported by one of the brain's arteries are not reaching some part of the brain, which in less than a minute will begin to shut down. And you will show signs of stroke.

The 50 professional groups forming the Brain Attack Coalition describe the signs of stroke as follows:

- ✔ Sudden numbness or weakness of face, arm, or leg, especially on one side of the body
- ✔ Sudden confusion, trouble speaking or understanding speech
- ✔ Sudden trouble seeing in one or both eyes
- ✔ Sudden trouble walking, dizziness, loss of balance or coordination
- ✔ Sudden severe headache with no known cause

Most of the time, a stroke victim feels no pain as the stroke is occurring — so there is not much evidence to clue you in that the reason your hand looks funny and doesn't move when you want is because there's something wrong in your head.

Most people who have a stroke don't know what is happening to them. Most people who see someone who's had a stroke don't know what is happening.

A stroke doesn't hurt (except if a headache accompanies it), and its most obvious effects are far from the brain where the problem is located. This means a lot of people don't recognize they are having a stroke and can't use the opportunities they have to get into the hospital quickly and be treated.

Damage in your brain, symptoms someplace else

So, why is it that a blocked artery in your brain causes you to lose control of your legs and fall to the floor? Suppose a small blood clot forms in your heart and flows with the blood up into your brain and plugs an artery that feeds a part of your brain near the top of your head. Normally, that part of the brain sends nerve impulses down threadlike fibers through the base of your brain and along your spinal cord down to a point a couple of inches below your lowest rib. There those nerve fibers connect to other nerve fibers that extend down to muscles in your legs.

But without blood flow, the affected part of the brain stops sending messages. Your leg muscles only work when they receive messages, so they stop working. But the other parts of your brain that *are* getting oxygen and glucose don't understand that the whole team's not on board and look at the leg in confusion, trying to comprehend why it's not cooperating, not realizing that the problem is right upstairs.

The brain is sensitive to the slightest touch of your skin, but completely insensitive to serious injury to itself. As remarkable as it may seem, the brain is very poor at recognizing when it has been injured. This makes it hard for you to figure out what is going on when you have a stroke.

Responding quickly: Time is brain

Your brain is completely unprepared when blood flow is cut off. The organ is so packed full of knowledge and memories that there is no room in the design for storing sugars and fats that could keep brain cells alive in hard times when blood stops flowing.

Most other cells in the body can survive for up to an hour without blood flow. The brain cells stop working in a matter of seconds and start dying after five minutes.

The brain counts on the heart to do its job. That's why when you have a heart attack it is so important to get the heart restarted quickly. Within seconds after your heart stops, your brain stops working. Within minutes of the heart stopping, the brain is permanently injured and can't recover even if the heart gets going again.

In stroke, you have a *little* more time than in a heart attack. Because the heart keeps pumping, some blood can often get around the obstruction or broken portion of the blood vessels, or seep in from areas of the brain that are still getting blood. *But get yourself to a hospital right away. Call 911.* If you are going to get the best treatment, you need to get to a hospital within 60 minutes.

Recognizing Types of Stroke: Same Symptoms, Different Causes

Doctors can typically identify stroke when a patient comes in with symptoms — they're even pretty good at knowing what part of your brain may be damaged by the stroke just by looking at you. With some scenarios, such as a bursting *aneurysm,* a doctor can guess what caused the stroke. With other cases, it is almost impossible to tell what caused the stroke, although there is little doubt that a stroke is in progress.

Sometimes, with severe headache, for example, it's hard to tell whether a stroke is happening at all because the symptoms are similar to those of a migraine headache. A stroke might cause dizziness that is difficult to distinguish from an inner-ear infection.

Fortunately, testing instruments such as CT or MRI scans can indicate if there is a stroke and what its cause might be.

Red or white: Color-coding stroke types

A friend of mine, a cardiologist, once told me that neurologists make stroke too complicated with their jargon and classification. He said he just thinks of stroke like wine: There's red wine and white wine — and red stroke and white stroke.

What did he mean by this? Basically, some strokes are caused by *broken* blood vessels — which results in blood in the brain or brain area (thus, the *red*); other strokes are caused by the *blockage* of vessels to the brain, so no blood gets there (hence, *white*).

I liked his use of the color-coding and have found that when I talk to patients and their families, this explanation helps them better understand the cause of the stroke and what is happening in the brain. So throughout this book, you'll see that I classify the five major types of stroke into two general categories based on whether they are caused by bleeding (red) or blockage (white).

Oh, don't worry — I promise to give you the complex, hard-to-pronounce terminology, as well! Throughout the book, you will find the most commonly accepted medical terms for the types of stroke.

If you're ready now to track it down in a medical textbook, you'll find out more about red stroke under the term *hemorrhagic* stroke or *intracerebral hemorrhage.* White stroke is covered under the term *ischemic* stroke, *embolic* stroke, or *thrombotic* stroke.

A stroke by any other name

Stroke means that part of your brain has suddenly stopped working because of a problem with its blood supply. It may help to think of strokes caused by blockage as *white* strokes; they're most typically referred to as *ischemic* strokes by doctors. But here are some other names for this type of stroke:

occlusive stroke

cerebrovascular accident (CVA)

acute ischemic stroke

atherothrombotic stroke

embolic stroke

small vessel stroke

lacunar stroke

large vessel stroke

cardioembolic stroke

Ischemic stroke and *CVA* are probably the most common terms used. Doctors usually know what all these terms mean and use them each in different situations to mean virtually the same thing. "Little white stroke" and "big white stroke" could probably replace all these fine technical terms just as well, and everyone would know exactly what they meant.

I refer to strokes caused by bleeding in or around the brain as *red* strokes. Names for these types of stroke are equally varied:

subarachnoid hemorrhage (SAH)

intracranial hemorrhage

intracerebral hemorrhage (ICH)

brain bleeding

brain hemorrhage

Understanding white stroke

As you age, your blood pressure, diet, and the ravages of time roughen the fragile lining of your blood vessels and heart.

Your blood-vessel lining is like the coating on your best cookware — it keeps your blood from sticking and clotting. However, as you approach senior status, that Teflon-like protection starts breaking down, and your vessels develop spots where blood and other buildup stick to them.

Blood clots block blood to the brain

The most common sign of blood-vessel damage is *atherosclerosis,* also known as *hardening of the arteries,* the condition in which a rough, scarred area called a *plaque* forms because of high blood pressure and high fat content in your blood. (There is more about atherosclerosis in the Glossary and in Chapter 9.) The roughness makes it more likely that blood inside your arteries will form clots that can block arteries in the brain or break up into smaller pieces that are carried downstream to lodge in small brain arteries. Sometimes blood clots can break off and flow downstream to form a blockage somewhere else, called an *embolism* (see Figure 1-1 for illustrations of atherosclerosis, blood clots, and embolism).

Figure 1-1:
Plaque building up in the blood vessel causes a blood clot to form, which can block an artery and cause a stroke. Clots can also travel and block vessels downstream.

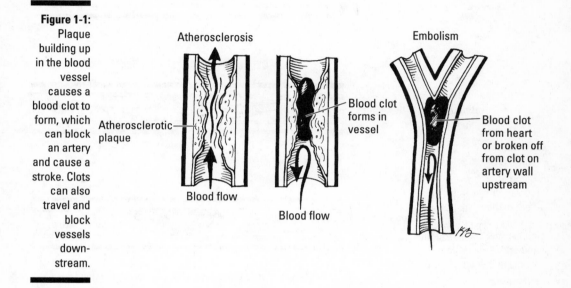

Atherosclerosis

Embolism

Atherosclerotic plaque

Blood clot forms in vessel

Blood clot from heart or broken off from clot on artery wall upstream

Blood flow

Blood flow

 JARGON ALERT

If the clot blocks blood to a part of your brain, you have a stroke. If the clot stays in place for even a short time, part of your brain dies, leaving a hole called a brain *infarction*. The affected area of brain turns from pink to white because there is no red blood flowing (another good reason to refer to this type of stroke as *white*).

Dissection: Blood vessel lining splits

White ischemic strokes are also caused by *dissection*. No, this doesn't mean somebody is practicing brain surgery on you. *Dissection* refers to the splitting of the blood vessel lining, typically occurring at a place where the blood vessel bends back and forth, such as in your neck. It can also happen where *atherosclerotic plaque* has built up in a brain artery. At the bend point or at the rough surface of atherosclerosis, a little flap of the vessel lining peels off and catches the blood as it flows quickly past. The blood dives under the flap and keeps tearing it. Eventually the blood can pack the lining against the other side of the vessel and stop blood flow completely. When the blood stops flowing, a white stroke occurs. Figure 1-2 shows how dissection causes stroke.

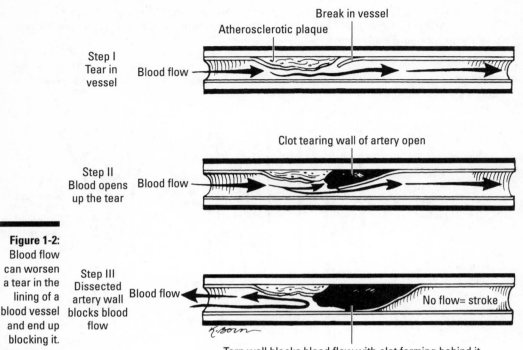

Break in vessel

Atherosclerotic plaque

Step I
Tear in
vessel

Blood flow →

Clot tearing wall of artery open

Step II
Blood opens
up the tear

Blood flow →

Figure 1-2:
Blood flow
can worsen
a tear in the
lining of a
blood vessel
and end up
blocking it.

Step III
Dissected
artery wall
blocks blood
flow

Blood flow →

No flow= stroke

Torn wall blocks blood flow with clot forming behind it

Transient strokes: Just as serious

White ischemic strokes may last just a couple of minutes and then clear completely. If the blood clot breaks up right away, the stroke is *transient* — so fleeting that no permanent tissue death occurred. These transient strokes are officially called *transient ischemic attacks.* Try to say that ten times fast. Doctors abbreviate it as *TIA.*

I don't like the term TIA or what it stands for because it doesn't tell you plainly that you had a stroke. A stroke is very serious even if it is transient, and you still need to consider it a medical emergency requiring a rapid response. After a TIA stroke, your next stroke may *not* be transient and you need to get busy to prevent it from happening. It could happen tomorrow.

You can have more than one transient ischemic stroke. As the number of these small strokes add up, your brain can just slow down generally, and you can suffer from dementia, as each small stroke erodes away more of your brain. Small white ischemic stroke dementia is often called *vascular dementia* or *vascular cognitive impairment.* This is the death of the brain by a thousand cuts.

Getting a handle on red stroke

Blood vessels can break and bleed into or around the brain, causing some of the most serious and deadly strokes. These type of strokes may result in similar symptoms to white stokes — although some are unique to red stroke — but in many cases, they should be treated differently.

Bleeding within the brain

A stroke caused by a blood vessel that breaks inside the substance of the brain is called _intracerebral hemorrhage, brain hemorrhage,_ or _brain bleeding._ The brain goes from pink to red. Hence, the term _red stroke._ The vessels that bleed are often damaged extensively by high blood pressure or diabetes (Figure 1-3). The blood vessels have thick, fibrous, but weak walls. They form little _blebs_ — bubble-like growths — from time to time. These brain vessels are very prone to break, especially when blood pressure is high.

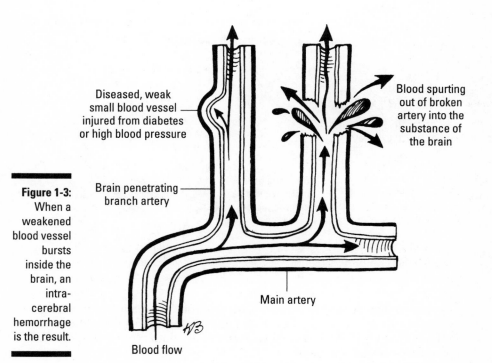

Figure 1-3: When a weakened blood vessel bursts inside the brain, an intra-cerebral hemorrhage is the result.

Diseased, weak small blood vessel injured from diabetes or high blood pressure

Blood spurting out of broken artery into the substance of the brain

Brain penetrating branch artery

Main artery

Blood flow

Bleeding around the brain

Sometimes red — or hemorrhagic — strokes are caused by bleeding just outside the brain, but still inside the skull (Figure 1-4). This type of red stroke is known as *subarachnoid hemorrhage.* The most common cause in this case is a little peanut or marble-sized bubble or pouch that forms at a Y-junction in a brain-bound artery. This bubble is called an *aneurysm.* It has tough, thin, rubbery walls and may actually be present for years before it starts causing trouble. Some never do cause trouble. But aneurysms may get larger as time passes and, as they do, doctors believe they are more likely to burst.

The result can be devastating as high-pressure blood from larger brain arteries floods into the space around the brain. If you aren't killed immediately, you have to survive weeks of recovery as your body tries to clean up the resulting mess. Further injury to your brain and rebleeding are likely, unless you get immediate medical attention.

Figure 1-4:
When a vessel bleeds into the space surrounding the brain, the result is a stroke called a sub-arachnoid hemorrhage.

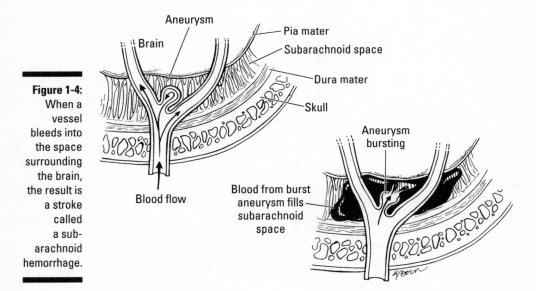

This type of red subarachnoid hemorrhage stroke is usually accompanied by severe headache. Many people also fall down unconscious when the stroke first hits. The pain and loss of consciousness are both strong warnings that something serious is happening.

When red and white stroke occur together

White ischemic strokes can turn red if a blood vessel is injured and breaks in the area where lack of blood flow caused a brain infarction. The bleeding can become a major intracranial hemorrhage or it may just be a small leak that doesn't do much more damage than has already been done by the ischemia.

In a stroke that starts out as subarachnoid hemorrhage caused by an aneurysm, white ischemic strokes can occur 4 to 14 days after the aneurysm bursts. This is a time when the blood around the brain irritates the brain's blood vessels and they clamp shut. Blood flow stops and ischemic stroke can result. This is of course bad news for someone who has just started to recover from the bleeding.

Five stroke scenarios

Blood clots and bleeding aren't the only causes of stroke — but about 99 percent of strokes can be attributed to one of these reasons. In this book, I've identified the five most common stroke scenarios and dedicate a full chapter to each type:

White strokes

- ✔ Ischemic stroke, caused by a blood clot (Chapter 3)
- ✔ Transient ischemic stroke (TIA), also caused by a blood clot (Chapter 4)
- ✔ Multiple small ischemic strokes causing dementia or vascular cognitive impairment (Chapter 7)

Red strokes

- ✔ Intracerebral hemorrhage caused by bleeding in the brain (Chapter 5)
- ✔ Subarachnoid hemorrhage caused by rupture of an aneurysm and bleeding around the outside of the brain (Chapter 6)

Assessing Stroke Risk

If you've suffered a stroke, let me assure you of one thing: You are not alone. In the United States, 750,000 people experience a stroke each year. Of these three-quarters of a million strokes, here's how they break down in our red and white categories:

✔ Eighty percent are white ischemic strokes, including TIA and dementia.

✔ Fifteen percent are red intracerebral hemorrhages.

✔ Five percent are red subarachnoid hemorrhages.

Survival rates by type of stroke vary greatly. Clearly, your chances of survival are much better with a white stroke than a red subarachnoid hemorrhage:

✔ 80–90 percent survival rate of ischemic stroke

✔ 60–70 percent survival rate of intracerebral hemorrhage

✔ 40–50 percent survival rate of subarachnoid hemorrhage

Taking steps to prevent stroke

Fact is, neither you nor I nor your doctor knows for certain whether a stroke is in your future. It's not really possible to predict with any certainty exactly who will suffer a stroke. To some extent, having a stroke is a matter of bad luck.

But we do know that certain characteristics place you at a greater risk for stroke. We know that you are more prone to this particular form of bad luck if you have high blood pressure, smoke cigarettes, and/or have heart disease, diabetes, or high blood cholesterol levels. Researchers have identified a number of indicators that can help predict the likelihood of stroke. Some you can influence; others you can't.

Risk factors beyond your control

Unfortunately, you may be carrying some genetic, hereditary, gender, or age baggage that you simply can't change, such as:

✔ You've already had a stroke.

✔ You are 65 or older.

✔ You are African American.

✔ You are Hispanic.

✔ Stroke runs in your family.

✔ You are a man.

✔ You have diabetes.

Risk factors you can control

So you can't change your age (don't we all wish we could?), your sex, your past, or your forebears' genetic makeup. But I can offer you plenty of ways to make changes in your life that will significantly reduce your risk of stroke. In fact, I devote four chapters of this book (Chapters 8, 9, 10, and 20) to stroke-prevention topics.

Some of the steps you can take to improve your outlook for a stroke-free future include the following:

- ✔ Treat high blood pressure with medication, if necessary.
- ✔ Reduce sodium in your diet to help control high blood pressure.
- ✔ Stop smoking.
- ✔ Lower "bad" cholesterol and raise "good" cholesterol through medication and diet.
- ✔ Maintain a healthy weight, which may reduce blood pressure and improve cholesterol levels.
- ✔ For women, consider the use of oral contraceptives or estrogen replacement therapy with the advice of a physician.

Treating Stroke: Fast Response Is Everything

Damage occurs quickly with the onset of stroke. Whether a brain artery starts bleeding or is plugged by a blood clot, in just minutes the symptoms become apparent. And in the next hours most of the damage will be done and the course set for the future.

In those first minutes and hours, a quick response and prompt course of treatment are critical in terms of reducing the amount of permanent damage and increasing odds for an optimal recovery.

Bottom line? Get to the hospital! If you're having the stroke, call 911. If you're watching the symptoms of stroke overtake an individual, call 911.

Once at the emergency room, the first course of action will likely be a battery of tests to verify which sort of stroke you are having. ER docs will likely take your blood pressure, start an IV, draw blood, check your heart, and perform a CT scan or an MRI to see your brain and determine what's going on. They'll gather this evidence as quickly as possible so they can start the appropriate course of treatment.

Treatment response for white stroke

In ischemic stroke, the goal is to dissolve or remove the blood clot as quickly as possible before the affected brain has gone from ischemia to infarction, or brain cell death. This is most often done with a drug called *tissue plasminogen activator* — or TPA.

TPA is a valuable drug and effective treatment, but it poses some risks. For example, it can aggravate bleeding — so it's critical to ensure that the stroke is a *white* stroke — and not *red.* Because of its risks, emergency-room physicians are cautious about using TPA. If they can't verify that the stroke onset was less than three hours prior, they will not prescribe TPA. After three hours has passed, the damage to the brain is mostly done, and the risks of TPA outweigh any benefit.

Treatment response for red stroke

Red stroke poses greater challenges to the emergency-room team. Treatments to stop bleeding are still being developed, and, currently, little can be done. However, your physicians will be keenly focused on keeping you alive through the first few days after your stroke. They will take efforts to lower your blood pressure, reduce any brain swelling, and keep you breathing.

The bleeding may cause you to stop breathing, or may make your brain swell. If we're talking subarachnoid hemorrhage — bleeding outside the brain — your doctors may consider surgery to patch an aneurysm or repair a ruptured vessel. I cover treatments for intracerebral and subarachnoid strokes in detail in Chapters 5 and 6.

Most people who find themselves in the middle of a stroke are unprepared — and being unprepared means losing precious time for treatment. The good news for you is this: Because you are reading this book, your eyes are now opened to the importance of fast response. Now's the time to research whether your community is one of the growing number of stroke-prepared locations where the emergency medical system and hospitals are fully prepared to respond to stroke. Stake out the best emergency center for stroke and have your "evacuation" plan in place. It's a minimal effort for maximum results.

Recovering from Stroke

If you've already had a stroke, improving your chances of recovery is as important as preventing the next one. And you can take many positive steps to increase your odds of a successful recovery.

Connecting with the best experts

You can prepare your own taxes and repair your car, but evidence is strong that placing your stroke care in the hands of a specialist will result in a healthier outcome than if you try to manage your recovery by yourself.

Stroke specialists from neurologists to physical therapists have a great deal to offer you, including the latest treatment opportunities when you first get to the hospital (quickly, we hope) and throughout your recovery. Some therapists are more experienced than others in taking care of stroke patients, however, and you want to seek out the best.

One of the best steps you can take is to find hospitals in your community that have special certifications as stroke centers. Check with your own doctor and with stroke patients in your community to find stroke specialists and experienced therapists.

Exercising your brain cells

You may have heard that your brain can't regenerate new brain cells to replace those that are injured by a stroke. For any practical application to your stroke, this is probably true. However, scientists are learning that the brain can change significantly in response to injury. Stroke studies of animals have established that new connections do form, and some evidence supports that this happens in humans, as well.

We don't know yet the extent to which exercise and physical and cognitive therapy can increase the extent of the restoration of function after a stroke. Exercising brain doesn't seem to build new brain tissue the same way that exercising muscle does. However, exercising muscles and joints does keep them flexible and strong so that they are more responsive to small improvements in brain function. And it is well-established that if you don't maintain your strength and flexibility after a stroke, you are less likely to regain as much useful function of an arm or leg.

Your full therapy program, developed and supervised by an expert, is likely to play an important role in your recovery. Adhering to the advice of your physical therapists and others on your recovery team will increase your results.

Asking for help

Stroke not only injures your brain and disables you, it also places stress on your family and your financial security. Often these stresses are more than a married couple or a family can cope with. Recovery can be more complete if you decide to take advantage of a wide array of community, employer, and government programs that suit your needs.

You can learn a lot about the different ways to organize and pay for all the care available after a stroke. It often takes two or more people to keep track of all the different medical, social, and financial interactions that are imposed on you by your stroke disability.

Several million people in the United States are living with the consequences of stroke. Getting to know some of them can help you recover from your own stroke — and perhaps provide emotional support as an added bonus. Community organizations, hospital social workers, and perhaps your own doctor may be able to put you in touch with support groups and helpful resources.

Letting "use it or lose it" be your guiding principal

The basic principle of stroke recovery is *use it or lose it.* Use your muscles or they won't be there for you — even if your brain is able to rewire or relearn old skills. Keep your joints flexible, or you won't be able to bend them when you do recover some strength. Use the opportunities to prevent another stroke, or the next one you have may destroy all the gains of your recovery from your first stroke. Use your community resources and the help of friends when you need it. They often don't offer more than once, if at all.

Living with Stroke: Reasons for Optimism

No doubt about it, stroke is a devastating event, a medical calamity that can leave its victims severely disabled — or worse.

But study after study has shown that patients recovering from stroke do indeed improve with time. They are better at three months than they were when they left the hospital — and further along at a year than they were at three months. Function returns, depression fades, and the skills to live independently are gradually regained by a significant proportion of patients. And as stroke survivors become more knowledgeable about stroke and how to prevent it, they follow treatment plans that can dramatically reduce the chances of a second stroke.

Just as there are a lot of people who have strokes, there are a lot of people who survive their stroke and learn to live with a disability. Life can return to normal after a very mild stroke, but even with residual disability, you can still have a meaningful life.

Stroke comes as an unexpected bolt from the blue and can dramatically change your life. There are many opportunities to take actions that will reduce the bad effects of stroke on your independence and quality of life. Arming yourself with as much information as possible will take you far in your recovery and improve your ability to cope with life after stroke.

Chapter 2

Understanding How the Brain Works

In This Chapter

▶ Touring the brain

▶ Reading the brain's roadmap

▶ Driving the brain: Blood vessels as energy highways

▶ Picturing the brain: From X-rays to ultrasound

The brain is arguably the most complex biological machine known. Buried within its folds of gray matter are operational mysteries that continue to confound the world's most brilliant minds.

Our brains are what make us *us*. Your dreams, daydreams, personalities, quirks, and unique points of view are all contained in your brain. Likewise, your philosophies, political ideas, prejudices, knowledge, and passions are buried inside your brain — though nobody really knows exactly where.

You can read a thousand books and travel a thousand miles, filling your brain with memories of sights, sounds, and smells. Yet it doesn't weigh any more for all the information you pack into it. We're just beginning to figure out how little we know about the brain. What other amazing capabilities do our brains have that we don't even know about yet?

In this chapter I describe basic brain workings — "The Brain 101," if you will — with as little complex theory and Latin terminology as possible. The basic facts are relatively easy to grasp — no more difficult, say, than learning the rudiments of car operation and maintenance.

The brain is a delicate structure, soft and pliable, easily injured, locked tightly and securely in a hard, protective skull that is well designed to protect it from the bumps and sudden twists on the highway of human life.

By understanding how the brain is put together and what makes it run, you'll have a better appreciation for the damage everyday mileage puts on it. And how, in some cases, that wear and tear can lead to stroke.

An Illustrated Tour of Your Brain

Information enters your brain, gets processed, and then comes out as behavior. The difference between what comes in and what goes out is what the world knows as you. Your brain — how you perceive data, process it, and react to it — makes you the unique human being you are.

Different areas of the brain are responsible for different cognitive functions, and these areas develop slightly differently in each person (see Figure 2-1).

But when it comes to the physical brain itself, one looks pretty much like the others. Yours isn't that distinguishable from Einstein's.

Figure 2-1: Different regions of the brain handle different jobs involved in perception and cognition.

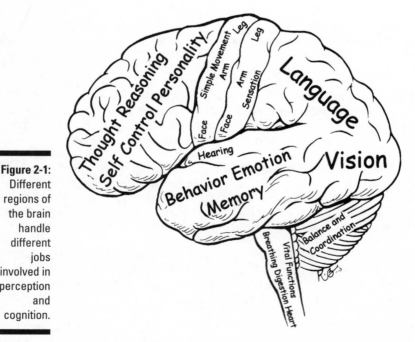

Parts of the brain

Figure 2-2 shows some of the parts of the brain.

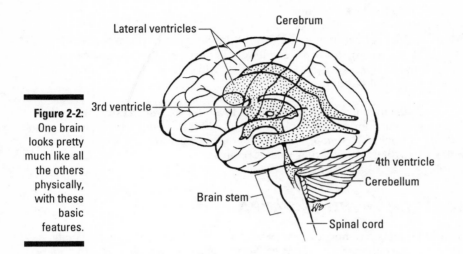

Figure 2-2:
One brain
looks pretty
much like all
the others
physically,
with these
basic
features.

Your *brain stem* is like the boiler room in a large industrial building. Maybe all the important things happen upstairs, but the temperature control, plumbing, and electrical circuits to keep the tenants in condition to work and live are all downstairs. The brain stem is where all the information flows in and out of your brain and also where all vital heart, breathing, and other vital functions occur.

Nerves to and from the eyes, ears, mouth, and throat emanate from the brain stem. The brain stem connects the thinking part of the brain to the rest of the body primarily through the *spinal cord,* the major carrier of millions of nerve fibers taking messages to muscles and organs of the body. The brain stem simply passes on most information with little modification.

The *cerebellum,* that little brain on the back, seems to be a little computer that smoothes things out, making us more graceful and less jerky as we move about. In women, the cerebellum is larger relative to the rest of the brain, interestingly enough. In strokes that damage the cerebellum, after you get over the unsteadiness, which can take several months, you can survive serious injury destroying large parts of the cerebellum.

Fluid-filled cavities called *ventricles* account for about 10 percent of your total brain volume, though nobody really knows what they are for. They are lined with special cells that produce a clear, protein-filled fluid. The brain's four ventricles are similar to the four ventricles of the heart. They are connected by narrow canals. The fluid produced in the ventricles flows from the largest two ventricles into the smaller two ventricles and finally out of the brain into the space surrounding it and the spinal cord. Once outside, the fluid is absorbed into the bloodstream.

Serious problems occur when the flow of the fluid out of the ventricles is blocked by blood clots or brain swelling that squeezes the narrow canals closed. Immense pressure can build up that will enlarge the ventricles and cause further brain injury or death.

The ventricles look like dark holes in the brain on a CT scan, similar to what appears in some kinds of stroke. You need to know about the ventricles when you look at your CT *(computerized tomography)* scan. Otherwise, you may think your stroke is a lot larger than it really is.

How the brain is wired

The brain consists of nerve cells, special support cells, blood-vessel cells, and blood cells all working together. Nerve cells occur in clumps and sheets that are organized the same in most human brains — yes, the same in men's and women's brains, contrary to popular belief. The surface of the brain is covered with around six layers of nerve cells, separated and held in place by support cells. The nerve cells look like a tiny forest, with their branches, twigs, and leaves touching each other at special connections.

The connection points between nerve cells are called *synapses.* Millions of synapses exist for just a few nerve cells. The number of synapses for the whole surface of the brain is truly staggering, almost unimaginable. There are a lot of them.

Ever try to stop thinking? Not so easy, is it? Your nerve cells are extremely active, chattering all the time like a flock of birds. Creating the chatter are little electrical charges that repeat several times per second, day and night, awake or dreaming. They never let up.

With all this electrical activity going on, it's a wonder your brain doesn't glow. The brain is constantly receiving and sending information from one area to another and directing it to and from the rest of your body. And this takes a lot of energy (more on the brain's energy later in this chapter).

Messages come into the brain from your sense organs: your skin, eyes, ears, nose, mouth, and tongue. These incoming messages rain on the brain every minute that you are awake. The brain depends on this raucous thunder of signals to know what's going on in your body and the world.

The brain's vineyard

The branches coming out of these central cell areas are amazing. Have you seen grapevines covering an arbor? Well, some nerve cells are like that. Although most connect to only a thousand or so nearby nerve cells, other nerve cells have long, threadlike branches that extend from your brain to the bottom of your spinal cord in your lower back. And some nerve cells in your spinal cord reach all the way to the surface of the brain *and then* stretch to the end of your big toe. How far is that? Could be five or six feet. Sending nerve impulses at a rapid rate down that long fiber consumes a huge amount of energy.

The brain reacts to signals you aren't even conscious of. It responds to a complex mix of speech and visual cues simultaneously. And from within, your body sends the brain signals — you're hungry, you're too hot, your blood pressure is too high.

Your responses to the incoming signals are formed all over the brain (Figure 2-3) and then routed out from the brain, usually as electrical signals to muscles, which obligingly move as instructed by the brain.

Of course, some of the outgoing messages go somewhere besides a muscle. For instance, your glands secrete tears, digestive juices, and all kinds of hormones in response to your brain's requests.

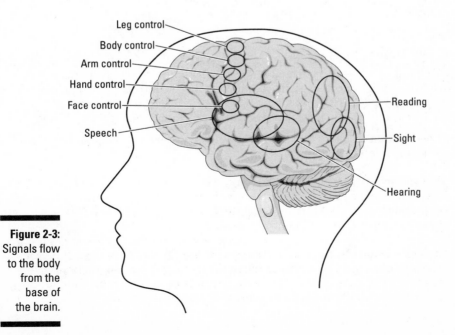

Figure 2-3:
Signals flow to the body from the base of the brain.

One thing your brain does well is *learn*. And it does so quite quickly. After you respond to the same stimulus a number of times, it takes a lot less time and energy for the brain to organize a response. Scientists agree that this learning requires the brain to form new permanent connections between nerve cells. Some of these connections between nerve cells apparently last a lifetime. This learning by forming new connections also takes a lot of the brain's energy.

So here's the summary of the brain's operating system:

1. The brain's nerve cells receive messages and information, mostly by electrical signals, from all over the body.
2. The nerve cells respond to the incoming messages by sending out messages to muscles and glands.
3. They also learn and remember by forming new connections.

But how does the brain process all these connections and signals? Next I look at how basic processing is organized.

The Brain's Roadmaps

The brain is like an atlas — full of roadmaps. The maps are organized in a logical way: The nerve cells that move your left index finger are located between the nerve cells that move your left thumb and left middle finger. The part of the brain that *feels* what the left index finger touches is situated right next to the part of the brain that *moves* the left index finger.

But the unusual thing about these brain maps is that they're reversed right to left. Many are even reversed up to down. In the two hemispheres — the largest part of the brain — the right hemisphere controls the left side of the body, and the left hemisphere controls the right side. These reversed maps are also found in other parts of your brain, including the brain stem and underneath the hemispheres.

How the brain manages all the different senses

The picture that you see as your brain peers through your eyes and out into the world travels to the *visual cortex* in the very back of the brain. The scene each eye picks up goes to the brain stem, to a little junction box. Nerve fibers from the junction box send this data across the middle of the brain stem and to the very back of the brain where it's projected on the opposite side. For example, what your eyes see to the upper left is shown on the lower right part of the map.

Hearing is presented on a whole series of little maps that arrange the pitch by frequency. The *hearing cortex* is located between the more straightforward mechanical areas that coordinate movement and the areas where more emotional functions are known to reside.

Ordinary touch is mapped according to the position on the body, just like the area responsible for simple movements.

Taste and smell have their own special locations in the brain stem and frontal cortex just above the nose.

Left brain, right brain

Although the brain appears to be similar from side to side (the left hemisphere looks the same as the right hemisphere), each half of the brain seems to specialize in certain functions. Large areas of the left side of the brain (between the area for simple movements and the area for vision) are related to language and language processing as well as mathematics. The left side of the brain is often referred to as the *logical* half.

Interestingly, there is some speculation that people with injuries to their left hemisphere are more likely to become depressed than those individuals with right-hemisphere injuries. Is the left brain happier than the right? Although there may not be a rigid division of emotional centers in the brain, experience indicates that positive emotions may be located on the left side of the brain.

What does the right brain specialize in? We tap into the skills of the right hemisphere when we listen to music, draw a picture, and approach complex spatial problems and abstract problem-solving. The right brain is associated with our imagination. Just as it appears that positive emotions may be tied to the left hemisphere, negative emotions may be associated with the right brain.

Numerous books delve into the differences between the right and left side of the brain, even offering exercises for developing your creative side or your analytical skills. There's even some speculation that the functions of the left and right halves of the brain are to some extent based on your culture and how you are raised.

The two sides of the brain work together to create a balance in perceiving and responding to the world. The following key concepts about the makeup, organization, and workings of the brain are particularly important when considering stroke:

- ✔ The major brain functions are spread over a large area on the outer upper surface of the brain.
- ✔ Nerves and nerve fibers for the same functions are concentrated in very small areas in the brain stem.
- ✔ The map of brain functions is quite similar for most humans with normal, uninjured brains.
- ✔ The brain functions related to one side of the body are generally located on the opposite side of the brain.
- ✔ After a stroke, by measuring the strength of your muscles in your face, arms, and legs, it is possible to make some guesses about the area of the brain that has been affected by the stroke from the weakness that you have.
- ✔ After a stroke, the brain injury may make it impossible to recognize that there is a brain injury or even that a hand, arm, or leg is part of your body.
- ✔ Language occurs primarily in the surface of the left brain. Problems with language almost always point to damage or injury on the surface of the left brain.

Fueling the Brain's Energy Highways

Ever try to concentrate on a difficult mental task when you were tired or hungry? Doesn't work very well, does it? It's kind of like driving your car on an empty tank of gas.

Your brain also needs fuel — in this case, that fuel is provided by the blood. Now that we've looked under the brain's hood, we understand a bit more how the brain's operating system works — how nerve impulses are transmitted to and fro, picking up data and sending messages. We've established that the brain and nervous system are extremely active and require a lot of fuel.

So let's take a look at how the brain gets that energy.

From superhighway to back road

Basically, your blood vessels are the delivery system for the food — oxygen and glucose — that the brain needs in order to function. Imagine your body's vascular system as a national highway system.

Four superhighway blood vessels move large amounts of blood to the brain. The two *carotid arteries* are the largest highways, with ten lanes each. They are in the front of the neck and pulse away your whole life. You can feel the pulse in the hollow on each side of your windpipe. At the back of the neck, threading through the bones, are the two four-lane *vertebral arteries.* They join to form the larger *basilar artery.*

The basilar artery then divides to create a large traffic circle called the circle of Willis that connects the four major arteries (the superhighways). Parts of this traffic circle are small or incomplete in a surprisingly high percentage of people. In general, though, it is hard to completely block traffic in this system at the base of the brain because it can usually reroute itself to reach almost any part of the brain stem and brain.

The blood vessels grow out from the traffic circle at the base of the brain and spread upward into the brain. Once away from the traffic circle — out in the country where most of the brain is — only one major blood vessel (like an old state highway) serves each area.

Branching off from the country highways are even smaller back roads and driveways — tiny blood vessels called *capillaries,* as small as a single red blood cell, which are about the same size as the smallest neuron — that deliver oxygen and glucose to the brain. This fuel simply oozes through the capillary wall and is absorbed by the different nerve and nerve support cells in the brain.

Sending fuel where it is needed most

One remarkable thing about the brain is more blood goes where the brain is more active. For example, if you start tapping your right index finger on the table as fast as you can, more blood will flow to the part of your (left) brain that has responsibility for moving that finger. This may be a small place — about the size of a dime — but more blood flows here as the brain sends thousands and thousands of extra electrical volleys out to the small muscles that move your finger.

You can even see the increased blood flow in special pictures of the brain. When you solve problems, plan activities, or look at complicated patterns, your brain momentarily shifts more blood flow to the areas of the brain that are associated with those actions.

When the main vessels to a certain brain area are blocked, the only alternates are very small routes that support hardly any traffic flow. In an emergency, these smaller vessels can widen and open up, but the process can take several days.

In the meantime, those brain areas normally served by the main vessel don't get needed supplies. Without fuel and oxygen, these areas can last only a few minutes or hours on supplies brought in along the small alternate routes. The longer it takes to restore the flow of energy through the main vessel, the higher the chances are that they will suffer ill consequences from the break in their main supply line.

Connecting blood vessel to brain area

The area of the brain supplied by a particular artery doesn't have just one purpose or affect function in just one area of the body. For example, blocking the *anterior cerebral artery* may affect movement and feeling in the opposite leg as well as make it more difficult for you to control your emotions and impulsive behavior. Cutting off blood flow in another artery can make you deaf *and* dizzy. This is because brain arteries travel through areas of the brain that aren't necessarily related.

In cases of stroke, the brain is damaged by a blocked or bleeding artery. One challenge for doctors is to figure out which blood vessel is causing the stroke. Dozens of blood vessels are associated with the right leg, for example. But fewer are connected to the right leg *and* the personality. Neurologists, therefore, can sometimes make a pretty good guess about which blood vessel is causing the stroke based on the patient's combination of symptoms.

(An MRI scan, CT scan, or angiogram may also help define which vessel is causing the symptoms. More about these procedures later in this chapter and elsewhere in the book.)

Consequences of Gridlock on the Vascular Interstate

Now that you have an idea of how your blood vessels carry food to your brain, just imagine the consequences of a breakdown in that delivery system. Consider the impact of a major pile-up on your route home from work — you can count on missing dinner. Likewise, when there's a blood clot or another blockage in a major blood vessel to your brain, it likely means your brain is not going to be fed. And a brain without food cannot last long.

How long? When you apply a tourniquet to your arm or leg, the maximum time the affected muscles can endure complete loss of blood supply without destructive injury is approximately two hours. Your brain is *far* more sensitive to lack of blood flow than your muscles. The maximum time your brain can survive without blood flow without sustaining permanent injury is approximately *five minutes.*

Why such a difference between muscles and brain? Muscles are designed to survive with limited oxygen and sugar fuel. When blood flow is halted, the muscle cells turn to their own internal stores of *glycogen* for fuel. They convert glycogen to energy through a chemical process that allows them to continue working. Thus, organs and tissues can buy a little extra time before damage occurs — organs and tissues, that is, other than the brain or spinal cord.

This is your brain on stroke

You know those scented candles in jars? The ones I am thinking of have quite a bit of space above the candles. You have to tip the jar to the side and reach down in to light the candle. The wick burns, and the jar acts as a reflector. When you put the top on the jar, the candle continues to burn for a certain number of seconds before it begins to flicker and then goes out as the oxygen inside is consumed.

Putting the lid on the candle is like cutting off the blood supply to the brain. You don't have much time after stopping blood flow before the brain cells cut off from that energy quit working and are permanently injured. This is what happens in many strokes, when a blood clot blocks the blood flow to your brain.

In white stroke — the topic of the next chapter — some brain cells can survive for one or two hours because the blood supply is not always *completely* blocked by the blood clot. As I mention, the main road can be blocked, but smaller side roads can widen a bit and allow for some flow. A very small amount of blood can flow in from nearby areas of the brain where the artery is *not* plugged by a blood clot.

The benefit to the brain cells that this backup blood flow provides can be critically important. But when symptoms of a stroke are apparent, backup flow is nothing you can count on. It certainly doesn't mean you should relax and take the time to pack a suitcase or call a family member. The sooner doctors start doing what they can to restore blood flow and protect the brain, the better. Just remember that *every* minute of delay is killing millions of brain cells. Call 911.

The nearby case history about the *clot-buster* drug called *TPA* illustrates what happens when a blood clot blocks the main artery to the left side of the brain — the left internal carotid artery — and causes a stroke. This case demonstrates many of the principles of brain structure and function discussed so far. The injury to the left brain stopped language and the function of the right arm and leg. The left side of the body wasn't affected. Because the blood flow was re-established quickly, the permanent brain injury was less than if the artery had remained closed.

TPA: Clot-buster to the rescue

One Saturday morning, a 75-year-old man was in his yard when he developed a headache, right-side weakness, and confusion. Neighbors called EMS. He was brought to the emergency department of a mid-sized Midwestern hospital. When first examined, he couldn't lift his right arm, the right side of his face drooped, and his right leg was weak. He was unable to talk and did not seem to understand what was being said to him.

He was taken for a CT scan immediately. No blood was seen on the CT. Because of his symptoms, the doctor taking care of him thought that the problem was probably in the left internal carotid artery or one of its main branches. Because there was no bleeding seen on the CT scan to suggest a red stroke, the doctor assumed this was a white ischemic stroke caused by a blood clot blocking an artery.

The doctor on call gave TPA, *tissue plasminogen activator,* a commonly used *clot-buster* for stroke patients, to dissolve the blood clot two hours after the stroke started. The patient had recovered the use of his right leg and could speak and understand words to some extent. This man owes a lot to his quick-thinking neighbors who got him to an emergency room so fast.

Your brain's response to injury

When your brain is injured by stroke, it mounts a significant response to repair the damage and clean up the mess. The result is similar to what happens anywhere when you injure yourself.

White blood cells are activated to absorb dead and dying cell debris and carry it away in the bloodstream. Some brain cells form a kind of scar tissue on the edges of the injury. When the stroke is larger than a few cells, a small cavity, which fills with a clear or yellow fluid, forms in the brain. When a red stroke (see Chapters 5 and 6) heals, it often stains the brain yellow because the white cells change the color of the red pigment of blood in the process of cleaning up the blood clot. This is similar to the yellow tinge that you may have seen as a bruise heals.

Evidence indicates that part of the healing process for the brain may include some sort of rewiring. The younger you are, the more extensive the rewiring is, and the more rapidly it occurs. What actually happens in the cells is something of a mystery. Whether new cells are formed as part of the process remains unclear, but we do know that new connections are formed.

One of the best-studied examples of rewiring is when patients with normal vision become blind. When their brains are studied several years later, it is clear that the part of the brain that used to respond to *visual* stimuli now responds to *touch* in the fingers as the patients read Braille.

After a stroke, brain function generally improves some with time. This is true regardless of the type of stroke. The improvement is more rapid in the first few weeks and months and is thought to be greater if other problems, such as muscle contractures and atrophy of muscles, are prevented. (Read more about rehabilitation and prevention of contractures in Chapter 13.)

Occupational, speech, and physical therapy all incorporate exercises to aid in rehabilitation. Recent research indicates that such therapy may play an important role in stimulating brain rewiring and regrowth. Naturally, the larger the brain injury is, the less you will be able to recover.

Medical Technologies for Peering into the Brain

A picture is worth a thousand words, and this is especially true when it comes to stroke. Pictures of the brain help neurologists and stroke specialists understand a lot about a patient's condition and how he or she has been affected by stroke. Until the invention of modern techniques to visualize the brain inside the skull, neurology depended almost entirely on a careful examination of the patient, plus a spinal tap reading, to diagnose brain problems.

In the past three decades, especially with the development of CT and MRI scans, doctors have been able to get a clearer picture of the living brain inside your skull. Today, a variety of tools allow doctors to peek inside the skull and learn more about the state of an individual's brain.

The CT scan

The *CT scan,* the most common scan used on the brain, involves X-rays, using about the same amount of radiation as a chest X-ray (refer to the next chapter's Figure 3-1 for an example of a CT scan).

CT stands for *computerized tomography.* A CT scan is also called a CAT scan. CAT stands for *computerized axial tomography.* Tomography is the process of getting the whole picture from a lot of different views from different angles. You don't have to remember or know what CT or CAT stands for. Many doctors couldn't tell you, either.

To have a CT scan of your head, you are placed on a large, movable table, and your head is positioned in the middle of a futuristic-looking metal-and-plastic donut. X-rays are taken from many different angles as the emitter orbits around your head. In about five minutes, the scan process is completed. A computer constructs an image of the brain inside the skull by adding together all the information.

Imagine slicing an orange horizontally into quarter-inch slabs. As you move through the orange the slices get larger, and then smaller after you pass the halfway point. The first slice may only contain peel, revealing a white center outlined by the thin orange skin. Progressive slices begin to include the segmented interior of the fruit, and you see a wagon-wheel pattern develop. Further toward the center you encounter the seeds.

That's what a CT scan does. Each slice is a picture of a thin part of your brain. The slices are usually arranged from the base of your neck to the top of your head. You can see more than the brain — often the eyes and part of the nose are visible. Typically, the images are taken at an angle that avoids the teeth because these interfere with the X-rays, especially if you have metal fillings.

On the CT scan, the brain appears gray. The ventricles and the spaces in the convolutions of the brain are dark gray or black. The bone of the skull and jaw appears white. Typically, the outer surface of the brain, the cerebral cortex, appears a little whiter than the rest of the brain.

Evidence of white stroke can be found on a brain CT scan only after several hours or days. This is because the damage caused by white stroke can take a while to show up. The first visible sign is most often swelling of the brain, then the part of the brain destroyed by the stroke becomes darker until it matches the ventricles. This is because after weeks or months the parts of brain injured by stroke are replaced by clear fluid.

Red stroke shows up as a white area in the brain. The white area is outside the brain, mostly at the base, in *subarachnoid hemorrhage.* The white area is inside the brain if the red stroke is caused by bleeding inside the brain. (Read about these two forms of red stroke in Chapters 5 and 6.)

The MRI scan

The *magnetic resonance imaging,* or MRI, scan can look a lot like the CT scan, but it uses magnetism and radio waves instead of X-rays to form images (check out Chapter 7's Figure 7-1 to see an example). Because of the strong magnets, you have to be careful about metal in the scan area. Tooth fillings aren't a problem because they aren't magnetic.

An MRI scan takes longer to perform and requires the patient to hold still in a very confined space. In this case, the "donut" encompasses your whole body, not just your head. The result, however, is a much more detailed picture of the brain than a CT scan provides.

In addition, the MRI scan can give a clearer picture of blood flow. Using an MRI scan, a white stroke is detected easily, even in the first hours after the stroke. The same stroke would probably not yet be visible on a CT scan. On the other hand, hemorrhage is not usually as easy to see early on an MRI scan.

So which scan should be used?

MRI scans give more information than CT scans — but take more time and cost more money. Under emergency conditions, the time it takes to do them may delay treatment. A CT scan is all that is needed in the emergency room to deliver the best care according to current stroke treatment guidelines.

The angiogram

Stroke, as you now know, is all about the blood and blood vessels. The best pictures of the brain's blood vessels come from a procedure called an *angiogram* (refer to Chapter 6's Figure 6-3 for an example). An angiogram involves the injection of a special dye into the blood vessels of the brain through a long tube inserted in the groin and run up through the body. As the dye pumps through the blood vessels, a rapid series of X-rays are taken.

The result is an easily read X-ray of the blood vessels. Several pictures have to be taken in order to get a good idea of what the vessels look like. What you get is a picture of the inside of blood vessels that are larger than a sixteenth of an inch or so.

Though rare, there can be complications during an angiogram. The tube can punch a hole in a blood vessel, which could cause a brain hemorrhage. The tube might knock a piece of blood clot loose, or a clot may form on the end of the tube. Doctors keep the patient awake during the angiogram so they can test brain function during the process.

Because of the risks of conventional angiograms and better alternative technology, angiograms are being done less often than they used to be. This is partly because the same machines used for MRI scans can also do MRA, *magnetic resonance angiography*. The images formed in MRA can be almost as clear as those obtained from conventional angiography. CT scan technology can also be used to obtain images of brain arteries, to some extent.

If there is any doubt about CT or MRA angiograms, then a conventional angiogram may be required.

The ultrasound

Surprisingly, sound waves often produce a telling picture of the brain's blood vessels. These waves, called *ultrasound* because their pitch is so high that they can't be heard, are emitted into and through you, and a computer analysis of the echoes from the sound waves helps doctors identify problems in your vessels.

Ultrasound is thought to be one of the safer methods of imaging. In fact, you are probably most familiar with the use of ultrasounds in taking pictures of unborn fetuses in pregnant women. An ultrasound can spot narrowing of the blood vessels in the neck. As ultrasound techniques improve, surgeons are increasingly eliminating the angiogram, which leads to certain risks, before doing surgery on the carotid artery in the neck.

A form of ultrasound called a *Transcranial Doppler ultrasound* can safely help diagnose narrow places in brain vessels inside the skull. The images that are formed are blurry and lack the clarity seen with angiograms. But then, there is almost no risk. And the ultrasound is portable and easily performed in the emergency room, stroke unit, or intensive care unit.

The brain is an extremely complex organ. Many of its mysteries remain hidden from even the most brilliant and knowledgeable experts. But a general understanding of the makeup of the brain, how it operates, and how it is fueled can benefit any of us. For stroke patients and caring family members, knowing more about the brain underscores the importance of doing all we can to prevent stroke and, if it inevitably occurs, respond quickly and effectively in treating stroke.

The PET scan

Well, since CAT scans aren't for cats, don't be surprised that PET scans are not for pets. A *positron emission tomography,* or PET, scan can actually show the chemical activity of the brain via the introduction of special radioactive compounds into the brain. This procedure results in more exposure to radiation, and it is almost impossible to do a PET scan in an emergency. The compounds used have a very short shelf life. The images are in color, but are not as detailed as CT and MR scans. For the present time, PET scans are for research purposes.

Part II
Types of Stroke

The 5th Wave   By Rich Tennant

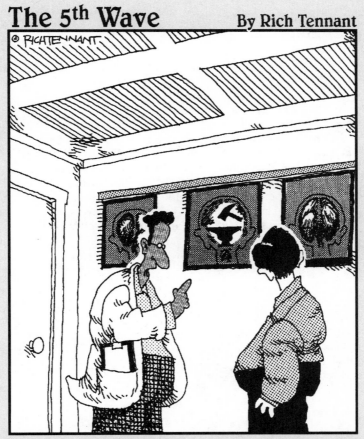

"Initially I was going to say your stroke was caused by a blood clot. But the X-ray indicates you actually have a tiny hammer striking an anvil in your head."

In this part . . .

There are five basic types of stroke, so there are five chapters in this part. Stroke is caused by two things that can go wrong in the brain. When a blood clot blocks an artery to or inside the brain, that is what I call a white stroke, because of the lack of blood. When there is bleeding inside the skull, that's what I refer to as a red stroke. These chapters take each type in turn and discuss each in detail.

Chapter 3

White Stroke (Ischemic): Blood Clots Block the Brain

*W*hat I term *white strokes* — technically called *ischemic strokes* or *acute ischemic strokes* (AIS) — are so called because they stop the flow of blood. White strokes are the most common type of stroke, representing four out of five strokes. They stand in contrast to *red strokes,* which, not surprisingly, cause bleeding in the brain. In almost every white stroke, a blood clot forms and *blocks* blood flow to a part of the brain. The result is a painless loss of brain function. Sometimes, the incident has little or no impact on a person's life; in other cases, it causes severe incapacitating disability. Most white strokes result in some kind of life-changing disability.

Strokes come suddenly. Few victims recognize what's happening as it strikes. The characteristic signs are weakness of an arm, drooping of one side of the face, and inability to speak, understand language, or walk. Usually with white stroke, the victim does not experience pain. Others nearby often report that the individual just appeared surprised or stunned. In the luckiest cases, someone calls an ambulance, and the victim is quickly taken to an emergency department of a large hospital with a stroke team.

Many are not so lucky. They don't understand what is happening and wait around to see if things improve. They may not want to make a big deal of the inexplicable and unusual feelings they are having. They may call a family member or a doctor's office. Instead of minutes, it takes these people hours or even days to get to the hospital — usually too late to get the best treatment. In other words, if you think you might be having a stroke, don't delay because of any doubts. Call 911.

In this chapter, I explain in detail how white strokes occur, what causes them, how they injure the brain, and how to help prevent further white strokes.

Getting a Handle on the Jargon

Like all doctors, I use a lot of jargon in my day-to-day dealings with the brain. I try to avoid that as much as possible in this chapter. The problem is, your doctor may *not* try to avoid it, and I don't want you to be intimidated when you hear "stroke talk." Most of the terms I define in Table 3-1 are relatively simple.

Table 3-1	White Stroke Jargon
Term	*Translation*
Ischemia (*ih SKEEM ee uh*)	Not enough blood
Ischemic stroke	White stroke (caused by not enough blood)
Cerebrovascular accident or CVA	Stroke (white or red, but usually white)
Acute ischemic stroke or AIS	Recent white stroke (within a week or so)
Infarction (*in FARK shun*)	Cells dying due to lack of blood flow by an ischemic stroke
Cerebral infarct	Dead brain area caused by an ischemic stroke

I'm kind of a purist, so I don't mix up the term *stroke,* which means the sudden loss of brain function, with *infarct,* which is the *result* of some white strokes. White strokes can be transient and not cause an infarct. Or, they can be treated soon enough to reverse ischemia before the process of infarction begins. Infarction is the process of cells dying because of insufficient blood flow. Initially, the brain area killed by prolonged ischemia — an infarct — contains dead brain cells. With time, the dead tissue is cleaned up to leave a hole in the brain that is filled with clear fluid.

Technically, it's not right to point to a hole in a brain and call it a stroke. That is an *infarct.* Many people have evidence of brain infarction with no recollection of ever having stroke symptoms. Does that mean a lot of people are running around out there with holes in their brain and don't even know it? Yes, it does. They have brain infarcts but have not had a stroke. They may have other symptoms (see Chapter 7).

You can also have a stroke, even a white stroke, without having an infarction. A blockage must last several minutes before brain cells start dying and an infarct begins to be formed. Some strokes are *transient* and, fortunately for those who have them, do not cause infarction. There's a lot more about transient strokes in Chapter 4.

How Blood Clots Cause Stroke

Understanding how stroke happens is pretty simple. What to do about it and how to recover from serious brain injury are not so simple, as you will see.

In Figure 3-1, notice that inside the white skull are gray areas, which are brain, and dark areas, which are fluid. Some of the dark areas are normal — they are usually similar on both sides of the brain. Some dark areas, however, indicate that a stroke occurred. In this scan, almost half of the brain has been destroyed by a stroke, and the dark area you see on the left is an infarct. The stroke happened a week before this scan was taken.

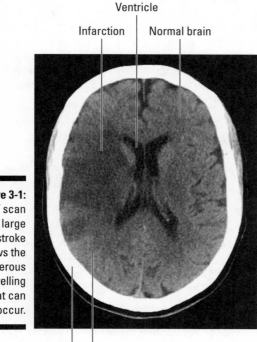

Figure 3-1:
A CT scan of a large stroke shows the dangerous swelling that can occur.

A quick response to stroke symptoms

A 68-year-old retired glass blower woke at 6 a.m. and came downstairs to read the paper and eat his breakfast. His wife was at the counter talking about the weather and looking out the window. She heard a spoon clatter to the floor and turned to see her husband looking bewildered. His mouth hung down on one side, and he was looking at his right hand, which had apparently just dropped the spoon.

When she asked what was wrong, he started to speak, but a garbled noise came out of his mouth. He stopped talking and looked at her, then his hand. His face seemed flat on the right side and he kept slowly clenching and unclenching his right hand. He looked down and tried to stand up. He slipped and put out his right hand to catch himself, but fell.

His wife realized he had had a stroke. She called 911, and he was taken to the emergency room. He received a drug to dissolve a blood clot and he improved somewhat by the next morning in the hospital. Three months later he is still retired at home. His speech has never quite returned to normal.

If you knick your thumb with a knife or bruise your hip on the edge of a table, you may bleed for a while, but eventually the bleeding stops. This is because blood has the amazing ability to stay liquid inside blood vessels, but turn solid and patch holes in the same vessels when they are cut or torn. The blood's ability to *clot* can save your life during childbirth or when you are injured in accidents. However, as with many wonderful things, there are times when blood clotting can be a big problem. Stroke is one of them.

Getting blood through the pipeline

Your brain weighs just a couple of pounds, yet it uses about a fifth of your body's energy — even when it seems to be idle. Solving problems, and other stress, significantly increase the brain's energy consumption.

The brain gets all this energy from the blood. The basics of blood energy are *glucose* (sugar) and *oxygen*. Unlike muscle tissue and other organs, brain cells don't store energy to be used if the blood doesn't provide enough. Some organs can even survive without oxygen on the short term. The brain is not among them. The brain can't adjust to lack of oxygen. It burns sugar so fast that without blood flow, it begins to fail within 30 to 60 seconds. You can hold your breath for a minute or more without injuring your brain because your heart is still beating and there is enough oxygen and glucose to keep your brain going. When *all* available oxygen is pulled out of the blood, you either have to take a breath or lose consciousness.

The brain needs about a pint and a half of good, oxygenated blood every minute to get its job done. All this blood has to travel north from the heart in four main arteries. These lines branch and branch again as they travel up into the brain. Eventually, tiny arteries branch into *capillaries* that hold only a single red blood cell. In the capillaries, the oxygen and sugar leave the blood and enter the substance of the brain. All this activity allows one to think, talk with a neighbor, play video games, and so on.

The key idea is that from main arteries as big around as your little finger, the vessels narrow down to such fine diameters that only a single red blood cell can get through. Anything that can't be squeezed through such a tiny pipe stops blood flow there, and some part of the brain is starved for oxygen and glucose.

Blood and clotting

Every day, blood clots repair blood vessel leaks that come about from the ordinary wear and tear of everyday life. Brushing your teeth, banging your knee on a table leg (which just happened to me this morning), and scraping yourself on a tree branch are all events that injure blood vessels. Their rapid repair goes unnoticed most of the time.

When I was a kid, I lived in Denver, where these little, thorny weeds growing out of sidewalk cracks were forever causing flat tires on my bike. One day, a man at Jenson's Hardware showed me NeverLeak Tire Fluid. You squeezed this remarkable stuff into the tire's valve and, miraculously, no more flat tires. It was a glue-like liquid that ran around inside the tire all the time, sealing the leaks as fast as they happened.

You see where I'm going with this. The blood is like NeverLeak, a liquid that is always just seconds away from becoming a gelatinous solid and minutes to hours away from becoming a tough plug of sticky gum. The balance between liquid and solid forms of blood is very delicate and can be shifted one way or the other by a number of different factors.

As you age, your clotting system tends to tilt more toward clotting than bleeding. These clots can form anywhere in the blood vessels, but do tend to accumulate most often in the heart and at rough spots in the blood vessels.

Breaking loose and forming in place

Blood clots begin as rather loose clumps of tiny blood cells called *platelets*. Platelets get sticky and adhere to each other and to the wall of the blood vessel near places where there is a break in the lining of the blood vessels.

Over time, these clots get harder. Some eventually become quite rigid without much to hold them together — like dried mud, they break into small fragments easily.

If a piece of a clot breaks off, it can travel downstream to the brain, where it can eventually lodge . . . and cause a stroke. The lining of the blood vessel where it lodges is usually intact and can activate processes in the blood to dissolve the clot. Because these broken-off clots were formed sometime earlier, they tend to be firmer, gummier, and harder to dissolve than clots that have just formed in place. As the clot gets smaller, it moves further downstream. As it moves downstream, it moves past openings into branch arteries that are then open to carry blood to more of your brain.

The result might be that someone in the emergency department might regain the ability to use their right hand, but still have difficulty saying words. In this case, the clot blocked blood flow to two branch arteries. When it broke up or was partially dissolved, the blood pressure forced it downstream past the branch that took blood to the part of the brain that controlled the person's right hand before any permanent damage had occurred. That part of the brain started working again. The clot was still large enough that it blocked flow to the language area of the brain, and speech was still abnormal.

Clots can also form at narrow spots in blood vessels where there is atherosclerosis. When they do, they can cause a stroke, but because the clots are relatively new, they are softer and may be easier to dissolve.

Bleeding into the vessel wall

Some experts suspect the cause of stroke is a little more complicated in a large number of cases. Suppose your *carotid artery,* which leads through your neck to the brain, develops a large *plaque* that nearly closes it off. The plaque looks like the craters of the moon: rough, with ridges and valleys where the artery lining has been torn and replaced many times.

As the plaque grows rougher and thicker, it also grows more fragile. The carotid artery is twisted and stretched whenever you move your neck. Eventually the top layer of the plaque may split open exposing the fat, calcium, and scar tissue underneath. The split in the lining can create a pocket in the surface of the plaque that catches the blood flowing past — like an umbrella turned the wrong way breaks in a strong breeze. Under high pressure, the blood catches the split edge. As the blood forces its way under it the edge, the plaque enlarges and closes against the opposite wall of the artery. The sudden enlargement of the plaque fills the artery and stops the blood from flowing past. A stroke results. Then the blood in the plaque clots, and you have a permanently blocked artery.

TIP

Hearing a "whoosh" in your head

Even a little bit of clot formation can cause a stroke in vessels where *atherosclerotic plaques* have built up so much that they nearly block the flow. In these cases, there is hardly any room for the blood to squeeze by. Because the passage is narrow, the blood tends to go faster — like whitewater through a narrow canyon. Sometimes it moves so fast that it causes a whooshing sound every time the heart beats. This sound is called a *bruit* (BROO-ee).

You usually can't hear your own bruit. Sometimes a doctor can hear it with a stethoscope on your neck next to the carotid artery. The sound is "whoosh . . . whoosh . . . whoosh" in your head or neck in time with your heartbeat. Don't worry if you hear this sound yourself while you are lying down with the side of your head pressing down on a pillow. Almost everyone hears this sound at one time or another when lying down. A bruit could mean that you have a very thick atherosclerotic plaque in your carotid artery. Your doctor will probably have it checked out with a special ultrasound test, because some of these thick plaques can be removed by a surgeon to prevent a stroke. A bruit is a sign of a narrowing vessel, which means more wear and tear on the vessels — they can be very rough, and the lining can be injured more often. And if a small clot forms in that narrow spot, it can quickly close off the already tiny space available for blood flow. Then you have a stroke. If it's a major blood vessel like the carotid artery, you have a major stroke.

White Stroke Risk Factors

Most of the factors that lead to forming blood clots can be related in one way or another to things you do — or don't do — that increase your chances of having a white stroke.

High blood pressure

Hypertension, or longstanding high blood pressure, is a disease that causes your blood pressure to be higher than it should be, even when you are relaxed and rested. Atherosclerosis is worse in people who have high blood pressure, simply because of the extra wear and tear of all that blood going by faster and pushing harder. Rushing fluid cut the Grand Canyon out of rock — imagine what it can do to the lining of your blood vessels.

High blood pressure quadruples your chances of having a stroke compared to people your same age. Having high blood pressure is like being someone who drives too fast and follows other cars too closely all the time. Chances of a crash are much more likely. Your car has a speedometer you can read anytime you want. You have to go to a doctor's office or drugstore to measure your blood pressure. Do you know how fast your blood pressure is wearing out your blood vessels?

Some people who have never shown any signs of high blood pressure in the past can increase their blood pressure by taking certain drugs such as decongestants, high doses of anti-inflammatory drugs like ibuprofen, prednisone and other steroids, or diet pills — or by being anxious or angry. Be sure you are checking your blood pressure if you are taking any of these medications on a regular basis.

High blood pressure injures the lining of your blood vessels, leading to a clot, which can result in a stroke. Usually the stroke is a white ischemic stroke.

High blood pressure is also a major risk for red strokes. Sometimes it causes a weak-walled artery to burst and bleed into the brain — a red stroke (see Chapter 5).

Fat and atherosclerosis

Blood vessels have a thin, delicate lining that keeps blood from clotting. But whenever there are rough spots, such as when this lining is broken, the blood comes in contact with the underlying muscle and protein that make up the wall of the blood vessel. Suddenly, just like NeverLeak in a tire, blood starts clotting right there, covering over the bare spot that has lost its lining. This happens while blood that doesn't touch the bare spot continues to rush on by. The clotting of the blood stimulates the cells of the lining to grow, and the patch is complete.

A couple of other factors also work together to create rough spots on the inside of your arteries where blood clots can form. One is the process of *atherosclerosis,* which seems to result in part from high fat in the diet. With atherosclerosis, for whatever reason, fat collects *underneath the protective lining* of the blood vessels and occasionally breaks through it. Result: blood clot, fat, and a new lining over the conglomeration of fat and clot. As this process continues, especially at places where the blood flow is under high pressure or where it turns a corner, hard little irregularly shaped nubbins called *plaques* form. Plaques can collect calcium and often become quite hard and crunchy. Hence, the term *hardening of the arteries* — also called *atherosclerosis.*

Large plaques can be removed by surgery. And some are reported to get smaller if you go on a diet very low in fats.

Why no finger strokes?

If 80 percent of the blood goes elsewhere, why don't people have strokes elsewhere — such as a finger, for example? Well, for one thing the blood vessels in the brain are much less interconnected than blood vessels in other organs. I have no idea why this is. For whatever reason — unlike the case with the finger — if you plug an artery to the brain, there are very few alternate routes for the blood. And other tissues tolerate the blockage longer, giving more time for the clot to dissolve on its own.

In muscle, for example, ... nate routes because the ve... together in a network. The ... that muscle or other tissue... because of an artery blocke... Sometimes, a black spot may for... ...er or a toe where skin dies because a... ...ry got plugged, but this is not nearly as common as in the brain.

Smoking tobacco

The chemicals that get into your bloodstream when you smoke tobacco apparently irritate the lining of the blood vessels and make atherosclerosis worse.

Millions of Americans are buying and smoking tobacco products, primarily cigarettes. They are paying to shorten their own lives. They usually worry about lung and mouth cancer. But a lot more harm comes from injury to your heart and blood vessels. Smoking more that doubles your risk of heart attack and stroke. Smoking also increases your blood pressure.

Some smokers seem to believe that the damage is already done and that stopping won't make any difference. The evidence is overwhelming that stopping smoking will reduce your odds for having stroke. After a year or two, your chances of stroke are reduced to the same as if you had never smoked.

Atrial fibrillation

The heart is designed to pump at a steady pace in order to maintain a strong enough pressure and keep the blood flowing smoothly. The contraction of the different chambers of the heart needs to be carefully synchronized. Otherwise, the blood doesn't flow smoothly.

In a condition called *atrial fibrillation*, the heart has an irregular beat that allows the blood to slow down, swirl in *eddies* against itself, and collect in pockets of the heart chamber called the *atrium*. A simple *electrocardiogram* (EKG) test of your heart — the one where they hook wires onto your chest, wrists, and one leg — can tell you if you have atrial fibrillation.

How does a clot in the heart cause a stroke in the brain? Simple: It grows, and a piece of it breaks off and is shot out of the heart under high pressure. There's a one-in-five chance it will hit the brain because 20 percent of the blood goes there. If it does, it's inevitable that it will clog an artery and usually cause a stroke. The smaller the clot, the smaller the artery that gets clogged and the smaller any stroke will be.

Estrogen: Pregnancy, the pill, and hormone-replacement supplements

Women face a unique risk of white stroke: *Estrogen*, a hormone that occurs naturally in women, has long been known to increase the occurrence of blood clots. Estrogen levels are especially high in pregnancy, when it is a good idea to be able to clot and prevent excessive bleeding. Many women also take estrogen orally in birth control pills or in hormone-replacement supplements during menopause.

Smoking is especially bad for you when combined with taking estrogen. When combined with other risk factors for stroke — such as high blood pressure or high cholesterol or smoking — the extra estrogen that comes from pregnancy, birth-control pills, or hormone-replacement therapy after menopause makes it important that you take other steps to reduce the chance of blood clot formation and stroke. I suggest you discuss this with the doctor prescribing the estrogen.

Other risks

Here are some other factors that some experts warn may further increase your chances of blood clots:

- **Dehydration:** *Dehydration* means not enough water in the blood. The blood is thicker and, therefore, more likely to clot. Many older people are dehydrated simply because they tend not to drink enough water. Alcohol, caffeine, and exercise dehydrate you, and people tend to become dehydrated overnight. Dehydration increases the chances of a blood clot forming in the arteries — hence more chance of stroke.

- **Stress:** Stress is related to blood pressure, but its impact is less understood. I'm a little hesitant to write about this — it seems like placing blame for a stroke where it doesn't belong. One hears stories: "He had the stroke right after his daughter said she was going to marry that biker." Sure, this may have raised Dad's blood pressure, but it could have been one straw out of the pile on the camel's back. I think it's unfair to blame the daughter. (Maybe the biker, though.) You could probably find a lot of upsetting things that happened a few hours before any particular stroke. Still, a couple of research projects have confirmed the association of emotional upset with stroke onset.

✔ **Certain medications:** As I mentioned earlier, some medications, even over-the-counter drugs, can increase your blood pressure suddenly, leading to blood-vessel injury and blood clot. Diet pills, prednisone, high doses of pain medications like aspirin or ibuprofen, and decongestants are examples. Read the fine print that comes with your prescriptions. Watch your blood pressure if there are warnings about the drug increasing blood pressure.

✔ **Changing blood-pressure medication dosage:** Many who suffer from high blood pressure feel secure that they are on medication to maintain a healthy blood pressure and stave off strokes, among other related problems. But they may not realize that carelessly changing dosages or switching medications may result in a sudden spike of high blood pressure. It's extremely important to monitor your blood pressure when changing medicines or dosage.

Other Causes of White Stroke

Blood clots are almost always the cause of white strokes. But there are long lists of very unusual causes of stroke. I won't burden you with all of them, but two are common enough that you should understand them.

Dissection

Dissection is a medical term for splitting something apart, usually along lines that are already there. It usually *doesn't* mean cutting. At least to a physician. So how does dissection cause stroke?

As I have mentioned, blood vessels are like tires with inner tubes. They are hollow and made up of strong layers of material that fit inside each other. Blood vessels have three basic layers, and each is a separate sheath. If you follow the line between the layers, you can peel — dissect — the layers of an artery just as you can peel the bark off a green tree branch. There is a natural line along which the artery breaks into two separate parts.

If the edge of a torn innermost layer faces upstream into the flow of blood, the blood can force its way under it and peel the vessel from the inside, in

An accident leads to white stroke

A 62-year-old news cameraman was carrying a television camera behind a reporter who was chasing down a story. There was a short hedge in his path. As he stepped over it, someone yelled and he turned his head quickly while still holding the camera on his shoulder. He had to twist his head very far and back because of the camera. And then he tripped on the hedge and fell. When he got up he had a strange burning pain in the back of his neck and within a minute or so began to feel extremely dizzy and nauseated. He felt as if he would lose his balance again when he tried to walk, but he managed to drive home.

Later, he noticed his face felt a little numb. He continued to have neck pain and was unsteady when he walked. The neck pain became a pretty severe headache. He didn't like doctors so he just stayed home for a few days. The symptoms got better and he returned to work, though he was still a little unsteady on his feet. He saw a doctor only after his company made him do it, because he had missed work. A very small stroke deep in the brain was diagnosed by MRI scan. He was told he couldn't carry the camera at work any more. He retired. The diagnosis was stroke caused by *vertebral artery dissection.*

much the same way you can pull the bark off a tree limb, strip the plastic off a wire, or peel a banana. As the blood forces its way under the edge, it makes a blister of blood on the inside of the artery. This blister swells and lengthens and can completely shut off the blood flow. This kind of stroke usually happens at the back of the neck in arteries going to the brain, called the *vertebral arteries,* meaning stroke can result. See the nearby sidebar called "An accident leads to white stroke" for more.

Red strokes

One kind of red stroke called subarachnoid hemorrhage can also cause white strokes. Chapter 6 deals with red stroke caused by subarachnoid hemorrhage — but I give you a little preview here so that you can understand how it causes white strokes.

The bleeding from subarachnoid hemorrhage can embed some brain vessels in a blood clot. These are blood vessels just outside the brain but inside the skull. For unknown reasons, the muscles in blood vessels just hate to be exposed to blood, and usually the vessel lining protects the artery muscle from contact with blood. After severe red strokes, though, there is blood all over the outside of some brain vessels. The artery muscles then contract and go into spasm, shutting off the blood flow downstream in the arteries and causing a white stroke.

The nurses may notice that a patient's red stroke caused by subarachnoid hemorrhage is getting worse. This may be due to a white stroke. The white stroke is said to be due to spasm in the arteries, *vasospasm* (*VAY zoh spaz um*).

How White Stroke Injures the Brain

So now you know that white ischemic stroke is caused by a blood clot blocking an artery to the brain. Either the flow is completely or partially cut off to some portion of the brain that depends primarily on that artery for blood. As time passes, brain cells in the affected region stop their usual function as they run out of oxygen. After a short time, if blood flow is not restored, the brain cells are not able to keep up with their basic needs for survival. When this happens, the cells begin to die, and their cell walls begin to break down.

For a while, the brain can hold its breath. Some cells in the brain can survive longer without oxygen than others. Some can steal enough oxygen from nearby blood vessels that are still flowing to keep themselves alive. However, others start dying within minutes of the first deprivation of blood. Most of the cells die within three to four hours.

It is very important to treat white stroke before three hours have elapsed. Because it takes time to get ready for treatment, you have to be in the emergency room as soon as possible — certainly within an hour — to get the most benefit from restoring blood flow. After enough time passes, unblocking an artery and restoring blood flow doesn't revive any cells. The area in the brain where cells die from lack of blood flow, as mentioned earlier, is called the area of *infarction* or an *infarct*.

Brain swelling

As the outer membranes of the brain cells in an area of infarction begin to fail, fluid rushes into the cells and they swell until they eventually burst open. As cells are dying, they attract white blood cells into the area — the cleanup crew. In addition, blood vessels in the injured area leak, and blood fluids are forced into the area. This is just like any other injury to your body. When there is injury, there is swelling and inflammation from white blood cells and leaky blood vessels.

Brain ischemia from a white stroke causes the brain to swell. In large strokes, the swelling can be so significant that the whole brain is distorted out of its normal shape. The swelling gets worse in the first few days after the stroke. It typically reaches a maximum at two to four days and then resolves as the injured brain area is cleaned up by white blood cells.

If the swelling causes the injured side to press across the midline of the brain into some of the space usually occupied by the other side, vital structures at the base of the brain can be crushed by the pressure. Brain swelling is one of the most common causes of death in stroke patients. There are several treatments for brain swelling, but they only help for a short time.

Brain bleeding

I already explained how one type of red stroke can cause white strokes. I will now tell you how white strokes can cause red strokes.

Brain blood vessels, unlike brain cells, can survive reasonably well without oxygen or glucose. Made of muscle and other components, they have their own energy stores on board. However, lack of blood flow begins to weaken them, lessening their ability to contain blood under pressure. Given enough time, though, the blood vessels may open themselves back up by dissolving the offending blood clot — but typically not quickly enough to stave off stroke effects.

If a blood vessel into an area of dead and dying brain happens to reopen naturally, then the part of the vessel downstream that may have been weakened while no blood was flowing through it can rupture. This can cause a real mess, with blood, dead brain cells, and fluid flowing into the area of infarction.

The body responds by sending in the troops — white blood cells — to clean up. They do a thorough job. We don't know yet whether they are a little *too* thorough and cause further brain injury in the cleanup process, but if they do, it isn't much. Nevertheless, over a few weeks, the brain infarction area is cleaned up until all that is left is a cavity filled with clear liquid. These cavities (infarctions) are usually pretty easy to see on a CT or MRI scan.

Seizures

Epileptic seizures sometimes occur after white strokes, typically when the stroke creates an infarction at or near the surface of the brain, where seizures start. Presumably, as the infarction heals, the brain is more vulnerable to the hyper-excitability that causes seizures. Just like a person under stress is more prone to an angry outburst, brain cells without sufficient oxygen are more likely to fire off an outburst of electrical waves. The reason for this is that a short circuit develops in the electrical control system. Left on its own, the unrestrained electrical system cannot hold back its surge of electrical activity. One result is that oxygen and glucose are used up even faster than usual. Another result can be a seizure. These seizures are often fairly easy to control with medication that restrain the production of electrical discharges in brain cells.

Different Sizes of White Strokes

Both blood vessels and blood clots come in a variety of sizes. This means that white stroke comes in many sizes, too.

One thing to realize is that the severity of the stroke doesn't always match the size of the hole — or infarction — that it leaves in your brain. The brain has small control centers, where a lot of information from all over the brain connects or passes through on the way someplace else. Even a small infarction in one of these critical information centers can cause severe disability.

Big strokes: Blocking a major artery

The biggest strokes occur when one of the four major arteries supplying the brain is completely blocked and there is little blood flow to make up for the loss from the other side. The availability of blood from the other side of the brain is somewhat a matter of luck. Some people have great *collateral* flow from one side to the other. For instance, if your right carotid artery is blocked by a blood clot in your neck, you might have a stroke on the right side of

---

Big stroke: Left side leads to communication problems

An 87-year-old retired postal worker was found by a student who was renting a room from her. She was in a chair in front of the television, breathing deeply and noisily, her mouth opening and closing. She was looking over to her left side. The student called 911. In the emergency room, she was found to be completely paralyzed on her right side. The right side of her face was flat and her mouth drooped. She was unable to speak and didn't seem to understand anything said to her. She drifted into sleep and noisy breathing whenever she was left alone for a few minutes.

After a few days in the hospital, she began to improve. She tried to speak and seemed to understand a few words. She was able to move the fingers of her right hand slightly. She still couldn't raise here right arm or walk on her own. With some help, she could support herself while standing.

One of her visitors was the student who found her. He told the doctor that she had had a spell a few days before her stroke. She had said she was in the bathtub and lost the use of her right arm for a few minutes. It returned to normal, and she apparently thought no more about it.

She had no immediate family. She was discharged from the hospital to a nursing home. She required a great deal of care. Her neurological condition improved, but her continuing difficulty with communication limited her progress. She had persistent difficulty with swallowing. She finally developed pneumonia and died several months later.

your brain. Often this doesn't happen because blood from the left carotid artery crosses over to the right side through the traffic circle of vessels at the base of the brain.

Both of the nearby case study sidebars talk about big strokes caused by blockage of the carotid artery to the brain, but in each case the carotid artery is blocked on a different side. A carotid artery blockage on the left side, as in the case of the elderly retired postal worker, causes weakness and numbness on the right side of the body, as well as difficulty with speaking. A big stroke on the right side of the brain paralyzes the left side, but leaves the victim capable of speaking and communicating. Typical with this type of stroke, though, is that the victim may not recognize that the left side is not working, as is the case with the retired insurance agent.

Medium stroke: Blocking branches of main trunk arteries

Most strokes are not as severe as the two described in the preceding two case studies. They may *start out* with quite severe symptoms, but often improve in the first few days. Patients with medium stroke are very likely to

CASE STUDY

Big stroke: Right side leads to left side paralysis

A 67-year-old retired insurance agent awoke early to go to the bathroom. He found he couldn't get out of bed and began talking to himself. The sound awakened his wife, a frequent visitor to a nursing home. She knew immediately by looking at him that he had had a stroke. He was not moving his left side and his face drooped on the left. She called 911. He didn't want her to make such a big deal out of it. In the emergency room, he was not treated with the drug TPA (*tissue plasminogen activator,* a drug that dissolves blood clots) because the time the stroke started could not be established. In the hospital, for the first few days after the stroke, he was sleepy and dozed a great deal. A CT scan showed some brain swelling on the right side of his brain. Further testing showed that his carotid artery was completely blocked, but that quite a bit of blood was crossing over from the left to the right side of the brain.

After three or four days, he became more alert and regained some use of his left arm and leg. He didn't seem to pay much attention to the fact that his left side was weak. He did complain of some discomfort from the numbness of his left arm. He had no problems with speech or communication. He was sent home with his wife without going to a rehabilitation unit. The fact that he didn't really care about the paralysis on his left side was considered an indication that he would not do well with rehabilitation.

At home, he became depressed during the first four weeks. His wife mentioned this to his doctor and he was given medication for depression. After that, he did remarkably well. He continued to socialize with his family and he learned to get himself around quite well using a cane and ankle brace to walk.

CASE STUDY

Medium stroke: Quick response and near recovery

One night, an 82-year-old retired teacher called her daughter who lived out of town. She said, "Something's wrong," in a strangled voice that was difficult to understand. Her daughter called the local police who notified EMS of the emergency. The woman arrived at the emergency room about an hour after she called her daughter. There, she exhibited moderate to severe weakness of her right arm, slight weakness of her right leg, drooping of the face on her right side, and difficulty pronouncing words — but no difficulty comprehending speech. When she finally got them out, her answers to questions were sensible. The emergency department doctors were able to determine what time the stroke started from her memory of the television show she had been watching. A CT scan of her head showed no evidence of brain hemorrhage. Blood tests were normal. She was treated with the drug TPA and admitted to the ICU.

The next morning her right arm was stronger, but not normal. Both her face and leg also still showed signs of weakness. It was difficult to tell whether her speech had improved. Physical therapy was started right away in the hospital. She remained outgoing and smiled a lot during the next few days. She spent one week in a rehabilitation unit working with physical and occupational therapists before returning home.

Three months later, her condition had improved so that most people did not notice the clumsiness of her right hand or her slight limp. When she walked, her right arm tended to bend at the elbow and her right hand formed a fist. Her speech was still noticeably different, but there was no problem understanding her. She did routine stretching exercises twice a day of all the muscles of her right arm and leg.

---

benefit from rehabilitation and typically are able to return home, though frequently they may not be able to continue working. Medium strokes are usually caused by blockage of just a branch of one of the main trunk arteries to the brain.

Small strokes: Cross circulation minimizes injury

The case here involved one of the four major trunk arteries to the brain — the left vertebral artery. Because of extensive cross circulation from the right vertebral artery and the two carotid arteries, the resulting stroke was pretty minimal.

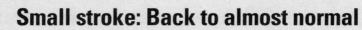

Small stroke: Back to almost normal

A 57-year-old maintenance worker was out walking his dog. He felt some pain in his head, became very dizzy, and was seeing double. He staggered when he walked. A neighbor started to help him walk home, but the man insisted that he just wanted to sit down for a while. After resting, he still was dizzy and seeing double. He thought he was a little better and started to walk again. He still had problems with his balance.

The neighbor called an ambulance and got the man to lie down on his porch. The ambulance took more than an hour to get to him. The EMTs suspected that he had dizziness due to a viral infection. They took quite a while evaluating him on the porch before deciding to take him to the emergency room. He waited in the emergency room for an hour before a physician saw him. His blood pressure was high at 170 over 120. He took no medication except B vitamins.

He was admitted to the hospital. He still had some difficulty with coordination, but his walking was much steadier and his double vision had resolved. He was able to leave the hospital three days later and returned home. His balance never felt quite normal again, but most people didn't notice this when they saw him walking. He continued to work and walk his dog.

Diagnosing White Stroke

The most serious problems encountered in white stroke are also encountered in red strokes. These include brain swelling, brain hemorrhage, blood clots in the legs, and pneumonia and other infections. Chapter 12 explores the treatment of all types of stroke in the hospital. Here, I provide a little extra detail on diagnosing white stroke in the hospital.

When no brain bleeding is seen on a CT scan in the emergency room, doctors will likely determine that a stroke was a white stroke by the time the patient is settled in the hospital. They will now concentrate on further testing to determine what caused the blood clot that led to the stroke. This is important because there are treatments that can reduce the risk of another stroke. In addition, they are as worried about brain swelling and bleeding into damaged brain and another white stroke. In order to monitor cause, severity, and potential for further strokes — both white and red — they may employ the following tests:

✔ **CT and MRI scan:** An X-ray CT scan performed earlier in the emergency room may have been normal (see Chapter 2 for more on CT and MRI scans). This is because an infarction may take days to appear clearly on a CT scan. So, another one may be done. An MRI scan can show the changes after just a few hours. After a few days, both CT and MRI scans can show the amount and location of brain injured by the stroke. And both can also give some idea of the condition of the major brain blood vessels.

✔ **Ultrasound:** You may be familiar with ultrasounds as a method of capturing images of unborn fetuses in pregnant women. These pictures produce images using sound waves instead of X-rays. The ultrasound is a less invasive procedure than an angiogram — in other words, no needle. Usually some form of jelly is applied on the skin and a probe is moved around until a good picture angle is found.

Ultrasound can give a good picture of the mainline carotid arteries and determine if there is a large atherosclerotic plaque. It can also get a fairly good picture through the skull of some of the larger arteries at the base of the brain. Finally, some very clear images of the heart can be obtained, especially if the patient is willing to have a tube placed in the throat (which apparently looks small to doctors, but may look like a garden hose to the patient — the truth is probably somewhere in between). If the test can determine where the clot came from, it may save you from having a second, perhaps larger, stroke.

✔ **Angiograms:** These invasive tests involve pumping dye into the brain arteries and taking X-rays to find clots. A large needle, placed into the big artery of one leg, feeds a long plastic tube through the arteries up toward the head, around a few tight corners, and then into the carotid or vertebral artery of choice. Then a special dye is pumped into the arteries at considerable pressure. The patient is sedated, the head held tight so it doesn't move.

Angiograms are not used very frequently, because similar information — some think better — can be gained from a non-invasive ultrasound. Another reason is that there's a slight risk — less than 1 percent — that an angiogram can *cause* a stroke (by breaking a piece of clot loose or by punching a hole in a brain artery).

✔ **Other tests:** If you've had a stroke, the chances are well over 50 percent that you have some combination of several other medical problems including high blood pressure, diabetes, heart disease, arthritis, or problems with memory. So, in addition to stroke, these other conditions may need to be evaluated and treated as well. Like when you take your car to get the oil changed and they tell you that the brakes are almost gone, the timing belt is about to break, and the shocks are finished. Whatever you decide about your car, when it comes to stroke, the repairs recommended are probably worth the expense. You definitely can't trade yourself in for a new model.

Treating White Strokes

Treating white strokes involves dissolving the clot that caused the stroke, treating complications from any brain injury that does occur, and preventing the next stroke.

Dissolving the clot

At the time of this writing, there is only one FDA-approved treatment for white ischemic stroke. This is TPA (tissue plasminogen activator), a drug that dissolves the blood clot that is blocking a brain artery and causing ischemia in part of the brain. If TPA is given early — three hours or less after the first symptoms of your stroke — the blood clot may be dissolved, and blood flow re-established soon enough to reduce the amount of injury to the brain.

TPA has been shown to increase your chances of going home with minimal or no disability by 30 percent. However, there are serious side effects of brain hemorrhage in about 6 percent of patients who receive the drug, usually in those with the worst strokes. Doctors have to be sure you are not prone to bleeding and that you do not have a red stroke caused by bleeding. TPA would only make a red stroke worse.

Using TPA requires a coordinated team effort to ensure your safety and the earliest possible treatment when the benefits are likely to be greatest. Many hospitals are just now getting around to organizing the teams that are required.

Treating the complications

Unfortunately, not many patients get to the emergency room soon enough to be treated. If TPA can't be given, there is still a lot that can be done, but nothing that will reduce the amount of brain injury from the stroke. The things that can be done fall into two categories: Preventing the complications of the brain hemorrhage and preventing another stroke. All of these treatments are described in later chapters in this book.

For white stroke, two of the most important complications to treat in the hospital are swallowing and blood clots that form in your legs due to inactivity from the stroke. Swallowing problems can lead to serious, possible fatal, cases of pneumonia. Blood clots in your leg veins can break loose and stop your heart or lungs. This isn't good either.

Swallowing problems can be treated by a speech therapist who can teach you ways to eat without choking or inhaling bits of food or drink.

Blood clots in your legs can be prevented by compression stockings or blood-thinning drugs. The choice depends on your other medical problems and the severity of your stroke disability.

Preventing another stroke

Each of the treatable risk factors can be addressed after you have a stroke. A second stroke may be even more serious that the one you just had, so it is definitely worth the effort. Stroke specialists know a lot more about preventing second and subsequent strokes than they do about preventing that first one. Ideas on prevention, in fact, are scattered all over this book because prevention is so important. But you should especially see the chapters in Part III for a lot of information on preventing strokes.

I present the following short list to summarize what you should be doing to prevent a second stroke while you are recovering from your first stroke:

- Control your blood pressure.
- Thin your blood if you have atrial fibrillation.
- Swear off tobacco.
- Take aspirin or a substitute.
- See if you would benefit from having a large atherosclerotic plaque cleared out of your carotid artery.
- Lower the cholesterol levels in your blood.
- Learn the signs and symptoms of stroke and teach your family to call 911 so that if you do have a stroke, you can be treated rapidly to reduce disability from a second stroke.

Chapter 4

Transient Stroke (TIA): Warning Sign

A 68-year-old retired postman was out walking his dog one morning. He noticed a fog forming in his vision and rubbed his right eyelid to see if it would clear. It didn't. He covered his right eye and the fog cleared. When he covered his left eye he could barely see anything with his right eye, as if his vision was grayed out. He stopped and sat down at a bus stop. Still his vision did not clear. He was beginning to worry now. He got up and decided to hurry home. By the time he got home his vision had cleared. He told his wife, and they decided to call an eye doctor. The receptionist scheduled an appointment in two weeks.

The morning after her boss's daughter's wedding party, a 61-year-old accountant was resting in the living room watching television and slowly drinking a cup of coffee. As she reached for the cup, she became aware that her right hand and forearm felt numb. Her hand seemed clumsy. She tried to pick up the cup but her fingers wouldn't wrap around the handle. She noticed her face felt funny as well. She thought about whether she had too much to drink at the party the night before. Then she remembered her blood pressure and wondered if she was having a stroke. She started to get frightened. She looked for the telephone to call for help but decided she didn't want to scare everyone or cause a lot of commotion. She tried to calm down and take a deep breath. The feeling was still gone in her hand, and her face felt heavy on the right side. In a minute or two, the feeling started to return to her hand. The whole episode lasted three or four minutes. She went to the hospital's emergency department that morning and insisted on being seen right away.

Both of these scenarios illustrate typical occurrences of *transient ischemic attack* (TIA), or transient stroke, a form of white stroke that is distinguished by its short duration and the fact that it passes without lingering symptoms.

How about a quick refresher: In Chapter 3, you found out that white strokes come in different sizes because blood clots and brain arteries come in different sizes. The symptoms depend on which artery is plugged. Blockage of the right carotid artery could leave you paralyzed on your left side; a clot in the left carotid artery might cause you to be unable to communicate or understand language. Strokes in smaller brain arteries cause other symptoms — not necessarily less severe — depending on what part of the brain that artery leads to.

This chapter explores another factor: the *length of time* the artery is plugged. If the vessel is plugged for a shorter amount of time, less or even no damage may occur. These "mini strokes" — in which the victim recovers from stroke symptoms in as little as a few minutes and has no lingering stroke symptoms — are considered transient strokes (or, by their official name, *transient ischemic attacks — TIA*).

Transient strokes typically last about two to seven minutes. Some last a little longer. You might read an official definition that transient strokes are all those that last less than 24 hours. But as a rule, they distinguish themselves from classical white strokes by being noticeably shorter events.

A type of stroke that neither lasts long nor leaves the victim with any debilitating after-effects? Should we be concerned at all? If there's one thing that you take from this chapter, let it be this: If you have a transient stroke, be concerned. Be very concerned. Why? Because a transient stroke can be followed by a serious disabling stroke within 24 to 48 hours. Roughly 10–20 percent of individuals who experience a transient stroke will suffer a bigger white stroke within 90 days. *Half of these strokes will occur in the first 48 hours.* And 15 percent of strokes are preceded by transient strokes. That amounts to at least 75,000 people per year in the United States. But experts estimate that these figures are actually higher — because many transient strokes are probably not reported.

In this chapter, I discuss transient strokes and why they are serious, even if they're often referred to as *minor* strokes. I cover how to respond to a transient stroke and suggest steps for preventing future strokes, transient or otherwise.

Defining Transient Stroke

Transient means lasting only a short time. Thus, a transient stroke is differentiated from the white stroke dealt with in Chapter 3 by its length. Recall the alphabet soup of names for white stroke: *cerebrovascular accident,* or *CVA,* and *ischemic stroke,* or *acute ischemic stroke* or *AIS.* You'll hear doctors and medical professionals refer to transient strokes as *transient ischemic attacks* — or, in their acknowledgment of how hard this is to say, *TIAs.* Why some strokes are *accidents* and others *attacks* has always baffled me. I prefer to say that some white strokes are *transient.*

So you have this little stroke. It's over in minutes and you're back to normal. Your arms and legs work fine, you walk without a limp, your speech returns, your mind is working, and you exhibit no sign that you ever suffered this strange episode. Are you free of brain injury?

Not necessarily. As explained in Chapter 3, if a brain artery is plugged for long enough, the brain is permanently injured, and the result is a hole in the brain called an *infarct.* If the infarct is big enough or in a critical location, then a permanent disability is the result — lingering symptoms such as impaired speech or walking with difficulty, for example.

Transient strokes present a different situation: a relatively short period of stroke symptom and no apparent disability after the episode clears up. This doesn't guarantee, however, that there isn't any brain injury. If the blood flow is stopped or slowed down for a long enough period of time, brain injury will occur, and the resulting infarct may be seen on a CT or MRI scan.

In a transient stroke, it's possible that no brain injury occurred. But it's just as possible that it *did* occur. Some transient strokes may cause brain injury, but that brain injury may not cause any abnormality noticed by the patient. Stroke comes, stroke leaves, brain is injured, but nobody could tell unless they observed the little hole revealed on a brain scan. It's like a scar on your leg: It's usually hidden, and no one notices because you don't walk any differently.

But how can it be that there are no symptoms at all, yet the brain is injured and an infarct can be seen on a brain scan? Well, it seems that some parts of your brain just don't cause obvious symptoms when they are injured. A lot of people live with small brain injuries they don't know they have. The only problem comes when all these small injuries begin to add up to a bigger, more obvious injury, called *vascular dementia,* that does cause symptoms.

Table 4-1 lists all the possibilities for white stroke.

Table 4-1	White Stroke: Symptoms and Brain Injury from Infarction	
Symptoms	*Brain Injury on MRI/CT*	*Description*
Don't clear completely	Yes	White stroke with infarction injury
Clear completely	Yes	Transient stroke with infarction injury
Clear completely	No	Transient stroke without brain injury
None	Yes	Brain infarction without stroke symptoms

How a Transient Stroke Occurs

A transient stroke begins just like any other white stroke. It may start when a blood clot forms in an artery and blocks it right there. This often happens at a spot where the artery, such as the carotid artery, is narrowed by a rough, raised *plaque* of cholesterol and scar tissue caused by *atherosclerosis* and high fat in the diet (see Figure 4-1). (See Chapter 3 for more information about *atherosclerosis* and blood clots.) Or a clot that has formed in an artery or the heart can break free and travel downstream to the brain or the retina.

Your carotid arteries, the pulses from which you feel around your voice box in your throat, are each about the size of your little finger. Near the angle of your jaw, each artery branches — one branch to your scalp and face, the

Transient stroke can cause vision loss

A transient stroke may result in loss of vision in one eye. One of the arteries to the brain is an artery that supplies blood to the retina of the eye, the seeing part at the back of the eye. (The blood supply of the retina is what causes the red eyes seen in flash photography.) When a blood clot plugs this artery, the retina stops working and a gray curtain falls on the vision from that eye. Often it will clear. If it does clear,

it is called *transient monocular blindness* or even *amaurosis fugax* (*fleeting blindness* in Latin). If it doesn't clear, it is called *retinal artery occlusion.*

Because technically the retina is part of the brain, I feel comfortable calling this a stroke. Others, perhaps most, don't.

other a mainline for blood to your brain. For some reason, this branch in the carotid arteries is prone to develop thick plaques of atherosclerosis.

The carotid plaques are particularly rough and cragged with craters and valleys. The plaques are composed of cholesterol, scar tissue, and calcium all mixed together. Because they are right in the path of blood headed to the brain, they are a common cause of stroke.

Such a stroke can occur a couple of ways:

✔ A clot can form on the plaque and close off the branch to the brain — this can be a major stroke affecting almost one third of the entire brain.

✔ A clot can begin to form on the plaque and then break loose in the bloodstream to travel toward the brain and block a smaller brain artery — this would also cause a stroke, but probably one not as serious as the clot blocking off the entire carotid artery.

In some patients, surgeons can remove the plaques to prevent strokes.

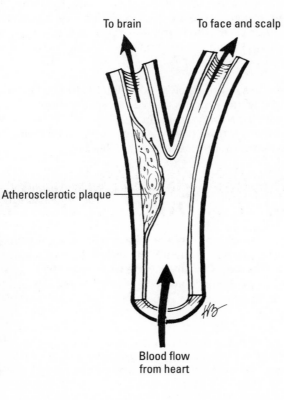

To brain

To face and scalp

Atherosclerotic plaque

Figure 4-1:
The carotid arteries are both close to the brain and prone to atherosclerotic plaque.

Blood flow from heart

In any case, the vessel is clogged, and you begin to notice one or several of those stroke warning signs discussed so far in this book: The left or right side of your body loses feeling; you can't hold an object with your hand; you have blurred vision in one or both eyes; you can't find the words for what you want to say; you don't understand what others are saying to you.

In a regular white stroke, these symptoms are likely to continue for quite a while, even while you're being taken to the emergency room. In a transient stroke, they're likely to clear up within 10 minutes — because in this case, your body is working efficiently against the clot.

As soon as blood flow is blocked, blood vessels all over the body spring into action to restore the flow. First, the small blood arteries that cross-connect with the blocked artery enlarge and increase their capacity to carry blood. Then *enzymes,* blood cells, and other molecules in the lining of the blood vessels are activated to dissolve and remove the clot.

In a white stroke that results in permanent brain injury, this process is not fast enough for the brain. By the time the blood clot is cleared and blood flow is restored, the sensitive substance of the brain is already injured beyond repair. In a transient stroke, however, the enzymes successfully attack and break up the clot quickly, and the blood flow returns. There can still be a brain injury — an infarct might be seen on a brain scan — but often there is no brain injury at all.

In transient stroke, the symptoms clear completely after the episode. The brain, puzzled by the whole process, heaves a sigh and thinks, "I wonder what that was?" Unfortunately, your brain also learns that maybe if you wait the next time you have a stroke, it may also go away on its own. That is not the right lesson to learn from transient stroke. Read on.

How to Recognize a Transient Stroke

Some people aren't sure whether they are having a transient stroke. If it goes away while they are still trying to figure out what is happening, they may not realize how serious it is. I don't want anyone who has a stroke to stay home confused or simply hope it will go away. On the other hand, I don't want everyone running to the emergency department just because their foot fell asleep.

If you have a little spell that starts out like a stroke but clears up, it could be a transient stroke. But it could also be a migraine headache, pressure on a nerve, a small seizure, or even low blood sugar. Sometimes, it might be hard to distinguish between, say, a dizzy spell and a transient stroke. Often people are confused and a little afraid of making too much of the episode and err on the side of timidity. They tell themselves they'll wait and see — and then never get around to going to the doctor at all.

But often, telltale signs distinguish a headache or a dizzy spell from a stroke.

Arm or leg falls asleep

If you sit on a hard surface for a long while, your leg may start buzzing with numbness. Tight straps or clothing may cause numbness in your arm or hand. This is because of pressure on a nerve going to your arm or leg. Having an arm or leg fall asleep is so common that most recognize this phenomenon for what it is. You know you have been in an uncomfortable position and you can often feel pain at the site where the nerve was pinched.

The numbness of stroke can be similar. But a few indicators might help you differentiate between an ordinary numbness and a transient stroke. If the numbness spreads to your shoulder, or hip, or elsewhere on the body, then this is a sign that the problem is more serious. If it spreads to include both an arm and a leg on the same side — and you have clumsiness or weakness of that arm or leg — then it's likely a stroke.

You better call 911 or get yourself to an emergency department soon, even if it clears up on your way or before you even leave for the hospital. Now you understand what is most likely a transient stroke that needs to be evaluated by a physician. Don't wait for it to go away. Even if it has before.

Dizzy spell

Dizzy spells are extremely difficult to figure out — especially when they clear up in a few minutes. There can be an episode of "wooziness" when the brain just doesn't feel right. There can be bouts of spinning vertigo with nausea and vomiting. A spell of lightheadedness, or vertigo, is usually not a stroke. There are many causes of vertigo: viral infection, an unusual form of migraine, even a benign condition that results in vertigo when you rise up from bed or move your head in certain ways.

But stroke is one of the causes of room-spinning vertigo, too. How do you know if that dizzy spell you just had is a sign of a transient stroke? Stroke-caused vertigo is often associated with other symptoms, including numbness or weakness on the side of the face, a droopy eyelid, or double vision.

Sometimes dizziness caused by a stroke can be associated with clumsiness or weakness of the hand. Likewise, you might have difficulty with balance while you are walking — or staggering, as the case may be — supporting yourself against tables and chairs.

Age is another indicator of whether your dizziness is likely to be stroke-related. A dizzy episode when you are 33 is probably not a stroke in progress. (It's not *impossible,* though, especially if you are taking birth-control pills and smoking cigarettes.) If you are 67, stroke is a more likely culprit — particularly if you also have high blood pressure, diabetes, and a history of heart trouble.

If you have a dizzy spell that clears up quickly — and you usually don't have them — then you may well be perfectly healthy. However, you might take this opportunity to assess your stroke risks and be sure you are doing everything necessary to prevent a stroke. See a doctor, especially one with a special interest in stroke.

Migraine headaches

Some migraines start out as strokes. The blood vessels of the brain constrict so tightly that blood flow is cut off to a part of the brain. The result is very similar to a stroke caused by a blood clot.

For individuals who've never before experienced a migraine headache, the severity of the symptoms often persuades them to go to the emergency room. The stroke-like symptoms usually fade and are followed by an incredibly painful headache. Those who periodically suffer from migraines are familiar with the feeling and can usually distinguish an ordinary migraine from a stroke.

If this is the first time you've had a headache like this, even if you suspect your sudden excruciating headache is a migraine rather than a stroke, go to the hospital to make sure it isn't some type of red stroke. Read more about headaches and stroke in Chapter 6.

Seizure

A seizure is one symptom of epilepsy, a convulsion involving a massive uncontrolled discharge of nerve impulses from all or part of the brain that causes muscles to jerk back and forth. Usually a person having a seizure loses consciousness.

However, there are times when only a small part of the brain loses control. In that case, only one limb may jerk back and forth. Sometimes the jerking is not as noticeable. When the seizure is over, the brain is completely exhausted and may not function for several minutes. Occasionally the brain doesn't get itself together for an hour or two. In the meantime, there may be temporary paralysis on one side of the body or another, one arm or leg. The result can be numbness, tingling, or weakness, just like a small stroke. Seizures may be caused by a number of factors unrelated to stroke: an old head injury, a tumor, a viral infection. In young children, they can even be the result of a sudden spike in temperature.

People can have a seizure in their sleep and not remember it. When they wake up or someone else finds them, all they may see is the paralysis from the seizure. Even during the day the seizure that causes the paralysis may not be witnessed by bystanders or remembered by the person who has just had a seizure. The person having a seizure isn't a reliable witness. He or she can't tell a stroke from a seizure, and who's to say someone with epilepsy can't have a stroke? Watch for shaking if you suspect a seizure, but go to an emergency room to see what's causing the problem.

Diabetes

If you are diabetic and take insulin to convert glucose into energy, you may experience stroke-like symptoms if you've taken too much insulin or some other medication to lower your blood glucose. At blood glucose levels below 80, your brain will begin to show symptoms. You will usually have the telltale symptoms of an insulin reaction: confusion, sweating, hunger, dizziness, confusion, and numbness or tingling of the lips.

If you don't have or don't heed these warning signs soon enough to get some sugar into your system, your brain may begin to shut down. Though you might expect the brain to turn off everywhere at once, only one part of the brain may in fact shut down. The symptoms may be paralysis on one side of the body or inability to speak or comprehend language that looks just like a stroke. It doesn't happen often, but every stroke specialist will tell you about a case that he or she was sure was a stroke until the blood glucose came back as 45, and the symptoms cleared up with the rapid infusion of glucose.

Sometimes the symptoms of low blood sugar can mimic a stroke by occurring on just one side of the body. Most stroke symptoms affect one side of the body or the other. Either way, your symptoms should clear rapidly when you drink some orange juice or other sugared drink. Otherwise, regardless of the cause of your symptoms, call for an ambulance. An insulin reaction is a life-threatening situation.

Responding to a Transient Stroke

You're *lucky* if your first stroke is transient. Some people experience a series of transient strokes, each similar to the last. This can go on for weeks or months. It's unusual, though. More often, a transient stroke is followed by a full-blown stroke that causes permanent disability.

If you take one thing from this chapter, make it this: *Transient stroke is a warning sign.* If you have a transient stroke, you are very likely to have another more serious stroke in the future. It's possible that a full-blown stroke could occur as early as 24 hours later. If you have a transient stroke, even if you feel completely normal, *you must do something!* You must *immediately* get yourself evaluated to find out what caused the stroke.

Get medical attention now

You had a close call. Your stroke lasted for a few minutes, then cleared. You were fortunate. But you may not be so fortunate next time. If you were really attuned to the importance of stroke, you would already have called 911 without waiting to see if your stroke was going to clear on its own. The ambulance is already on the way and will take you to the emergency department. If you have delayed, then start acting now to take advantage of the warning your transient stroke has given you.

The problem is that not everywhere is set up to treat transient strokes as emergencies. It can be hard to take get others to pay attention to your problem. You can ask your emergency room whether they have an emergency protocol for stroke.

The majority of stroke experts now believe that you should be admitted to the hospital the first time you have a transient stroke (TIA). In the hospital, you should be quickly evaluated so that any treatment you require can be started right away before you have another stroke that leaves you disabled.

In the ideal situation, you have your condition rapidly evaluated by stroke specialists and are admitted to the hospital. Some hospitals can run the tests you need while you are in the emergency room. In addition to blood tests, these would include a CT or MRI scan, a carotid ultrasound test, and an electrocardiogram.

Your other medical conditions and medications you are taking would be evaluated. Your history of stomach ulcers and other bleeding problems would be considered because that may influence whether you are given aspirin or a substitute. If you weren't already taking aspirin, then you might be started on aspirin. You would be given instructions on the symptoms of stroke and told to call 911 immediately if the symptoms returned.

Be proactive in getting treated

There are always scary stories in the newspapers and medical journals. One study recently suggested that even if you go to an emergency room, there's no guarantee that you will leave with the best recommendations. If you are sent home without being told whether you should be taking medication to prevent stroke, you might want to get to another physician more interested in stroke.

Because you are essentially "back to normal" after a transient stroke, it may be hard for emergency-room doctors who are responding to serious and urgent medical trauma to perceive your problem as critical. It is critical, *however,* and if you don't get the attention you require, you could be back in the emergency room sooner rather than later. Insist on getting the attention immediately — and don't stop until you get it.

If you aren't satisfied with the way things go in the emergency room, then try calling your physician's emergency number. Ask to be seen in the emergency room to be evaluated for stroke or TIA. If he/she says to come into the office in the morning, say you are worried about a stroke in the meantime. Ask if a stroke expert can be called in to see you or to talk to you on the phone.

If you are standing there reading this while your significant other is browsing travel books, and you are figuring out that you just had a transient stroke four days ago, then you need to know you have an opportunity here to prevent a real disaster. We are not talking about your car or your house, but your brain and your life as you know it.

Checklist for your check-up

Whether you get to an emergency room after your transient stroke or are able to see your physician immediately, you'll want to be sure that certain tests are considered and relevant health issues are addressed.

Here are the basics to consider:

- **Blood pressure:** Your blood pressure should be checked to see if it needs treatment or if treatment is effective.

- **Atrial fibrillation:** You should be checked for *atrial fibrillation,* a condition in which your heart pumps irregularly, causing ineffective blood flow, pooling of blood, and clots inside the heart that can break free and cause a white stroke. This check requires an EKG. (See Chapter 8 for more on this.)

- ✔ **Cholesterol levels:** Your cholesterol levels should be read. If you have high cholesterol, you are a candidate for *atherosclerosis* — the condition in which plaques form inside your blood vessels. (Several chapters in this book address this topic. Check out Chapters 9 and 10.)

- ✔ **Listen to the neck:** The doctor should listen to your neck with a stethoscope in order to determine whether you have an audible bruit in your neck that is a sign of a large carotid atherosclerosis plaque. Surgical removal of the plaque may reduce your risk of stroke. The doctor may not do this if an ultrasound test is going to be done immediately.

- ✔ **Carotid ultrasound:** The carotid artery in your neck should be checked to see if it is partially obstructed by a thick atherosclerotic plaque.

- ✔ **CT or MRI scans:** A CT or MRI scan is advised. This may reveal brain infarctions and injuries, indications that you have had brain infarction previously and not known it, or perhaps that your transient stroke wasn't as transient as you thought it was.

- ✔ **Heart exam:** Your transient stroke may be a sign that you have serious heart disease. A doctor should examine your heart as well.

- ✔ **Blood tests:** These are to check your blood glucose level and other tests to determine the cause of your symptoms. The clotting status of your blood will be evaluated as well.

Preventing the "Big One"

Once you've had the work-up following your transient stroke, you may have confirmed some stroke risk issues that you can now address more effectively. Perhaps you learned that you have atrial fibrillation, high cholesterol, heart disease — or maybe other conditions were detected that require follow-up.

In any case, now that you know you're at high risk for another stroke — one that might be permanent and disabling — it's high time to decide whether you are going to use this opportunity to take steps to reduce your risk.

Avoiding blood clots with medication

Perhaps the most important step after a transient stroke is to determine whether you should be taking aspirin or another drug to slow down your blood's tendency to form blood clots that cause strokes. If you have an ulcer or stomach problems, that's no reason not to treat your clotting risk. Aspirin is known to aggravate stomach problems, but there are other drugs that are as effective as aspirin in preventing clotting. Clinical trials have shown time and again that aspirin and other similar drugs reduce the number of in patients who have had a transient stroke. See Chapter 8 for more de about aspirin and other medications that reduce the risk of clotting.

Considering surgery

For some, surgery is the best way to prevent a follow-up stroke after transient stroke or a small white stroke. If you have a thick plaque (atherosclerosis) blocking one of the carotid arteries to your brain, then you may benefit from having the plaque surgically removed if the plaque is in the portion of the artery in your neck. Surgery has its risks: There's a 2 to 5 percent chance that you could have a major stroke during the procedure. But several clinical trials support that the odds are in your favor if you have the surgery.

Clinical trials have shown that the thicker the plaque, the more you have to gain from surgery. The thickness of the plaque is measured in terms of the percentage of blood flow that is blocked. The blockage is called *stenosis,* or narrowing of the blood vessel. If your carotid artery stenosis is more than 50 percent, then surgery is probably beneficial if you have just had a transient stroke. If it is more than 70 percent, the benefits are greater. For lower degrees of stenosis, less than 50 percent, surgery is not usually helpful.

The risks of surgery are serious stroke and even death. The percentages are low, but after a TIA you are completely normal. Be sure you have a clear understanding of the risks and want to go ahead. It's a little like seatbelts in a car. In most accidents, they will protect you. In a small percentage of cases, they may cause more harm than good.

The surgical procedure to remove a carotid plaque is called *carotid endarterectomy.* It is one of the most common stroke-related surgical procedures done. But, as always with major surgery — especially when it involves the brain — it's important to consider your decision carefully. Whatever the degree of stenosis, you should get a second opinion and find out about the track record and success of the surgeon making the recommendation.

Should you choose to proceed with surgery, be sure to verify that your surgeon is experienced with the procedure. Ideally, you would like a surgeon who does dozens of these procedures every year. The surgeon should also be able to tell you the percentage of patients who have a stroke or die within 30 days of the surgery. This percentage should be less than 5 percent. This may seem high — keep in mind that it is not the result of poor surgical technique, but the fragile medical condition of many patients. Remember that for patients with a large plaque and a history of transient stroke, the percentage who have a stroke without surgery is much higher at one year than those who did have surgery.

alternative to surgery

...to consider *stents* instead of surgery. *Stents* are devices
...ide your carotid artery to hold it open. This alternative
...new and still being tested in clinical trials. To some,
...ause there's no scar on your neck. That doesn't seem
...to choose how to protect your brain from stroke.

...ents is not free of serious problems, however. The stent procedure
...cause strokes, just as surgery can. There are devices that are supposed
to keep blood clots and pieces of plaque from breaking loose and flying up to
the brain while the stent is being placed, but there is only limited evidence
that they work as advertised. There is more information on surgery and
stents in Chapter 8.

A reminder list

There are many steps you can take to reduce your risk of future stroke.
Chapters 8–10 explore many of them in detail. But here's a reminder list of
the most important preventive measures that will arm you in your war
against stroke.

- ✔ Monitor your blood pressure.
- ✔ Stop smoking.
- ✔ Lower your cholesterol — through diet and/or statin drugs.
- ✔ Thin your blood if you have atrial fibrillation.
- ✔ If you've had a stroke, even a transient stroke, take aspirin or a substitute daily if your doctor agrees.
- ✔ Prevent diabetes if you don't have it, treat it to the max if you do.

Answering the Wake-Up Call

When a transient stroke happens, you can think of numerous excuses for not
doing anything. It could be this. It could be that. You're just tired. You're
upset because of something and if you just settle down, everything will be
okay. You'll call your daughter — she always knows what to do.

We all make excuses and hope something terrible will just go away. Sometimes
it does. But often it doesn't. It's your brain. Your life of memories, your love,
your personality, your get-up-and-go. Take action when you need to. Don't be
fooled by one lucky turn of fate.

A transient stroke is like the red engine light on your car that blinks on while you are driving. The car is running fine — the road is smooth ahead. There hasn't been any other sign of trouble. Maybe the red light is malfunctioning? Unlikely.

Isn't it amazing that people actually burn up their car's engines? I wonder what they tell themselves. "I thought I could make it to work." "I didn't want to stop on the interstate." "If I stopped, I would be late."

If you have a transient stroke and keep on driving, you're taking a good chance of burning up the engine of your life. A transient stroke is a red light — a serious warning that you have problems. You can ignore the opportunity and very likely live to regret it. On the other hand, there are relatively simple actions you can take that will greatly increase the likelihood that you will live a longer and better life.

Chapter 5

Red Stroke (ICH): Bleeding Inside the Brain

Red strokes are the opposite of white strokes. White strokes are caused by blood clots in the brain arteries, but red strokes are caused by *bleeding* of the brain arteries. The two types of red stroke are differentiated by where the bleeding starts. One type involves bleeding in the areas surrounding the brain, called *subarachnoid hemorrhage* or *aneurysm;* this type of stroke is dealt with in Chapter 6.

This chapter covers the other type — called *brain hemorrhage* or *intracerebral hemorrhage* (ICH), which occurs when the bleeding is within the brain itself. I prefer the less technical term *brain hemorrhage*. Brain hemorrhage produces the same signs and symptoms as a white stroke. This includes paralysis of the face, arm, or leg on one side of the body, difficulty speaking or understanding speech, loss of sensation on part of one side of the body, dizziness, and clumsiness in the use of the arms or legs. However, a red stroke caused by brain hemorrhage often continues to get worse as the minutes and hours pass, eventually progressing to coma in many cases. A typical white stroke, on the other hand, stays the same or even improves on its own during the first few hours and coma occurs much less often.

Brain hemorrhages are more often fatal and cause more severe disability than the more common white ischemic stroke. The chances of someone dying in the first few days after a brain hemorrhage (ICH) are about 40 percent — double the rate for white strokes, which is about 20 percent. This is primarily because of the catastrophic consequences of brain swelling that accompanies brain hemorrhage.

Victims of brain hemorrhage are typically between 55 and 60 years old —
younger than those who suffer from white strokes. The good news is brain
hemorrhage is a less common type of stroke, striking approximately 15 percent of all stroke sufferers. This equates to an estimated 70,000 individuals
each year in the United States.

In this chapter, I identify the causes of brain hemorrhage, explain how the
brain reacts to bleeding, review a variety of treatments for this type of red
stroke, and, finally, cover steps to prevent further brain hemorrhage.

Although white strokes and red strokes result from different causes, the same
advice for preventing white strokes applies to this type of red stroke. Prepare
yourself now — you'll be reading a lot about high blood pressure and the
importance of getting it in check. (If you want to escape that altogether, try
one of the chapters on nursing homes or rehabilitation. I think I only mention
it in passing there.)

High blood pressure, among other factors, can increase your risk of brain
hemorrhage.

I would hope that, by now, it's understood that at the first sign of stroke, you
should call 911. It is *critical* to get to the ER *as soon as possible.* Early arrival
allows the stroke team to do a better job of controlling your blood pressure,
containing your brain swelling, and keeping you breathing if you lose consciousness. The earlier you receive treatment for brain hemorrhage, the
better your odds of reducing disability — and surviving.

The CT scan shown in Figure 5-1 shows a medium-sized brain hemorrhage
that started on the patient's left side (remember, right and left are reversed
on the CT scan) and pressed the brain to the patient's right across the front-
to-back midline. Those bright white spots in the ventricles are normal
deposits of hard calcium. The gray-colored brain has also swollen to press a
little more tightly against the white-colored bony skull on the left side: You
see fewer of the usual convolutions of the brain, which typically appear as
distinct creases on a CT scan. This is because they have been squeezed flat
against the skull.

Why the Brain Bleeds

High blood pressure — particularly longstanding high blood pressure — is
the leading cause of brain hemorrhages, being responsible for nearly half.
Still, that leaves many other possible causes. Unlike white stroke, which is
almost always caused by blood clots blocking arteries and reduced blood
flow, brain hemorrhage may be the result of anything from abnormal blood
vessels to a bladder infection. Sometimes the cause may be clear — in other
cases, it's a mystery until further testing can be done. If a patient survives

CASE STUDY

A fatal brain hemorrhage

A 62-year-old successful businessman was dancing at his youngest daughter's wedding. He had been diagnosed with high blood pressure and took his medication infrequently. (No one could verify whether he took the medication the day of the wedding.) While he was dancing, he noticed a headache and sat down for a rest. Gradually the headache got worse. Someone noticed that he was speaking abnormally. He reached for a drink of water and spilled it on the table and floor. When he tried to stand up, he found that he couldn't and lost his balance. Some thought he just had too much alcohol to drink. His oldest daughter, a nurse, recognized that he was having a stroke. She called 911. The ambulance EMTs started him on an IV and took him to an emergency room.

In the ER, it was noticed that his right arm and leg were very weak. He spoke, but the words were garbled and did not make sense. He was drowsy. His blood pressure was 220/160. He was given medication to lower it. Blood tests were ordered. The stroke team got a history from the family. One of the daughters was a physician. She was very concerned because the hospital did not have all the resources of a major big-city hospital. Other physicians,

including a neurology specialist, were called in. Meanwhile, the patient lost consciousness.

The specialist ordered a CT scan while the family discussed transferring the patient to another hospital. The scan showed a large ball of blood on the left side, centered deep in the middle of the brain. The blood had gotten into the ventricles of the brain. Already, swelling on the left side of the brain was pushing across the midline into the right brain. When the physician daughter saw this, she knew the story was over. The patient had been placed on a respirator and was being prepared for the intensive care unit. His breathing alternated between slow and fast. Soon he stopped breathing on his own and the ventilator began breathing for him.

In the next few hours, his condition worsened as his coma deepened and his brain stopped functioning. He had told his family he never wanted to be kept alive for a prolonged time when there was little or no chance he would survive. The immediate family, all gathered at the hospital, asked that he be taken off of life support. He died about eight hours after the first signs of his stroke.

the initial hours of the brain hemorrhage, a variety of tests may be done to determine why the stroke occurred.

Longstanding high blood pressure

Over the years, high blood pressure, particularly if aggravated by diabetes, wears out and weakens the walls of small blood vessels deep inside the brain. These vessels are connected directly to high-pressure mainline arteries to the brain. They are exposed to greater stresses than other small blood vessels in the brain. After years of strain, the blood vessels develop dilapidated, patched, and repatched walls. In some places the vessels are so weak, they form tiny *blebs* that can easily break under high pressure.

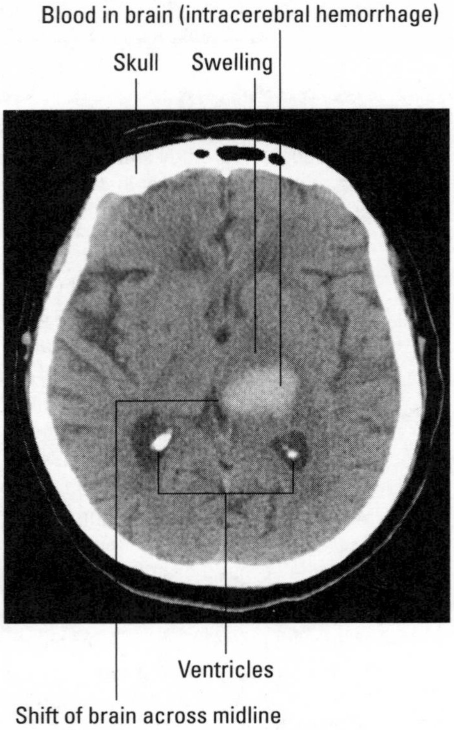

Blood in brain (intracerebral hemorrhage)

Skull   Swelling

Ventricles

Shift of brain across midline

Figure 5-1:
CT scan
of a red
stroke (ICH).

Blebs? Yes, blebs. Blebs are little blisters on the walls of these blood vessels, about the size of the head of a pin. These tiny blebs are also called *micro-aneurysms,* but they are not to be confused with the much larger *berry aneurysms* that cause *subarachnoid hemorrhage,* the type of red stroke discussed in Chapter 6.

If blebs break, blood pours out of the ruptured artery. The extensive damage that can be done by blood gushing out of one of these pencil-lead-thin arteries is amazing. It shows how hard the arteries work to contain the pressure. Think about that the next time you consider skipping your blood pressure pills.

When white stroke leads to red stroke

What starts out as a white stroke caused by a blood clot blocking an artery can turn into a red stroke with bleeding into the brain. Most experts think this happens because the brain blood vessels are injured when their blood supply is cut off by a blood clot upstream. The vessels are starving for glucose and oxygen. When they don't come in time, the vessels begin to fall apart. Then later — perhaps hours or even a day or two — the blocking clot may be cleared by the normal processes that keep blood vessels free of clots and wide open for the flow of blood. Then the blood rushes from the site of the clot that caused the white stroke into blood vessels that have been weakened and injured by lack of glucose and oxygen. Sometimes the vessel walls are so weak they can't contain the new rush of blood. This brain bleeding can worsen the original white stroke disability and can be fatal. This process is called *hemorrhagic conversion* of a white ischemic stroke. It happens more often when your blood is thinned with a drug like warfarin, heparin, or TPA.

Medication that thins the blood

It seems ironic that trying to prevent a white stroke can cause a red stroke, but warfarin and heparin, two drugs used to slow down blood clotting for sufferers of white stroke, must be carefully monitored. Blood tests must be done regularly to be sure that blood clotting isn't slowed down too much. But even when the clotting time is acceptable, brain hemorrhages can occur. Heparin is mostly used in the hospital since it must be dripped into a vein. Warfarin (also called Coumadin) is taken when you are not in the hospital.

I don't think anyone is exactly sure how the hemorrhages start. Perhaps there are tiny breaks in the blood vessels all the time that are repaired rapidly by the clotting mechanism. When blood clotting is too slow, these tiny leaks become larger until they are too large to contain. Perhaps it is like the first trickle over the top of an earthen dam that quickly washes the dam away.

Although there are treatments that help reverse the effects of warfarin and heparin, often the damage from hemorrhage is done before the effects can be reversed.

Should you risk treating white stroke with a drug that could lead to red stroke? Probably. Clinical trials have shown that the odds are still in your favor if you take warfarin when you have *atrial fibrillation,* a condition that can lead to white stroke (see Chapter 8 for more details), even though it does increase risk of brain hemorrhage. The potential benefits outweigh the risks. When dealing with something as serious as stroke, most people are willing to take greater risks. A closely monitored drug and treatment strategy ought to balance the benefits with the risks.

If you are on Warfarin or Heparin to treat white stroke, you're wise to keep an eye on your blood-clotting time through frequent blood tests. Don't miss scheduled blood tests, and let your doctor know if you change medications or notice any change in bruising so that extra tests can be scheduled. You should also watch your diet to avoid sudden changes in the amounts of foods with vitamin K and in the timing of your eating relative to when you take your medication. Also be careful when you change any other medications, because stopping or starting a drug and changing your diet can affect blood clotting time.

Blood-vessel abnormalities

Have you seen people with large, red patches or birthmarks on their skin? Those are caused by abnormal blood vessels. Sometimes they can enlarge, but other than their appearance, they cause no problems. Abnormal blood vessels can also occur in the brain. They are more problematic. The knots and tangles of arteries and veins, which can become quite large, are intertwined in the substance of the brain. Because they are abnormal, they often have weak walls that tend to break and bleed. Some never bleed.

One of the most common blood-vessel abnormalities, *arteriovenous malformations* or AVMs, are formed from brain arteries and veins. Brain bleeding from AVMs is generally not as severe as the more common type of brain hemorrhage from a broken artery. High blood pressure increases the risk that an AVM will bleed, but they often bleed when the blood pressure is normal.

You should know that many specialists recommend that you do nothing at all to get rid of an AVM. In fact, an AVM may bleed several times before some doctors think it is worth the risk to treat them. They are quite rare, and not all of them cause brain hemorrhages. Some cause epileptic seizures, as well, but that is for another book.

What to do about AVMs?

Testing for AVMs requires MRI scans or a procedure called an *arteriogram* or *angiogram*. A large needle is poked in the groin, a spaghetti-sized hollow plastic tube is threaded into a main brain artery, and the brain is blasted with a special contrast agent through this tube to make the AVM light up on an X-ray. The pictures show all the blood vessels at once and reveal a lot of detail that is needed to figure out the best way to treat the AVM.

Some specialists recommend doing nothing to treat the AVM. Others recommend brain surgery, radiation therapy, or blocking off the AVM from inside the blood vessels — or a combination of these. We really don't have evidence

from good clinical trials to help you decide about treatment of AVMs. You will have to go by the recommendations of your physicians.

Any of these procedures present risks, and there are frequent complications. A patient who is advised to undergo any of the treatments should seek out a second — or even third — opinion. If you choose to proceed, confirm that the surgeon or radiologist has experience with this procedure *successfully*. I would suggest going with the most experienced surgeon you can find. The AVM may be treated during the same hospitalization as the brain hemorrhage or after the patient is transferred to a more comprehensive stroke treatment center.

Infections from tooth to bladder

On occasion, something as seemingly unrelated as a bladder infection or the infection resulting from a dental procedure can lead to a brain hemorrhage. Some infections can get into the blood, where the bacteria grow and are carried to the heart and valves. The infected blood can collect in clumps in the smallest blood vessels in the brain. Lodged there, the infection continues to multiply and eats away at the blood vessel walls, potentially breaking through to cause a hemorrhage. Usually, though, the brain can contain the hemorrhage, and a relatively small hemorrhage is the result.

It is important to determine whether a hemorrhage is caused by bacteria, because antibiotics will cure the problem. If a stroke victim survives, the antibiotic should clear up the infection and eliminate the risk of future brain hemorrhages. Without antibiotic, more hemorrhages and serious infection can develop in the brain. Simple blood and urine tests can determine whether infection is the cause of a brain hemorrhage.

Other causes of brain hemorrhage

As I said earlier, brain hemorrhage claims a lot more causes than white stroke does. Here are several others that doctors may test for:

- ✔ **Aging of blood vessels:** When some people get to be more than 70 years old, their brain arteries are weakened by a rubbery substance deposited among the muscle fibers of the artery wall. The substance is called *amyloid* (AM uh loyd), and the weakening of the artery wall is called *amyloid angiopathy* (ann jee OPP uh thee). Bleeding from these weakened arteries is usually near the top surface of the brain. It is probably the second most common cause of brain hemorrhage.

- ✔ **Tumors in the brain:** Tumors growing in the brain may go unnoticed until they start bleeding and cause a stroke. The tumor itself may be hidden within all the blood. If it is a small tumor, it may not be noticed in the emergency room — after all, the ER team is more focused on treating the stroke and keeping the patient alive until the bleeding stops. Later, as doctors try to figure out what caused the brain hemorrhage, further testing may reveal what remains of the tumor.

  Surviving a brain hemorrhage only to find a brain tumor is not a happy series of events. However, it may turn out that the tumor is entirely treatable. So it's important to explore this possibility.

✔ **Cocaine and stimulant drugs:** The use of cocaine and stimulant drugs is associated with a higher incidence of brain hemorrhage. Some hemorrhages may occur because of sudden increases in blood pressure associated with the drug; others, by some type of reaction of the brain blood vessels to the drug.

✔ **Blood-clotting deficiencies:** People who have conditions such as hemophilia, leukemia, cancer, and liver failure also have abnormally slow clotting of the blood, making them more prone to brain hemorrhages. And because the blood doesn't clot normally, these brain hemorrhages are usually more serious and more often fatal.

✔ **Extremely high blood pressure:** A sudden and severe increase in blood pressure is called a *hypertensive crisis.* The lower of the two blood pressures (the diastolic pressure) goes over 120. The longer the blood pressure stays up, and the higher it is, the greater the risk that a brain artery will rupture under the strain. The result is bleeding into the brain. The most common cause of hypertensive crisis is an unexplained sudden blood pressure increase in someone who already has high blood pressure. Suddenly stopping some of the less common blood pressure medications like clonidine can precipitate a crisis. Hypertensive crisis also can occur during pregnancy as part of the problem called *eclampsia.*

✔ **Red strokes due to subarachnoid bleeding:** As explained in Chapter 6, *subarachnoid hemorrhage* is when bleeding occurs in the fluid surrounding the brain. Occasionally, this bleeding occurs in such a way that the jet of blood goes *into* the brain. Subarachnoid hemorrhage caused by rupture of a blood vessel outside the brain is much worse if it is accompanied by bleeding into the brain.

✔ **Head trauma:** If you bang your head hard enough, all the padding and fluid cushions that protect the brain will fail. The result can be a few tiny, torn vessels deep in the brain. Or it can be a brain destroyed by a skull-crushing blow. Brain trauma is not a stroke, so I don't discuss it in this book.

Because this book, to a certain extent, is like a brain owner's manual, I can't help but say to you that brain hemorrhage occurs a lot more often than most people realize. Over the years, all the bumps on the head and resulting minor hemorrhages begin to accumulate. So, wear a helmet when you are supposed to and buckle your seatbelts when you are driving.

How the Brain Reacts to Blood

The brain hates blood that isn't where it is supposed to be. And when blood gets outside of brain blood vessels, by whatever means, the brain reacts strongly. Although eventually the bleeding stops on its own as the clotting process kicks in, the repercussions can be extremely destructive. In this section I list some of the challenges.

Brain swelling

Blood gushing from an artery into the substance of the brain makes it swell up just like any bruise under the skin or in a muscle. The extra blood alone causes the brain to swell. But the reaction also causes white blood cells to release special chemicals to respond to the blood. More white blood cells are drawn to the area. The blood vessels in the surrounding area begin to leak fluid around the blood clot. Injured brain cells also leak fluid into the substance of the brain. The result is that the brain swells even more as it reacts to the release of blood within the brain.

Often on CT or MRI scans, you can see a darker area around the white area of hemorrhage. This darker area represents a part of the brain that is swollen and filled with water (mostly) as a result of the brain's response to the blood. This extra water filling the brain is called *edema*. You may notice a little dark rim around the white clot areas in the brain CT scan shown back in Figure 5-1. The more blood in the brain, the more brain edema is produced.

Pressure mounts, blood flow stops

The problem with all this swelling is that the brain is trapped inside the skull. If the brain swells, then something else has to shrink. For a while this can be the clear fluid around the brain and in brain ventricles. But if the brain continues to swell, something else has to give.

As bleeding continues to increase the size of the brain inside the skull, the pressure in the skull goes up. It's as if the brain is pushing against the skull and all the holes in it. As the brain pushes out, the heart has a harder time pushing the blood into the skull. If the pressure gets too high, the heart will fail to push enough blood into the brain to sustain brain function.

This is a total disaster. First, the brain shuts down, leading to unconsciousness. Then before too many minutes, the brain starts to die from lack of blood flow. Sometimes there is so much blood and swelling in the brain that nothing works. Within a few minutes or hours, death occurs. Fortunately, in most cases, either the pressure doesn't get so high that blood flow stops, or the pressure inside the skull can be controlled so that blood flow continues.

Deforming the brain

The swelling from the bleeding happens on just one side of the brain, but the imbalance in pressure squeezes against the side of the brain that is not bleeding. If you look carefully back in Figure 5-1, you can see in the center of the skull where the blood (which appears as the white splotch on the right) has pushed the right side of the brain into the left side and deformed it.

The brain is flexible only to a certain extent. The spinal cord and nerves at the base of the brain still have to exit from the holes in the skull. They can stretch a little, but they pull back on the brain as it is deformed by the pressure. The brain can actually push part of itself down into the space in the neck where the spinal cord usually is.

There are a few really tight places where vital brain structures that keep a person alive and breathing are squeezed so hard that the nerve cells are crushed and torn. The victim loses consciousness, but this time because of actual physical injury to the brain. Injuries to the base of the brain are not easy to fix, and they are the most common cause of death for patients with brain hemorrhage.

Unconsciousness

Sleep is good. Unconsciousness is bad. *Unconsciousness* is due to a failure of vital structures in the brain to respond to stimuli that would ordinarily keep someone alert. There are different degrees of unconsciousness, but in the deepest levels of coma, the brain is not able to keep the lungs breathing. The patient may easily choke and becomes more prone to infections. Obviously, people in this state cannot feed themselves.

Here come the tubes. Tubes to help you eat, tubes to help you breathe, and tubes to help you eliminate waste. As more and more of the brain is permanently injured by brain hemorrhage and swelling, the closer a patient comes to brain death — the vegetative state that most of us consider to be unacceptable.

It's hard to predict whether someone who remains unconscious and accumulates brain injury will survive and recover. If the hemorrhage is unusually large, if there is blood in the ventricles, if the person is very old, if there is shift of the brain across the midline, then meaningful survival is unlikely. Overuse of technology can certainly keep people "alive" — even if they have no chance of meaningful life after the brain swelling is brought under control.

Treating Brain Hemorrhage in the Hospital

Treating bleeding inside the brain is difficult. The bleeding is tightly enclosed in the skull where broken blood vessels can't easily be reached. Even if a surgeon cuts through the skull, the source of the bleeding is usually farther inside the brain itself. Eventually the bleeding stops on its own — by clot formation and increasing pressure inside the skull. But doctors must deal with the effects of the bleeding, including brain swelling and unconsciousness and other conditions that may slow the clotting process.

Hyperventilating to reduce brain swelling

The goal of medical treatment for brain swelling is to keep the blood flowing and to control the swelling so that the brain doesn't crush itself. Serious brain swelling means the sufferer is already unconscious and a machine is breathing for him or her.

It is remarkable but true that during hyperventilation the brain shrinks. Someone on a ventilator machine is given drugs that paralyze the muscles and keep the patient from fighting to control breathing. By simply setting the ventilator to go a little faster than normal, the patient can be forced to hyper-ventilate, and, hence, the brain shrinks. But there are certainly risks to this tactic. Lots of expensive blood tests have to be done to control the breathing once the brain is no longer being allowed to do that.

Using drugs to reduce brain swelling

Another way to reduce swelling in the bleeding brain is the use of drugs. Mannitol, barbiturates, and steroids are all drugs that can help reduce swelling. Like hyperventilation, though, they only work for a while, and then only produce a relatively small effect. But a small amount of extra space in the skull at a critical time can save a life.

Brain drain

Increased pressure inside the skull is more of a mechanical problem than a medical one. However, it is a *difficult* mechanical problem, and MRI and CT scans are needed to map out the best solutions. One surgical treatment physicians may consider in order to bring down swelling is to place a tube in the brain to drain the fluids.

In some cases of brain hemorrhage, blood breaks through into the ventricles of the brain. It's bad news if this happens, for several reasons. For one thing, when the blood in the ventricles clots, it blocks the usual flow of the fluid from one ventricle to another and eventually out of the brain into the space around the brain and spinal cord where it is absorbed. In the CT scan shown in Figure 5-1, three of the four ventricle spaces are filled with blood (it's really red or reddish black, but on the CT scan it looks white).

If the blood clots and prevents the escape of the fluid out of the ventricles of the brain, pressure builds up, and the ventricles expand. As you might imag-ine, this isn't good. Fortunately, there is a relatively easy way to deal with this. A surgeon can drill a hole in the skull and press a soft plastic tube through the brain and into a ventricle to relieve that pressure. This is called a *ventriculostomy,* and it can potentially cause infection and more bleeding. Neither is good — but sometimes there isn't much choice.

Removing the clot: Risky business

Well, you may say, if it's so easy to put a tube in the ventricle and relieve the pressure by draining fluid, then why not put a tube in the clot and let the blood escape? Believe me, it's been tried. Problem is, it's just not clear whether it helps or hurts.

The blood doesn't stay fluid very long. Contact with the substance of the brain tends to make it clot quickly.

So when a surgeon puts a tube in the center of the bloody area, blood doesn't gush out like the clear fluid from the ventricles. Sucking the blood out with vacuum pressure doesn't work that well either. Attempts to dissolve the clot before sucking it out through a tube have not been very successful in saving lives or reducing disability. Nevertheless, when things are not going well, some neurosurgeons are willing to accept high risks rather than do nothing at all.

Another approach is to open up a larger hole in the skull and expose the clot. This is easy to do on smaller brain hemorrhages near the surface — not so manageable for deep hemorrhages, such as shown in Figure 5-1. Once the clot is exposed, the surgeon can remove it and stop any bleeding. This approach has its problems, too. For one thing, clots near the surface are often those caused by bleeding from old blood vessels weakened by *amyloid angiopathy.* They bleed easily — so this process can actually make the problem worse. Also, there is some potentially good brain mixed in with the clot. You can't always remove the clot without injuring some brain.

There is one situation in which surgical removal of the clot can be beneficial. If the bleeding is in the *cerebellum* (refer to Chapter 2's Figure 2-2), a brain hemorrhage can be rapidly fatal, because a large clot here presses the brain against a sharp edge that cuts into vital brain areas that keep someone alive. Emergency surgery in this somewhat rare situation can be life-saving.

All in all, except for the larger hemorrhages in the cerebellum, surgical removal of a blood clot in the brain is pretty dicey. Some surgeons claim they can make things better in specific situations. Often, the situation is so dire that the family and other doctors may think taking any chance is better than having no chance at all. In other cases, the clot may be small and in a place that's easy (for a neurosurgeon) to reach. In that case, risk of further injury seems less, and possible benefits from clot removal may seem worthwhile.

The patient is going to be sound asleep or unconscious, so the neurosurgeon is going to be talking to someone in the family about the risks and benefits of doing the surgery. This isn't a situation in which there is a lot of time to get a second opinion from another surgeon. If the surgeon at hand is experienced and thinks it's worth the risk, then it's probably wise to go ahead with the understanding that the surgery could make things worse.

You don't think I sound convinced? Well, I'm not, and you should know that a lot of doctors have their doubts about surgical removal of clots.

Reducing blood pressure

High blood pressure causes the bleeding for nearly half the incidents of brain hemorrhage. Why not just drop the blood pressure? If there is anything doctors are good at, it is raising and lowering blood pressure. But it isn't that simple. High blood pressure has benefits as well as disadvantages. We still don't have a good way to keep the blood pressure in *just* the right range, not too high and not too low.

Slowing the bleeding . . .

When a brain hemorrhage is caused by a blood clot that pushes high-pressure blood into weakened brain vessels that break, the bleeding can continue because of the high blood pressure. Most physicians agree that it's critical to lower the blood pressure to help slow the bleeding and perhaps reduce the size of the eventual blood clot.

. . . but strangling the brain

On the other hand, lowering the blood pressure can reduce the amount of blood going to the brain. The higher blood pressure may be needed to push harder against the growing pressure inside the skull. If you lower the blood pressure too much, the brain gets less and less blood flow as the size of the hemorrhage grows. The whole brain can start to die from lack of oxygen and glucose in the blood. This isn't good either, obviously.

Because of the risks, the lowering of blood pressure is done *cautiously* with drugs chosen to have a slow and gradual effect. Dropping the blood pressure suddenly can cause serious problems, so it's not uncommon for a patient on such a treatment to be placed in an intensive care unit just to control and monitor the blood pressure.

Getting the blood to clot

If your brain is bleeding, you want your blood to clot, and the sooner the better. So if blood tests show that for some reason the blood isn't clotting well, doctors will undoubtedly take steps to fix that. First, they try to determine why the blood won't clot. Sometimes, the problem may be a drug — warfarin, heparin, even aspirin — prescribed to prevent blood clotting. As mentioned, drugs given to prevent white strokes may cause very serious red strokes. Other conditions also result in blood-clot problems:

- ✔ **Kidney failure:** Those who are on dialysis sometimes receive heparin to keep the blood from clotting inside the dialysis machine.

- ✔ **Liver failure:** The liver makes vitamin K, required for healthy clotting. If the liver is compromised, vitamin K production may be down.

- ✔ **Cancer:** Some cancer drugs reduce the number of blood platelets. These cells are necessary for clotting.

Medical treatment to increase the ability of the blood to clot is relatively straightforward. Vitamin K counteracts warfarin or the effects of liver failure. There are drugs that reverse the effects of heparin. An alternative solution is to give a special transfusion of blood that contains all the clotting factors. Or if the problem is a shortage of platelets, platelets can be transfused.

Treating infections

If a brain hemorrhage was caused by an infection in the bloodstream, then it is likely that massive amounts of antibiotics will be administered along with treatments for brain swelling and unconsciousness. If the brain recovers well, the treatment of the blood infection can takes weeks or even months to complete. If a heart valve or implanted device becomes infected, surgery may be required, though it usually can be postponed until after stroke recovery.

Relying on life support

Keeping someone alive who is deeply unconscious raises complex issues — not to mention hospital bills. Yet the wonderful capability of modern medicine has saved many folks for long and productive lives.

A stroke patient who has drifted into unconsciousness may require life-support measures to maintain basic body functions. The family needs to be aware that after the worst is over, the patient may *appear* more unconscious than he or she is. Many treatments in an intensive care unit make it impossible for someone to move or speak. Because being agitated and awake raises intracranial pressure, patients are sedated while connected to a ventilator. This may result in a groggy state in which the patient can hear, but may have a hard time responding. Nurses are usually aware of this and often talk to the patient. Family members may be encouraged to do the same.

All the tubes and electronic machinery can be frightening. The family may feel that their loved one is suffering, not realizing that the individual is not feeling much of anything. Doctors and nurses are used to seeing people in this condition and know that they can survive with little or no complications. For this reason, they may seem a little insensitive. But just because the surroundings look like Dr. Frankenstein's lab doesn't mean anyone should give up hope. What really makes a difference is the condition of the brain. No one should give up hope until the doctor does.

Preventing More Red Strokes

Someone lucky enough to get out of the hospital after a brain hemorrhage needs to take action to prevent more strokes. A red stroke puts you at increased risk of white strokes. Here are some preventative measures:

- ✔ **Treat your blood pressure:** It's your first priority. Remember, longstanding high blood pressure causes nearly half of all brain hemorrhages. This means check your blood pressure regularly, see the doctor more often, take medication if appropriate, and make lifestyle changes (diet, exercise) as necessary.

- ✔ **Monitor your warfarin:** If your red stroke was the result of a white stroke, and you are being treated for white stroke, you want to make sure that your dosage of warfarin (for reducing blood clotting) is closely monitored. This may mean more check-ups with your stroke doctor.

- ✔ **Manage blood lipids, diabetes, and heart disease:** High blood pressure is intimately connected to other blood-related conditions, including high cholesterol, diabetes, and heart disease. You can read more about this in Chapter 10. Being healthy may mean giving up favorite pastimes and taking more pills than you want to. Tough luck. Work hard to live long.

Chapter 6

Red Stroke (SAH):
Bleeding Outside the Brain

....

....

*T*his is a tough chapter to write without using the ridiculous tongue-twisters of medicine, but there is simply no way around them when discussing this form of red stroke. If I don't let you in on terms such as *subarachnoid hemorrhage* and *aneurysm,* you may be lost when you hear doctors talk, I won't be able to clearly explain how such strokes occur, you may not be able to understand the situation if you or a loved one suffers from this serious condition. We just don't have everyday words to describe the complex goings-on of the brain, its blood vessels, and the occurrences inside the skull.

So, just be patient and focus on two terms you don't hear every day. The first is *aneurysm,* pronounced "ANN yur ism." The second is *subarachnoid* (will you ever forgive me?), pronounced "sub uh RACK noyd." For those who know that *arachnoid* has something to do with spiders, I can only say that the people who came up with these terms must have had overactive imaginations.

But doctors soon tire of saying *subarachnoid hemorrhage* (who wouldn't?) and chop it down to SAH. This may not be much help to patients — *SAH* is as mysterious as *subarachnoid hemorrhage,* even if it is easier to say.

Whatever you call it, this form of red stroke — involving bleeding *outside* the brain — is the least common of the four major types of stroke, afflicting just 3 percent of all stroke sufferers. Each year, though, some 50,000 people in the United States suffer a subarachnoid hemorrhage. Though they attack at all ages, SAH strokes are most common in adults between 55 and 60 — a bit younger than the average stroke victim.

SAH strokes are some of the most catastrophic events in medicine. About half the people who have an SAH stroke die, many before they get to the hospital. The good news: Those who do arrive alive have promising odds. Several effective treatments support an 80-percent survival rate.

Like other types of stroke, certain behaviors increase the chances of SAH stroke. So once again, be aware of the importance of not smoking, controlling blood pressure, and reducing other risk factors.

This chapter examines the cause of SAH stroke, identifies warning signs and symptoms, reveals treatments, and more.

How SAH Strokes Happen

In order to get a handle on the cause of subarachnoid hemorrhages, let's peek beneath the skull to see how the brain fits into its casing and how it is wired into the circulatory system.

The brain's brilliant packaging

Even a linebacker's brain is delicate and fragile. If it wasn't for excellent packaging, you would have wrecked yours years ago. Fortunately, your brain is packed neatly inside your skull to protect it for a lifetime of inevitable bumps on the head.

The double-wrapped brain

First, the surface of the brain is wrapped with a tightly fitting layer of clear tissue, like plastic wrap. This waterproof jacket covering all the surface of the brain is called the *pia mater*. At the base of the brain, behind your eyes and above the back of your throat, this layer is penetrated by blood vessels and nerves.

A second layer of clear tissue is wrapped around the brain and all the blood vessels and nerves leading to the brain. But this layer is loose. It is called the *arachnoid*. The arachnoid presses tight against the leatherlike lining of the skull called the *dura mater*. Imagine putting two plastic gloves on your hand — one bigger than the other; one tight, one loose. That's what's inside your head: a double-wrapped brain positioned loosely inside the skull.

Shock-absorbing fluid

Despite its double wrapping, the brain would still flop around in the skull and be injured if it wasn't for this: The space between the two layers of tissue is filled with approximately one half cup of clear fluid, called *cerebrospinal fluid*.

That's right, your brain is floating! (Have you ever thawed ice that had been frozen inside a container? As the ice melts against the container's sides, you can spin the ice because it floats in the small amount of water spread out against the edges of the container. This is how the brain floats, protected, inside the skull.) Though it is tethered like a hot air balloon by the blood vessels at its base, your brain can sustain quite a bit of jostling because of this shock-absorbing liquid padding. In fact, this protective fluid covers your spinal cord as well, extending down all the way to your tailbone.

The space between the two clear layers of membrane is called the *subarachnoid space.* (Ah, there's that term again!) In addition to the fluid, branching arteries, veins, and nerves run through the subarachnoid space from the skull into the depths of the brain.

The role of arteries in SAH

Now, as we consider the network of arteries that spread through the subarachnoid space and into the brain, we get closer to understanding how SAH occurs here.

Your arteries are mighty tough and rubbery. They can stretch to take the force of your heartbeat, yet contain your blood and deliver it at high pressure everywhere in your body. These blood vessels are built like high-quality tires or garden hoses with three-ply construction. Layers of tough protein, muscle, and a delicate lining won't let blood stick or clot.

Weak spots lead to aneurysms

For a variety of reasons, sometimes weak spots are present in arteries. They can be caused by defects present at birth, the wear and tear of aging, or disease of the arteries. These weak spots can be anywhere.

Years of blood pressure pounding on the weak spots can lead to stretching of the artery where it is weakened. The stretched-out parts are called *aneurysms.* The entire artery balloons out, like a snake that just had dinner. This often happens in the aorta where the weakness is all around the entire diameter of this thumb-width blood vessel in your abdomen. If the weak spot is smaller than the whole artery, the bubblelike spot that forms is called a *bleb.*

Aneurysm in the brain

In the arteries of the brain, the weak spots typically form where they branch into smaller twigs. They begin as small blebs, like little buds on a tree. Through the years, some of the weakest blebs can stretch out to form small pea-sized bubbles. With time, they can continue to enlarge. As they grow, they stretch thinner and thinner and then, like a bubble-gum bubble, they run the risk of bursting.

Warning signs from enlarging aneurysms

Evidence indicates that aneurysms start out small and enlarge over time. Depending on where they are, aneurysms may reveal their presence — before they burst — through a variety of warning signs:

- **Face and eye pain:** Sometimes enlarging aneurysms cause pain in the face or around an eye. This type of pain can have many causes, making diagnosis difficult.

- **Large pupil in one eye:** The pupil of one eye may become much larger than the pupil of the other. If you look in the mirror and see a small difference in the size of your pupils, don't immediately go to the emergency room. Many are born with a difference in pupil size. An old picture can often show that a difference has been present for years. Contact lenses and eye irritation can also affect pupil size.

- **Headaches:** Before it bursts, an aneurysm may have a small leak that seals itself off before major damage occurs. The leak causes a headache, typically in the front or back of the head. The headache is severe. Such a headache can be mistaken for a migraine headache, though, particularly among those who do not often get migraines. People who suffer from migraine headaches can probably tell the difference.

- **Neck pain and stiffness that come on suddenly:** Headaches caused by leaks from aneurysms may be associated with neck pain and stiffness.

- **Sudden pain between the shoulder blades:** This is another symptom, though more unusual than neck pain and stiffness, that results from a headache brought on by an aneurysm leak.

When brain aneurysms rupture

So, we have our well-packaged brain floating in a layer of protective fluid, and within that shock-absorbing padding, we have arteries threading in from the base of the skull and into the brain. Arteries sometimes develop aneurysms — those stretched-out sections — from weak spots. These spots sometimes leak and seal themselves off, causing uncomfortable side effects such as a severe headache, unequal pupil size, and other pains.

But what happens if an aneurysm actually bursts (see Figure 6-1)? You have a brain catastrophe. A subarachnoid hemorrhage. SAH. Bleeding in the space between the brain and skull. Red stroke. Refer back to Chapter 1's Figure 1-4 for another illustration of this.

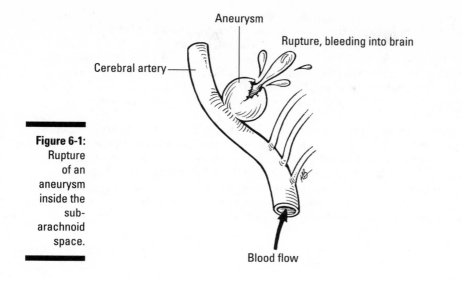

Aneurysm

Rupture, bleeding into brain

Cerebral artery

Blood flow

Figure 6-1:
Rupture
of an
aneurysm
inside the
sub-
arachnoid
space.

When an aneurysm bursts, blood rushes at high pressure from the artery into the surrounding space. In most cases, the rupture spews blood into the subarachnoid space that surrounds the brain. In a few cases, the rupture directs a high-pressure stream directly against the surface of the brain. Blood goes into the subarachnoid space but also can tear holes in the delicate tissue of nearby brain and force itself into the substance of the brain.

The problem with headaches

When headache is the only symptom, sufferers and doctors alike may be challenged to diagnose it immediately. Only one in ten patients who complain of a sudden, severe headache actually has subarachnoid bleeding. Severe headache is quite common in the ER, and, unfortunately, the telltale neck stiffness common to this form of stroke takes several hours to develop.

The consequences of missing a bleeding aneurysm are so bad, though, that it is usually considered worthwhile to do expensive tests when someone comes to the ER with a sudden, severe headache. A CT scan may be done. If it doesn't show blood or any other problems, a simple spinal tap may be in order. Spinal taps have an undeserved bad reputation — they're relatively safe and cause minimal discomfort (discomfort is medical talk for pain). The presence of clear fluid from a spinal tap is the best evidence that a headache is not caused by subarachnoid bleeding.

No test — CT scan, spinal tap, or even MRI scan — is 100-percent accurate. Some subarachnoid bleeds cause such mild or unusual symptoms that no one can be blamed for missing the diagnosis. Fortunately, the diagnosis is missed most often in the least severe cases.

Bleeding into the subarachnoid space can slow the normal blood flow to the brain. This is because the pressure inside the subarachnoid space is usually lower than the blood pressure in arteries. When blood leaks into the subarachnoid space, its pressure goes up, squeezing the brain, making it harder to pump blood into the brain, and the result is the blood does not flow in fast enough to meet the needs of the brain. This is why some people drop to the ground unconscious when their red subarachnoid stroke first happens.

In Figure 6-2, you can't see the aneurysm, but you can see all the white areas around the outside of the brain filling all the nooks and crannies where the convolutions of the brain are. In a week or so, the blood vessels on the top and bottom surfaces of the brain that are surrounded by this blood in the subarachnoid space may start going into spasm and cutting off the blood flow to areas of the brain. No one knows why the spasm occurs, but there are several treatments given to try to repeat it.

Blood around base of the brain

Skull   Eye   Lens of eye

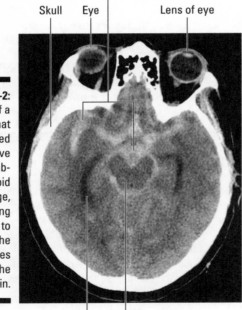

Figure 6-2:
CT scan of a brain that has suffered a massive subarachnoid hemorrhage, causing blood to flow into the spaces around the brain.

Ventricle

Brain stem

What does the individual experience when an aneurysm bursts in the subarachnoid space? Here are a few of the common symptoms:

- ✔ **A pop:** A few patients report hearing or feeling a pop inside their head when an aneurysm ruptures.

- ✔ **Unconsciousness:** Right after the rupture, about half of the patients become unconscious and remain so for more than an hour. Many are unconscious for less time. Some patients do not regain consciousness for several days. Some die before they awaken.

- ✔ **Headache:** Almost all victims who don't fall immediately unconscious complain of severe headache. Vomiting may accompany the headache. Sometimes there is a brief moment of sudden and severe headache before someone becomes unconscious. Those who lose consciousness don't report a headache, of course, but they often show signs of severe pain. After they awaken, they almost always have a severe headache.

- ✔ **Brain injury:** Approximately one third of patients who suffer an SAH stroke experience signs of brain injury immediately after rupture. These signs may be the same as almost any other stroke. They include abnormal eye movements, paralysis on one side of the body, language difficulties, and memory loss.

Can I post this warning too many times? If you note *any* of the symptoms listed for SAH in yourself or anyone else, call 911 immediately! Remember, 50 percent of all individuals who experience a subarachnoid hemorrhage die before they get to the hospital. *There's absolutely no time to delay.*

After an SAH Stroke

The initial bursting of the aneurysm is only the start of the problems with subarachnoid hemorrhage. If the victim makes it to the emergency room alive, then the bleeding has probably stopped. But plenty of other grim prospects face the survivor, from rebleeding to brain swelling, from seizures to white strokes. This section takes a closer look at these risks.

Rebleeding

In the hospital, the doctors' first concern is to prevent the aneurysm from bleeding again. As many as 30 percent of aneurysms rebleed, and when they do, the result is often fatal or causes severe disability. The symptoms of rebleeding are much like those of the first bleed. Needless to say, if the patient is still unconscious from the first bleed, the symptoms may not be apparent. Rebleeding is a greater likelihood the first day of the stroke. Thereafter, the risk of rebleeding reduces each day after the stroke.

Brain swelling

Two types of brain swelling threaten the SAH patient: *hydrocephalus* (hy drow SEFF uh luss) and *brain edema* (uh DEEM uh). Both cause the pressure inside the skull to increase. Increased pressure makes it harder for blood to flow into the brain, which can cause further brain injury — and greater likelihood that the aneurysm will start bleeding again. The good news: Both hydrocephalus and brain edema are treatable.

Hydrocephalus

Normally, fluid flows from cavities inside the brain out to the subarachnoid space. The fluid is generated inside the brain and percolates out through small openings into the subarachnoid space. When there is a lot of blood inside the subarachnoid space, the blood can clot and plug these openings. If it does, then the fluid inside the brain has no place to go. It builds up in the cavities and presses the brain tightly against the skull. Sometimes this condition improves on its own. Otherwise, drowsiness and inability to move the eyes may develop as the brain is crushed against the skull. Eventually, the swelling can result in death.

Brain edema

The brain tissue itself can swell up when it is injured. This usually occurs in two situations. When the aneurysm bursts with bleeding into the substance of the brain, you get the same kind of brain swelling that you get with red stroke brain hemorrhage. The blood in the brain draws white cells and fluid as a response to the injury — similar to your ankle swelling after you sprain it. The swelling goes down as the blood is cleared out by the white cells.

Edema is also a complication of severe spasm of the arteries irritated by the blood in the subarachnoid space. The brain swells because a white stroke has occurred. If the white stroke caused by spasm of arteries is so severe that there is brain edema, then the injury is very severe. Because the edema comes from dying brain cells, this type of edema is very hard to treat.

Heart problems

SAH sometimes causes heart problems. The heart is controlled by areas deep in the base of the brain, where most aneurysms are found. Perhaps the blood injures the brain's control mechanism for the heart. One of the heart problems that may develop is abnormal rhythm. The heart skips beats or contracts in a frantic, disorganized rhythm that pumps no blood. This can be fatal. Evidence of injury to the heart resembling a heart attack is also found in some people with subarachnoid hemorrhage.

Seizures

You have a 25-percent chance of having a *seizure* in the first 24 hours after a subarachnoid hemorrhage. Most seizures occur immediately after the bleeding starts. Brain seizures are thought to be caused by the blood irritating the surface of the brain. When blood escapes from blood vessels, it provokes an intense response to the organs and internal mechanisms it contacts. Seizures result in the case of contact with the brain; spasms occur when the blood contacts the outside of the brain arteries.

Among all the complications from subarachnoid bleeding, seizures are probably the least disabling — patients who suffer SAH strokes are prone to experience seizures after their release from the hospital. They are dramatic and frightening, but do not seem to predict a bad outcome if everything else goes well. Drugs can successfully treat and prevent further seizures.

White strokes

For reasons no one understands, arteries inside the blood-filled subarachnoid space may go into spasm. This means that the muscles in the wall of the artery constrict and make the artery smaller. If the spasm is severe, the blood flow can be cut off completely. As you probably know by now, decreased blood flow in an artery can cause a white stroke someplace in the brain downstream. Red strokes, then, may lead to white strokes.

Spasm of brain arteries is the major cause of brain injury and death *after* you make it to the hospital. This spasm occurs in about 30 to 40 percent of SAH patients. It starts to occur between 3 and 21 days after the stroke, usually between days 4 and 14.

For a few days after admittance to the hospital, the patient may start to improve, as with most strokes. However, after six or seven days, vasospasm of the brain arteries may cause a new stroke of the white type that paralyzes the face, an arm, or a leg and makes language difficult. This stroke is sometimes more devastating than the original red stroke.

Behavioral changes

Aneurysm ruptures almost always occur at the base of the brain. When an aneurysm bursts toward the front of the brain, you can expect behavioral changes because the resulting vasospasm of the large arteries here supply the front part of the brain that controls behavior.

The stroke sufferer may not notice the changes. Family members may find him or her more emotional, both laughing and crying more. They may report a change in personality.

Other behavioral changes may be less noticeable at first, especially in the hospital. However, once home, the patient may have difficulty performing tasks that were manageable before the stroke. Balancing a checkbook, filing taxes, or sending out birthday presents to grandchildren may be too much for the stroke survivor. Though free of any obvious disability, the individual must make more of an effort to concentrate and complete routine tasks. This may put a lot of pressure on relationships with family and friends.

The good news is that there is good treatment available that can reduce the extent of brain injury to some extent. Since behavior changes can occur with all the different types of stroke, how to cope with this problem is discussed later in Chapter 17.

The end result

Without treatment, the outlook after subarachnoid hemorrhage is pretty grim. Even if you live to make it to the emergency room, the death rate approaches 25 percent over the next three months because of the risk of rebleeding and artery spasm, which may lead to further red and white strokes. About 40 percent of patients will have some impairment due to resulting brain injury. Treatment, then, becomes an urgent priority.

Treating SAH Strokes

Subarachnoid hemorrhage is one of the worst types of stroke. It typically happens to younger individuals than other strokes — most SAH victims are 55 to 60 — and it is usually entirely unexpected. This form of red stroke results in more fatalities than other types of stroke, and the resulting brain injury among survivors can be more severe. So far, no treatments are available for help in the first few minutes after the aneurysm bursts. This type of stroke gets people's attention, and most victims are taken to the emergency room immediately by ambulance.

The good news is that, if the patient survives the initial onset, SAH is one of the most *treatable* forms of stroke. A stroke team may make the initial evaluation, but when it comes to treating red stroke — especially SAH red stroke — a neurosurgeon will be called in. This is because some of the most critical treatments for subarachnoid bleeding involve surgical procedures to the brain. Other treatments for SAH complications such as brain swelling and artery spasm may involve drugs.

Not every hospital has a neurosurgeon or the facilities needed to manage subarachnoid bleeding. In this case, the patient is transported immediately to another hospital for admission. Sometimes, the stroke victim may be stabilized in an intensive care unit for a short time before transfer is arranged.

Measuring the severity of the stroke

Many treatment decisions depend on an estimate of the severity of the stroke. Treatment always means some risk, and some treatments for SAH stroke have pretty high risks. It's no surprise, then, that treatment may be postponed or avoided if the stroke is less severe.

How bad is the brain injury?

Neurosurgeons give subarachnoid bleeds a score from one to five. One is the best, five the worst. The major determinant of the score is how alert and awake the patient is. One means awake, alert, and no signs of brain injury such as a paralyzed arm or abnormal eye movements. Five means essentially deeply unconscious.

How bad is the bleeding?

A CT scan can provide a good estimate of the extent of bleeding in the subarachnoid space. The presence of thick, dense blood clots and blood predict a more severe stroke. Blood spreading into the internal brain cavities is also a bad sign. Early brain swelling seen on the first CT scan is also bad news. Blood localized in just one area is better. But if more blood shows up in later CT scans, this predicts a difficult time controlling the bleeding.

Emergency treatment

Subarachnoid bleeding often affects brain stem. If you'll recall, this is where all the body's vital functions are regulated. It is the Houston Mission Control for the body we're talking about here, and when things go awry, a lot of bad things can happen. In SAH, the heart rhythm is most commonly affected. Blood pressure can also be affected with unexpected increases or drops in pressure. As prevention, emergency personnel utilize as much medical technology as needed, connecting the patient to tubes, wires, and catheters that can maintain those vital functions — perhaps even breathing — until the brain's central control system recovers and takes over again. If the patient is conscious, he or she will hear plenty of beeps, hums, and intense technical discussions as physicians evaluate the case. Blood tests, cardiograms, X-rays, CT scans, and special X-rays to look at blood vessels may all be scheduled in short order.

All this expensive machinery and testing may seem futile. After all, if an SAH stroke is so severe, perhaps death — or a life with severe brain injury — is inevitable. Why bother? For some types of stroke, that may be an appropriate question. However, victims of subarachnoid hemorrhage are generally younger, and a good recovery is possible with treatment.

I encourage stroke patients and their families to go for a full-court press — the odds are too good to pass up the possibility of a good outcome. Tough decisions to pull tubes and unplug machines should be put off for a few days in most cases.

Finding the aneurysm

After the SAH sufferer's condition is stabilized, he or she is put through tests to find the aneurysm that caused the bleeding. The methods for finding aneurysms are changing. The tried-and-true test, called an *angiogram* (ANN jee oh gram), injects a dye under high pressure into the brain arteries. Virtually all aneurysms can be identified this way, but a few patients may be injured by it.

Figure 6-3 is not a picture of some strange plant. It is an angiogram of the blood inside the blood vessels of someone who has a half-inch diameter spherical aneurysm at a branch of one of the arteries to his brain. The aneurysm is inside the skull but outside the brain in the subarachnoid space. You can't see either the brain or the skull. All you can see is the dye that has been injected into the brain arteries. Usually an angiogram is only done after an aneurysm ruptures and bleeds to cause a stroke. The purpose of the angiogram is to plan sealing the aneurysm so it doesn't leak again.

Safer tests have been developed. New tests use special CT (X-ray) or MRI angiograms. The downside is they miss 5 to 15 percent of aneurysms. If confidence in the accuracy of these new techniques continues to develop, fewer patients will need the older, more risky and uncomfortable angiogram.

Usually, just one aneurysm is found. Sometimes more than one is discovered. The odds of having two or more aneurysms are about one in four. Often, the aneurysm that bled can be identified, but sometimes this can't be proven. What to do about extra, unruptured aneurysms is uncertain. I can tell you that the bigger the aneurysm, the more likely it will rupture and bleed. If it is more than a centimeter (the size of a small marble), some doctors would recommend sealing it off from its artery so it can't bleed if it is easy to reach. Remember, these waters are full of dangers from surgery and radiological procedures. They are not well charted. Taking the opportunity to get a second or third opinion gives you more chances at a good outcome.

Middle cerebral artery

Aneurysm

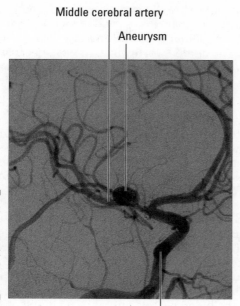

Figure 6-3:
An
angiogram
can find just
about any
aneurysm.

Internal carotid artery inside skull

Occasionally, no aneurysms are found. Not all subarachnoid bleeding is caused by aneurysms. In fact, 15 percent of subarachnoid bleeding has an unusual or rare cause. If an aneurysm isn't found, the patient may be at risk for further bleeding, and artery spasm can still be a risk.

Sealing off the aneurysm

No one denies that it's a good idea to seal off the ruptured aneurysm so it can't rebleed. Almost all agree that it should be done earlier rather than later, circumstances permitting. But when it comes to *how* to seal off the aneurysm, the debate heats up. Neurosurgeons have two choices: *clips* or *coils,* two simple and similar words for two vastly different procedures.

Clips pinch off the aneurysm

Clips are the traditional means for sealing off aneurysms. The procedure for placing a clip (it looks like a tiny ice tong) around the base of an aneurysm requires cutting a hole in the skull, lifting the brain up out of the way, and threading the clip between dozens of tiny blood vessels to reach around and pinch off the neck of the aneurysm. After surgery, your head is usually wrapped in a bandage that looks cool to your grandchildren, and you get the most expensive and complete haircut of your life.

Clipping is not a job for amateurs. One slip and disastrous bleeding from a torn blood vessel can destroy any chance of a good recovery. Even the most experienced neurosurgeons encounter problems in a significant number of cases. The risk is generally considered worthwhile, though, because clips have a good track record for preventing rebleeding. Not all aneurysms can be clipped, however.

Coils: No holes in the skull required

Coils are the new guys on the block, and their use is increasing. One large clinical trial suggests that when they can be used, coils may be the safest and most effective way to go. With coils, all the action takes place inside the blood vessels. No holes in the skull. No fashionable haircut or bandage-wrapped head.

Typically, radiologists who specialize in brain procedures put coils in. They almost always work in close cooperation with neurosurgeons. If a coil fails, a clip may be required. Some neurosurgeons are doing coiling themselves.

The straightened coil is introduced through a plastic tube inserted into a large artery in the groin. The physician weaves the tube through the body, turning and twisting along the blood vessels until the end of the plastic tube is actually inside or right at the mouth of the aneurysm in the brain area. Then the straightened coil is pushed out into the aneurysm. It springs back into its coiled shape inside the cavity of the aneurysm. The coil is made of a material — platinum, for instance — that causes the blood to clot around it. In this way, the clot seals off the aneurysm from the inside.

The coiling procedure can also result in serious complications if the aneurysm ruptures again or a hole is accidentally punched in an artery. But these complications are generally less frequent than the complications from clipping. Clipping also avoids all the complications of cutting a hole in the skull and lifting the brain out of the way. Because this method is the newer of the two, it's not certain yet whether coiling will last as long as clipping. Not all aneurysms can be coiled, but more can be coiled than clipped.

Which method is best?

I'm glad I'm not a surgeon. Surgeons know what they are doing and yet they have to put up with someone like me, who is always second-guessing them. They understand that experience is critical, and that experienced surgeons have the best results — whether it be by clip or coil.

Yet you still hear "Get a second opinion." This doesn't necessarily mean get a *better* opinion or get a different surgeon. It just means that every case is unique, and each one is worth some discussion among experts to be sure the best procedure is chosen.

It is important to seal the aneurysm quickly, so there isn't much time to consider all the alternatives. A hospital that offers only one approach may have to refer patients to another hospital for the other method. But the major determinant of success is the rate of complications of the procedure to place the device. Coils usually have a lower rate of complications.

My advice? Be sure both a neurosurgeon and radiologist have a chance to offer opinions, especially in the case of more than one aneurysm. Experience is important for success in both clipping and coiling. It's better to go with the most successful experience, regardless of coil or clip.

Relieving brain swelling

Treatment depends on which of the two types of swelling occurs. For persistent severe *hydrocephalus*, the fluid is vented out of the brain through a small plastic tube about the size of a ballpoint pen refill. It is threaded through a half-inch hole in the skull and pushed right through the brain into the cavity filled with fluid. *What? Pushed through the brain?* Believe it or not, yes, and it is done with almost no risk of brain injury. The tube is very soft, pushing aside blood vessels rather than breaking them (in most cases).

Brain edema is treated with drugs and hyperventilation (rapid breathing). If the swelling is severe, the success of the treatment may be monitored by screwing a pressure gauge into the skull to measure the pressure inside. This pressure is significant for a number of reasons, the most important being that high pressure can slow the flow of blood to the brain.

Dealing with artery spasm

It's possible to reduce the risk of spasm of brain arteries following subarachnoid bleeding. If the aneurysm has been coiled or clipped, the risk of bleeding is decreased. Therefore, the blood pressure can be allowed to rise to the higher levels required to push blood through narrow arteries. Maintaining good hydration with careful management of fluids is critical.

Drugs that prevent artery muscles from contracting, called *calcium channel blockers*, have been shown to improve the outcome from subarachnoid hemorrhage by reducing severity of vasospasm. The most common drug used is nimodipine. The pills are usually given six times a day for three weeks.

Artery spasm may occur despite maximum efforts to prevent it. When signs of brain injury become apparent, another stroke is happening. This time, though, it's a white stroke — caused by *lack* of blood flow rather than bleeding. Several treatments address this problem. No good evidence exists to prove that the treatments actually help.

One treatment is to increase the blood pressure and put a lot of fluid into the veins to thin the blood and force the most blood possible through the narrow arteries. This treatment has its risks. It puts a tremendous strain on the heart and kidneys. If you have diabetes, heart disease, or are simply in poor shape, the stress can cause heart attack and heart failure.

Some centers are trying another unproven treatment to open up arteries in spasm by pushing plastic tubes through the narrowed arteries. In some cases, it seems to work well. In others, there have been problems — mostly bleeding when the plastic tube tears open an artery.

I don't have any really good advice to offer once artery spasm starts. The treatment varies widely, and there is little knowledge from clinical trials that allows one to know whether the different treatments really are good for you.

Predicting SAH Stroke: It's a Family Affair

Brain aneurysms tend to run in families. About 20 percent of patients who have subarachnoid bleeding from an aneurysm have a family member who has evidence of an aneurysm. Should everyone in your family be tested to see if they have aneurysms? And if aneurysms are discovered, what do you do about it? The answers to these questions are still somewhat uncertain.

Most aneurysms never rupture. If there is a family history of aneurysms rupturing in more than one person, then there is more reason to consider evaluating other family members.

With an unruptured aneurysm, there is more time to think things over and get additional data and recommendations from several physicians. In general, the real worries are about the minority of aneurysms that are a centimeter in diameter or greater. Many agree that smaller aneurysms can be monitored. Coiling or clipping larger aneurysms comes with an undeniable risk. However, once an aneurysm grows to the one-centimeter size, the risk of rupture increases significantly and grows over time.

If ongoing measurements of the aneurysm show growth, then this might move me toward taking the risk of the coiling or clipping operation. If the aneurysm looked "easy" to coil, then that should also increase interest in having it sealed off.

Headache reveals aneurysm

A 56-year-old company president was playing handball when he began to experience a severe headache. He couldn't ever remember such a severe headache, but he did remember that his grandmother and fathers had died of a stroke. He stopped playing and sat down. The headache got worse. His friend called 911, and an ambulance took him to a nearby emergency room. In the ER he was a little confused and frightened but remained conscious. A CT scan of his head was normal. An MRA *(magnetic resonance angiography)* scan was inconclusive. However, 6 hours later, a lumbar puncture spinal tap did show the presence of blood in the usually clear cerebrospinal fluid. Special testing showed the yellow tinge to the fluid that indicated the bleeding was not due to the lumbar puncture procedure itself and had been present for several hours.

An angiogram was performed the next morning, and a small half-inch aneurysm was identified. Several physicians discussed possible treatments. Finally, because of the position of the aneurysm, a coil was placed to close it off so that it would not rupture in the future. He was scheduled for a repeat angiogram in one year. He was back to work within two weeks.

It is important to note, though, that if you decide to postpone sealing an aneurysm, you have a responsibility to get regular tests to see whether it is enlarging. You should also take measures to reduce other risks as well. Stop smoking, obviously. Get your blood pressure down through diet or medication. If you are a woman, avoid taking estrogen or birth-control pills and take extra precautions to control your blood pressure during pregnancy.

I know, I know. Eat right, exercise, stop smoking. That's a lot to ask from someone who's just received the bad news that they have aneurysms that could result in a devastating red stroke. But trust me. You do not want to hear that "pop" in your head, or find yourself reeling from a sudden and severe headache, or lose consciousness — or your life — before you even get to the emergency room. These necessary precautions are a small price to pay to improve your odds of a stroke-free future.

Chocolate, as far as I know, is not a risk factor for SAH.

Chapter 7

Dementia (Vascular Cognitive Impairment)

*Y*ou may be having a stroke right now and not even realize it! In fact, evidence supports that individuals can suffer a *series* of small white strokes over time and never even notice anything, or have only slurring of speech, or vague numbness or clumsiness on one side after an episode. But the bad news is that the cumulative damage from these undetected strokes may lead to *dementia*.

Typically linked with aging, *dementia* is a condition in which damaged brain tissue results in severely impaired memory, cognition, and loss of other brain function, which becomes progressively worse with time. Alzheimer's disease is a form of dementia. There are many causes of dementia, but approximately 10 to 20 percent of cases are the result of a series of small strokes. When small strokes are the cause, we refer to the dementia as *vascular cognitive impairment*. Many of the strokes that cause vascular dementia are the smallest and least noticeable of all strokes, but — make no mistake — they're still a serious problem.

It's challenging to get accurate data about the prevalence of stroke-caused dementia. These small strokes typically go unreported — no trip to the ER, no diagnosis. But it's estimated that this type of white stroke makes up about 25 percent of all white strokes. And those who suffer from one are looking at a one in ten chance of suffering another stroke within the year.

In this chapter, I explain exactly how a series of small, imperceptible strokes can lead to dementia, how to recognize stroke-caused dementia, and — most importantly — how to reduce the risk of vascular dementia.

Is There a Bright Side to Stroke Dementia?

Here's the good news about vascular dementia: *You can take steps to prevent it!*

Many in the medical world are concerned with the aging process of the brain and how to slow it — no one has yet figured out how to do this. Some are hung up on Alzheimer's disease, and much of our research and energies are focused on this devastating condition. But we've acted as if solving Alzheimer's will solve all the problems with the aging brain. It's becoming clear that it won't. In fact, there isn't even a test that can tell whether an individual has Alzheimer's with any certainty. And you can't treat Alzheimer's disease, at least not yet.

But you *can* treat your blood-vessel problems. Doctors are discovering that the blood vessels have a great deal to do with the health of the aging brain. Disease of the blood vessels may not be the entire problem, but it is part of the problem. A big part. And good care of blood vessels could help prevent the problem.

If you want to scrape every bit of quality you can out of your life, don't waste time worrying about what you can't treat; tackle what you *can* treat. High blood pressure and high cholesterol in your blood can injure your brain. Treat these conditions aggressively.

If you are experiencing memory loss or other symptoms of brain impairment, you *may* have Alzheimer's. Or you may have had a series of small strokes. Instead of getting discouraged and giving in to loss of brain power, take steps to protect your brain from further deterioration by reducing your blood pressure and cholesterol, among other things. (See the section "Preventing Stroke Dementia," later in this chapter.) Even if the symptoms *are* due to Alzheimer's, it's been shown time and again that Alzheimer's patients do better if they don't have high blood pressure, diabetes, or high cholesterol. So, no matter how you look at it, assuming a proactive role in taking care of your blood vessels can't hurt.

Small Strokes and Dementia

We've been talking about "small" strokes. Indeed, it's possible and perhaps even more common than we realize for individuals to have a small stroke — or many small strokes — and never know it. But let me emphasize this: Doctors don't like to give you the bad news. If you have a stroke and ask your doctor about it, you may hear something like, "It was only a small stroke." Well, no stroke is insignificant. A small stroke can be just as danger-ous to your health as a big stroke.

Small strokes, small blood vessels

Blood clots and blood vessels come in all sizes. So far in this book, I have talked about white strokes that occur when large clots block large blood vessels. This type of stroke definitely lets you know it's happening. You feel weakness or numbness in an arm or leg. You are unable to talk or communi-cate; you have difficulty understanding others — dramatic symptoms you can't fail to notice. These attention-getting white strokes — large-clot, large-artery blockages — send you to the emergency room.

But in addition to the larger arteries at the base of your brain, there are tiny blood vessels that carry the blood to and from the brain. These miniscule vessels are like fine, hollow hairs. They perforate right into the substance of the brain and carry blood deep into the core.

The pressure is on

Because these delicate vessels come right off the larger main arteries at the base of the brain, they are subjected to very high blood pressure, which causes a lot of wear and tear over time. Most of the wear and tear occurs in blood vessels near the origin of the arteries, where the pressure is highest.

The result of this high-pressure wear and tear is *plaque* — hard deposits of fat and scar tissue near the mouth of these small arteries. This process is called hardening of the arteries, or *atherosclerosis*. The vessels get stiff and hard. The nodules of atherosclerosis can narrow these small vessels so that little blood can flow past them. When blood clots form at these hard, rough spots, the whole small artery becomes plugged. Atherosclerosis can also attack larger arteries. It can lead to heart attack when the coronary arteries are attacked, and stroke when the carotid arteries in the neck are blocked. This hardening process and the blockage it produces is thought by most to be the most common cause of small strokes. Small vessel atherosclerosis *(microatheroma)* is worse in patients with high blood pressure, elevated LDL, and diabetes.

Deep in the brain, grape-sized holes

Whether caused by atherosclerosis or thickened artery walls, clots in the small, penetrating arteries of the brain can lead to injuries deep inside it. When they heal, the injured space is cleared out and a pocket of clear fluid is left in its place. The size of these small white stroke areas of infarction may be as tiny as a grain of rice or as large as a grape.

So what is it about this high-blood-pressure environment that can produce *so many* small strokes and so much blood vessel scarring with atherosclerosis in the brain? Remember, there are hundreds of branches of tiny vessels coming off the larger arteries at the base of the brain. They are all similarly affected by the flow of the blood. If an individual has risk factors such as high blood pressure, high cholesterol, smoking, and diabetes, all the vessels — not just one or two — are at risk.

This translates to the following: Have one small stroke deep in your brain and you're likely to have another.

The end result: A shrinking brain

After years of high blood pressure, even one small stroke every couple of months has a major impact on the brain. Most of the damage occurs in the deep core areas of the brain, which rely on small, penetrating arteries for their blood supply. In severe cases, there are so many little holes that the brain begins to look like a sponge. The brain itself shrinks, drawing away from the skull. The normal fluid reservoirs enlarge. In advanced cases, a CT scan or MRI scan shows that the brain has begun to shrink and the ventricles are enlarged (see Figure 7-1).

The small infarctions shown in the figure are called *lacunes*. As more and more accumulate over time, the patient becomes more and more impaired. In this MRI scan, the bone appears dark like the fluid in the ventricles and the area of infarction. This scan is early in the process. The ventricles are not much enlarged, and the brain has only just begun to atrophy, mostly on the sides where you can see more dark fluid around the convolutions than in the front of the brain.

A shrunken, spongy brain can function surprisingly well. Every day, a CT scan somewhere reveals a brain that shouldn't be expected to rub two sticks together, yet the patient is active, productive, and functional. This is a tribute to the adaptability of the brain. And also to luck.

But, trust me, you don't want to take the chance. There is almost no doubt that the cumulative effect of small strokes is to impair the brain, causing vascular dementia.

Ventricles

Small infarctions

Skull

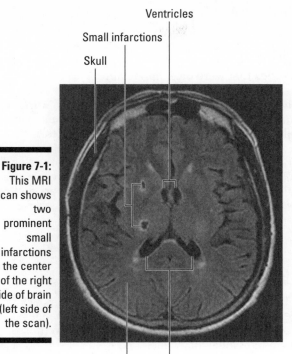

Figure 7-1:
This MRI scan shows two prominent small infarctions in the center of the right side of brain (left side of the scan).

Ventricles

Normal brain

Recognizing Stroke Dementia

How can you tell whether someone is suffering from stroke-caused dementia? It's often easy to miss the signs — or confuse it with the normal loss of mental acuity with aging or to assume that Alzheimer's is the cause. Here are some warning signals of brain failure:

- Loss of memory

- Confusion in complex situations

- Loss of control of emotions

- Problems with communication or expressing self

- Trouble paying attention

- Difficulty following a conversation

- Struggling to work finely with hands

- Disorganization in plans

✔ Failure to recognize things seen

✔ Straining with calculations

✔ Inability to solve problems

✔ Loss of interest in activities that were once important

All too often, we jump to the conclusion that many or most of these warning signals are signs of Alzheimer's. They might be, but they are the same symptoms suffered by individuals who've experienced small white strokes.

Then again, we have to expect some loss of mental function as a normal part of aging. Although lots of older people are likely to experience a few or more of the symptoms just listed, the symptoms are typically not very severe and/or occur infrequently. So between these two extremes, how do we recognize and distinguish stroke-related dementia? Sometimes it's a challenge.

Dementia is a gradual process

The onset of dementia is often so gradual it's hard to recognize at first. Day-to-day or even week-to-week changes may go unnoticed. But the changes month to month and year to year are more apparent, particularly to those who haven't seen the afflicted individual in a while.

Sometimes, especially around holidays like Thanksgiving, family members get together for the first time in months or even a year. It may be clear to those who haven't seen Mom for awhile, that something is wrong when she lets the turkey burn to a crisp. Or that Dad isn't his old self when he forgets how to play chess.

The normal loss of mental function that occurs with aging is gradual, too. But dementia accelerates the mental changes of normal aging. Comparatively, dementia is much faster and more extreme. It is thought that everyone over the age of 90 has some degree of dementia, but this is considered a normal part of aging. When we figure out a way to slow this down in the future, any mental changes with aging may be considered abnormal.

Loss of memory: The hallmark symptom

Memory loss, particularly short-term memory, is the most noticed symptom of dementia. This may be because memory is one of the most complicated and sophisticated functions of the brain. Memory involves integrating information from all over the brain.

Do you know how the long-distance telephone network is organized? Whenever you place a call, you might think that the connection follows the shortest pathway to the phone you are calling. But actually, your call to Illinois from New York may go through California, depending on which phone lines are busy or under repair. You dial. You talk. You never notice the many problems that divert your call out of the shortest pathway. As more and more lines become busy or broken, the time it takes to connect may be longer and longer. Eventually, when all the lines into Illinois are broken, you may not be able to call your friend in Chicago anymore.

Similarly, the failing brain may re-route the traffic of memory until, after more and more injuries, you can't recall a particular memory at all. What you experience is slower service from your brain, then one day something you think you should know is suddenly gone altogether. It's not so much gone as inaccessible.

Loss of other brain functions

The dementia caused by several strokes is likely to have a pronounced effect on movement and language — more so than Alzheimer's disease. Just like the sudden and dramatic types of stroke that send you to the emergency room, small strokes cause similar damage only at a less perceptible level. So, in addition to problems with thinking and memory, a series of small strokes may leave you with hand weakness or difficulty speaking. You may begin to have trouble walking or driving. Balancing the checkbook may become a challenge. Emotions may be harder to control. Because the brain is not receiving all the information it is used to, the sufferer may become less trusting and more suspicious of others.

Diagnosing Stroke-Related Dementia

If you have a stroke, you call 911 and go to the emergency room because of the sudden and dramatic signs that define a stroke. How, then, would someone with the gradual downhill course of stroke dementia end up in the emergency room for treatment? Well, he or she could have a *big* stroke instead of one more small one. In that case, they would probably be treated just like any other stroke patient in the emergency room — until tests showed that the patient had had a lot of other strokes already. Sometimes, family members or friends who haven't seen you in several months may visit and recognize that something is seriously wrong and insist on taking you to the doctor or even the emergency room. It may be sorted out that the problem is longstanding. No treatment may be recommended. A follow-up appointment with a physician may be suggested.

The problem is that the appointment is not considered an emergency and, if you feel better later, you may cancel. An opportunity to identify the problem and start preventing further brain damage may be lost.

Checking in for a check-up

It's unlikely that you'll discover in the emergency room that your failing memory is due to small strokes. There may not be a crisis event that provokes you to go to the ER — at least not for a long time. But the sooner you identify small strokes as the cause of your memory loss and other impairments, the earlier you can forestall further damage.

Maybe you forget why you're in the grocery store. Maybe your spouse has been noticing that you fail to remember plans you've made. Perhaps your children have expressed concern about you after a recent visit. You confused the names of your grandchildren, or just forgot them.

If you have any evidence that your memory and brain power may be failing — especially if you also suffer from high blood pressure, high cholesterol, or diabetes — make an appointment for testing. Are you just going to sit there while your memory fades and you keep having these funny spells? Boxing is a sport that virtually guarantees brain injury. If you know you're at risk for stroke and don't do anything about it, that's a little like boxing without the chance of the prize.

Tools for identifying small stroke damage

A big stroke is a lot easier to diagnose than stroke dementia, because so many things can cause dementia. The good news is that many of these things are treatable. Other causes of dementia include depression, thyroid disease, vitamin B-12 deficiency, and diabetes.

Although some doctors get a little hung up trying to rule out Alzheimer's, it may be more productive to test for the many treatable causes of vascular dementia as well.

Looking at the pictures

MRI scans and CT scans may show the tracks that small strokes leave behind. They aren't all as obvious as the ones in the CT scan shown back in Figure 7-1. Sometimes, just some increased darkness (or lightness) around the brain ventricles is the only indication of brain damage. Often the brain looks shrunken, and the ventricles — the series of connecting cavities — are larger.

If the scan is normal — no scars, shadows, or signs of shrinkage — then there is sure to be more talk of Alzheimer's and more tests to be sure there isn't a treatable cause of the problems you are having.

Psychological tests: Are they worth it?

Sometimes, a doctor may recommend a battery of psychological tests to get an estimate of how severe the brain failure is. These tests are expensive and can take a lot of time. Some love taking these tests — others find them upsetting, fearing that they can reveal some psychological trait that can get them committed (they can't).

I'm not a big proponent of such tests for determining small stroke damage. Except for depression and some other psychiatric problems, I don't believe that psychological testing can do much to diagnose the problems. But if you agree to any formal psychological testing, you might state up front that you don't want it to last more than an hour. Most of the really important testing can be done in an hour.

Ruling out other causes with blood tests

Blood tests can be very important in identifying and confirming other causes of dementia, such as vitamin B-12 deficiency, syphilis, AIDS, brain fungal infections, and thyroid disease. These treatable causes of dementia are not common, but if you have one of them, a blood test can reveal it.

Don't forget that many people have Alzheimer-like problems *and* risk factors for stroke dementia. Just because you may have one or both of these, it doesn't mean you don't have another treatable medical or psychiatric problem that makes the symptoms worse. Your first priority is how well you think, not why you don't think well. Anything you can do that might possibly make your condition better without a lot of risk is probably worthwhile.

The blood tests include

- ✔ CBC, a complete blood count
- ✔ Electrolytes in the blood such as sodium and potassium, as well as glucose
- ✔ Chemistry panel, 12–18 blood tests to see how your liver and kidneys are functioning
- ✔ Thyroid tests
- ✔ Diabetes tests
- ✔ Vitamin B-12 tests
- ✔ Blood tests for specific infections including syphilis, AIDS, and rare brain fungus infections
- ✔ Sedimentation rate, a non-specific test to determine whether you have an infection that is not obvious or some abnormal immune function

Spinal tap

The spinal tap was mentioned with regard to subarachnoid hemorrhage in Chapter 6. The procedure can be done in an office. It is also called a *lumbar puncture*. Done by an experienced physician, it is usually a relatively pain-free and simple process. However, there can be serious headaches afterward, and serious infections are possible though very rare. The idea is to get some of the clear cerebrospinal fluid that surrounds the brain and fills its ventricles. This fluid can be analyzed to see if there is evidence of infection or inflammation.

Fortunately, you can get the fluid from inside the spine in the lumbar region at about the level of your belly button. You usually lay on your side and a long needle is slowly pushed between the bones until the cavity containing the fluid is pierced. The fluid is withdrawn and the needle removed. The needle is three inches long. To someone who doesn't like needles, it looks more like a knitting needle although it's no thicker than the needles used to start intravenous lines in your arm.

If my thinking and memory were going seriously bad, I think I would want to have a spinal tap as well as blood tests. These are usually described as difficult and potentially risky (and they can be). But before I surrendered to diagnosis, I would want to be sure there wasn't some rare infection or other inflammatory process going on. A spinal tap is the only opportunity to detect these.

Be sure special spinal fluid cultures for fungi and tuberculosis are ordered.

Second opinion

You might think I only recommend second opinions for surgical problems. Not so. For a difficult diagnosis like dementia, I suggest it may be worthwhile to get more than one opinion. Most cases of dementia are accurately diagnosed, and most are Alzheimer's, but many doctors know of some case that was missed for years before the correct cause of the dementia was determined.

I suggest taking the opportunity to see two doctors in different specialties before a final diagnosis is accepted. Neurology and gerontology are two such specialties.

Addressing the risk factors

If you believe your memory impairment may be the result of small strokes and you don't already *know* if you have some of the risk factors — particularly high blood pressure, high cholesterol, diabetes, or atrial fibrillation (an irregular heartbeat determined from an EKG) — now's the time to find out. It's pretty easy to test for these conditions: Have your blood pressure taken.

Add simple blood cholesterol and blood lipid tests (for diabetes) to the battery of other blood tests you're taking to rule out other causes. And, for atrial defibrillation, have an ultrasound test of your carotid artery — the artery in your neck. This test will indicate if the blood is ineffectively pumping to your brain.

So what if you discover that you have any or all of these risk factors? And you rule out other potential causes of dementia? Plus your CT or MRI scan shows some damage or brain shrinkage? Chances are likely that your doctor may conclude that you have been suffering from small stroke dementia — and that, unless things change, you're likely to experience more small strokes and problems with brain impairment.

Preventing Stroke Dementia

As with most white strokes, the damage caused by a small white stroke tends to improve some on its own, especially with good rehabilitation. You can treat small strokes as you treat large strokes. The problem is, as I pointed out previously, it's rare to have just one small stroke. The more strokes you have, the greater the problems. So the best action is to do everything you can to *prevent* them. And, yes, you prevent small strokes the same way you prevent large strokes. Read Chapter 8 for more about how to reduce your risk of stroke. Here's a quick review of the tried-and-true stroke-preventing steps:

- **Lower your blood pressure:** Just picture the damage that pulsing blood can cause to the small arteries of your brain: plaque deposits and scarred and thickening walls. It should make you want to do everything you can to keep your blood pressure in check. In addition to checking your blood pressure regularly — and going on medication to lower it if your situation demands it — you can make some adjustments to your lifestyle to help, too. Evaluate your diet and reduce or cut out salt, which can aggravate high blood pressure. Regular exercise can also help.

- **Fight blood clots with drugs:** Aspirin and a drug called clopidogrel are anticoagulants or blood thinners — they slow down the formation of blood clots and may help prevent stroke. If you have atrial fibrillation, your irregular heartbeat puts you at an even higher risk for stroke. Warfarin is a treatment for this condition. It involves frequent blood testing, however, and careful adjustment of the dosage to prevent severe bleeding. But it sure beats having a stroke.

- **Get in shape:** Diet and exercise can't hurt. Obesity can aggravate many conditions that lead to strokes, including diabetes, heart disease, high cholesterol, and high blood pressure. By keeping your weight down with regular exercise and a healthy diet with minimal fats and sodium, you may improve the other conditions — and lower your risk of stroke.

✔ **Bring down your cholesterol and lipids:** The more fat in your blood, the higher your chances of atherosclerosis. The first place to look for reducing your blood cholesterol and lipids is your diet. Whether fast-food favorites (French fries) or all-American classics (T-bone steak or Southern fried chicken), your choice of sustenance may be increasing your risk of stroke. Your condition may require some radical dietary changes. Your doctor can tell you what your total fat intake should be.

But eating right may not be enough. If a low-fat diet doesn't reduce your blood lipids and cholesterol, you may need the help of medication. If your doctor thinks you should be taking statin drugs, then don't put off starting drugs for months and months while you struggle to do what most other people find almost impossible to do.

More and more doctors are prescribing lipid-lowering drugs for preventing stroke. There is some evidence to suggest they help prevent stroke in patients with high blood pressure or diabetes, but definitive proof of their ability to prevent vascular cognitive impairment is not at hand. Lipid-lowering drugs are not generic at this time. Cost is high, so you had better think of this as a long-term investment. Read more about the pros and cons of statins in Chapter 10.

✔ **Get your diabetes under control:** Do the best job you can of controlling it. Get your weight down. Exercise. Take your medication. Test your glucose frequently. Have regular check-ups. A lot of advances have been made in treatment for diabetes in the past few years — make sure you're taking advantage of them.

✔ **And please don't tell me you still smoke:** Those chemicals in cigarette smoke travel through your blood vessels, you know, to your heart and your brain. One of them — nicotine — causes blood vessels to constrict. Others cause the blood to thicken, and many do damage to the inside walls of the vessels. Not exactly what you want to happen if you're prone to stroke.

The word on wine

There's a lot of publicity out there that a glass of wine every day may actually reduce the risk of stroke and heart disease. It's amazing to hear that something enjoyable might actually be good for you. I haven't yet seen any clinical trials that show that drinking a glass of wine per day makes any real difference. Alcohol has a lot of other effects that are not accounted for in the studies I have seen. I would be especially concerned about your trying this if you have any liver problems, problems with numb feet or hands, or history of problems with alcohol. Until I see solid proof that it is good for the brain, I'm afraid I will tend to think alcohol is *not* good for the brain.

Blood pressure: To treat or not to treat?

There is some controversy about the value of lowering blood pressure in those who've suffered several small strokes. Does lower blood pressure result in fewer strokes? In general, there is good reason to believe it does. Blood pressure seems to cause both types of small artery problems: wall thickening and atherosclerosis.

If you have had a major stroke or a transient stroke, at least one clinical trial has shown that lowering your blood pressure, even if it is within "normal" or "high normal" limits, is a good idea. This trial, however, did not focus on patients who had small strokes.

Some experts speculate that higher blood pressure may help force more blood through small, narrow arteries, thus preventing further brain injury. The assumption is that blood pressure has already done most of the damage it can do. So it might be better to treat the problem rather than the cause. Right now, we don't have any definitive studies that support lowering normal or even "high normal" blood pressure. So you'll find most physicians will encourage small-stroke patients to lower their high blood pressure.

Planning for When You Can't Remember

If you are beginning to lose memory or other brain functions, it's time to get your life in order. If your condition keeps getting worse, you won't be making good decisions and will need someone else to act on your behalf. Now is the time to decide who you want to call the shots if you can't.

I am not the person to be telling you how to plan your financial and medical future. However, I do know from experience that your failure to make adequate plans, even in the simplest case, can cause you and your family an amazing amount of stress and even animosity.

Have you given or do you plan to give someone power of attorney and medical power of attorney? Do you have a will? If there is a chance you are going to lose your mental competence or the ability to make decisions, then you should make these arrangements now, when there is little doubt about your competence to do so.

Your children or even your spouse may hesitate to bring up questions about what your intentions are for your home or other real estate and investments should you have to go into a nursing home or other long-term care situation. Get an expert in planning for this possible outcome. Planning for a time when you *cannot* plan is extremely difficult — perhaps even more so than planning for a funeral. But it's an important obligation. While you are still able to, take as much responsibility for your future as you can, so that if the time comes, the job of your loved ones will be easier.

Part III
Preventing Stroke

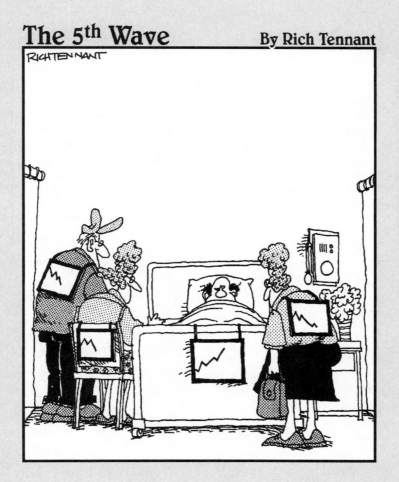

The 5th Wave   By Rich Tennant

In this part . . .

There are ways to increase your chances of avoiding a stroke, and that's what this part is all about. These three chapters are devoted to reducing risk of stroke in the future — whether or not you've already suffered one. The two most important factors are avoiding high blood pressure and reducing the amount of cholesterol in your blood. And there are other steps you can take to help avoid stroke — all of them are thoroughly covered in these chapters.

Chapter 8

High Blood Pressure

. . . .

In This Chapter

▶ Understanding how high blood pressure leads to stroke

▶ Learning who's at risk for high blood pressure

▶ Lowering your blood pressure to reduce stroke risk and improve health

▶ Exploring medications that treat blood pressure

. . . .

*H*igh blood pressure, or *hypertension,* means high stroke risk. Treatments that reduce high blood pressure reduce the risk of stroke by 40 percent. It can't get much simpler than that. If you've had a stroke or transient stroke, reducing your blood pressure will decrease the chances of having another stroke.

High blood pressure is a national epidemic. At least 40 million Americans have high blood pressure — at least 140/90. The older you are, the more likely you are to have high blood pressure, particularly if you are black. Until age 50, men are more likely than women to have high blood pressure. After the age of menopause, women are more likely than men to be hypertensive.

Some estimate that 40 percent of those who suffer from high blood pressure don't even know they have it. In a society where stress, obesity, and a landscape of convenience-food offerings high in sodium work against healthy blood pressure, it may be no surprise that hypertension is on the rise. But what is surprising is that so many folks don't know they have the condition when it is so *easy* to test blood pressure. Even if they receive a bad blood-pressure report card from their doctor, some still don't do anything to treat the condition.

Maybe it's because high blood pressure kills so slowly. It might be years before you suffer the consequences: damaged blood vessels, heart disease, stroke. In the meantime, you may continue to add up the work stress and salted French fries and cut out most physical activity. And all the while, your blood is pounding through your vessels at a high-pressure capacity, battering and scarring the walls and building up atherosclerotic plaque.

ng your blood pressure early is like investing in retirement. The earlier
art, the healthier your future will be. Monitoring and controlling your
pressure at 30 will reap greater health rewards than if you begin at age
jury to your blood vessels begins early and gets worse with time. So
enting high blood pressure before the wear and tear begins will serve
well.

That said, treating blood pressure later is better than never. Even if you are
older and have suffered a heart attack or stroke, the steps you take to reduce
your blood pressure may save your life. Read on to learn just exactly how
blood-pressure problems lead to stroke — and how you can take control of
your condition and reduce your risk.

Stalking the Silent Killer

High blood pressure is sometimes called the *silent killer.* You can have high
blood pressure for years before you have any sign of problems. As the heart
strains to push the blood at high pressure through arteries, it enlarges, and
the arteries start to show signs of wear. Although you can have *atherosclerosis* (a build-up of plaque on the blood vessel lining) without having high
blood pressure, atherosclerosis is usually much worse and gets worse faster
when accompanied by high blood pressure. And as I have said throughout
the book, high blood pressure is the number-one risk factor for stroke, and
atherosclerosis can cause stroke by formation of blood clots (Figure 8-1).

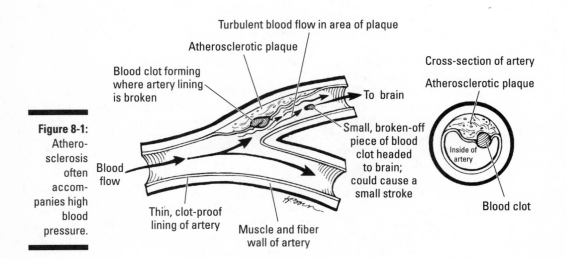

Figure 8-1:
Athero-
sclerosis
often
accom-
panies high
blood
pressure.

Turbulent blood flow in area of plaque

Atherosclerotic plaque

Blood clot forming
where artery lining
is broken

To brain

Cross-section of artery

Atherosclerotic plaque

Inside of
artery

Small, broken-off
piece of blood
clot headed
to brain;
could cause a
small stroke

Blood clot

Blood
flow

Thin, clot-proof
lining of artery

Muscle and fiber
wall of artery

After several years of untreated high blood pressure, you may notice some changes: You may suffer from headaches and dizzy spells, or you may have more frequent nosebleeds. As the atherosclerosis worsens, you may develop poor circulation in your feet.

The condition of your brain generally reflects the poor condition of your heart and blood vessels. As your vessels are repeatedly injured and continue collecting cholesterol and calcium in atherosclerotic plaques, clots form at these sites . . . clots that may be breaking free and traveling downstream to the brain to cause a stroke. You may begin to have trouble thinking and remembering as small brain arteries battered by high blood pressure fail. These arteries, weakened over the years, may even burst, causing a red stroke.

Understanding blood pressure

Young blood vessels are quite rubbery. When the heart beats, the blood is forced into the blood vessels under pressure. Like a thick-skinned tree-shaped balloon, the vessels stretch out and expand a little as the blood moves through them. When your heart beats, blood is forced through the vessels at the maximum pressure, called *systolic blood pressure*. Between heartbeats, the tight rubbery girdle of the blood vessels squeezes back down on your blood and keeps it moving through your arteries. Your blood pressure never drops to zero between heartbeats because of your elastic blood vessels. The lowest pressure is called the *diastolic blood pressure*.

As you get older, atherosclerosis and age make your blood vessels less elastic. That means it is harder for your heart to keep the average pressure up. The result? The heart has to beat much harder, creating a higher systolic pressure and a lower diastolic pressure. What's interesting is that older people with high blood pressure have a high *systolic* pressure, whereas younger individuals with high blood pressure have a high *diastolic* pressure.

Defining high blood pressure

Blood pressure is recorded as two numbers: the highest (systolic) pressure during a heartbeat *over* the lowest (diastolic) pressure between beats. For instance, your doctor may tell you that your blood pressure is 120 over 80 and write it down as *120/80*. (That, by the way, would be good news for you — as this is an average blood pressure reading.) The highest number, the systolic pressure, is given first. If you accidentally reverse it, doctors will smile at you like you said goodbye instead of hello.

Can blood pressure be too low?

It is possible that low blood pressure can put you at risk. Doctors worry that if you've had a stroke, your blood vessels may not be as flexible and may be narrowed by a great deal of atherosclerosis. Hence you may need more blood pressure to force your blood into your brain. Lowering your blood pressure too much, though, might cause brain injury from low blood flow.

We just don't know for sure what the lower limit is. It probably varies from person to person. Many believe that the lowest blood pressures aren't measured because they occur when you are asleep. You might discuss this with your doctor to see if 24-hour blood pressure monitoring might change the way your blood pressure is treated. If so, the cost might be worth it.

If your blood pressure is consistently high after several measurements when you are not being treated, then you have high blood pressure. But what is considered high blood pressure? Well, various levels of blood-pressure readings set off different alarms:

✔ **Pre-hypertensive:** If your blood pressure is higher than 120/80 but lower than 140/90, then you are said to be *pre-hypertensive* and likely to develop hypertension if you don't take measures to stave it off. National guidelines recommend that you walk more, lose weight, and reduce sodium in your diet.

✔ **Bad and really bad:** If your blood pressure is higher than 140/90 but lower than 160/100, you have Stage 1 high blood pressure (bad). If your blood pressure is higher than 160/100, you have Stage 2 high blood pressure (really bad).

Averaging your blood pressure

Some doctors think the important number is the *average* blood pressure.

You can estimate your average blood pressure by finding the difference between the highest and lowest blood pressure and adding one third of that to the lowest blood pressure.

(You can see that this means that the lower blood pressure is twice as influential in determining your average blood pressure. Don't you hate it when I say "you can see" and it isn't obvious at all? Well, I leave it to the engineers and accountants to check my math.) The point is that the diastolic blood pressure is a better measure of how much work your heart is doing to keep your blood pressure as high as it is and a better estimate of how much wear and tear there is on your blood vessels.

Getting your blood pressure checked

It's simple to determine whether your blood pressure is high. You're familiar with the little Velcro sleeve the nurse slips on your upper arm. As the nurse presses the rubber pump, the sleeve tightens, and you watch the needle swing up and tick down before it rests at the magic number.

You don't have to wait till your next doctor appointment to check your blood pressure — just walk into your local drugstore, sit down at the blood pressure booth near the pharmacy counter, and take your blood pressure yourself. Don't cross your legs when you are taking your blood pressure. Just crossing your legs can sometimes raise your blood pressure a few points. I don't know why.

If you're taking care of someone who can't make it to the drugstore, you can buy your own machine. Best things about getting your own machine: portable, private, easy to use, and available for daily use in a convenient place. Disadvantages: the cost and inaccuracy if you get the cuff in the wrong place or don't get the machine set up correctly.

Battling a life-long threat

So far, most cases of hypertension are never cured. Blood pressure is controlled, not fixed. It is absolutely amazing to me that so many people take one bottle of blood-pressure pills, find out their blood pressure is better, and stop, thinking the job is done. They act as if it was an infection that has been treated.

This isn't the way it works. You need to take blood-pressure medication *every day for the rest of your life* — unless you have an unusual, treatable cause of the high blood pressure, or a miraculous new treatment is found. Your efforts will be well worth it in preventing not just heart attack and stroke, but a number of other life-threatening health conditions (Table 8-1).

Table 8-1	The Effects of High Blood Pressure
Effect	*Risk*
Hardening of arteries (atherosclerosis)	Heart attack, stroke
Bulges in blood vessels (aneurysms)	Bleeding ruptured aneurysms
Enlarged heart	Heart failure, heart transplant
Injury to kidney blood vessels	Kidney failure and dialysis
Burst arteries in retina of eye	Blindness, vision loss

Who's at Risk for High Blood Pressure

High blood pressure isn't the result of a single cause. Some circumstances you can't control — your age or your family history, for example. Others may require lifestyle changes or medical solutions. In any event, you'll benefit by knowing the range of conditions that may lead to high blood pressure.

Keeping it in the family

If you have high blood pressure, chances are pretty good that someone else in your family does, as well. If you *don't* have high blood pressure, and a family member does, then, regardless of your age, it's important for you to check your blood pressure *now* and keep a close watch on it through the years. It is also good motivation to start exercising and keeping your weight under control now. This can help delay the onset of high blood pressure and all its problems.

Whether you are hypertensive or doing what you can to prevent high blood pressure, you can benefit from the experiences of your family members. They may have tried different drugs, diets, or exercise programs. The drugs and diets that they find work best may also work best for you. Their experience is particularly valuable because of their genetic relationship to you.

African Americans

African Americans as a group have a very high rate of high blood pressure. It starts when they are younger, and they have very high rates of heart attack and stroke — higher than other groups with the same blood pressure. The reasons for these differences are not known. For example, it is estimated that about 36 percent of African Americans have high blood pressure compared to 25 percent of white Americans. African Americans have approximately 50 percent more strokes than white Americans.

African Americans have a higher prevalence of other risk factors, including diabetes and obesity. There are differences in the care that they receive and differences in culture and diet. These explain part of the increased stroke rate in African Americans, but not all of it.

Fortunately, African Americans can be successfully treated for their high blood pressure. Ask your doctor about different medications. Successful treatment can usually be achieved with persistence.

Diet and lifestyle

Extra fat requires your heart to pump extra blood. Time and again, studies support that losing weight reduces blood pressure. There is a problem, though: Many people who are overweight have difficulty losing weight. They may postpone starting medication too long, thinking they will eventually get their weight under control. In the meantime, the high blood pressure is injuring their arteries.

I am not saying that you should start taking pills and stop worrying about your weight. Carrying extra weight can also increase the likelihood that you will develop diabetes and high cholesterol. I am saying that treating your high blood pressure is critical even *before* you reach your ideal weight. Additionally, people within normal weight ranges have high blood pressure, so there is no guarantee that losing weight *will* get your pressure under control.

Adding unhealthy sodium through table salt

Fast-food fries are the worst of all foods. Not only are they high in calories and the worst of all kinds of fats — *trans fats* — but they also contain massive amounts of table salt, which can raise blood pressure. Salt that you eat goes into your bloodstream and is excreted by your kidneys. When the concentration of salt increases in your blood, water is drawn into the blood from other tissues to dilute the salt until your kidneys have time to excrete it. The extra blood volume and extra work for the kidneys increases your blood pressure.

Try restricting salt to see if your blood pressure comes down. If you are living with someone on a low-salt diet, join in. You get used to the change of taste in just a few weeks. Throw away your salt shaker and substitute healthy herbs and spices to enhance the flavors of your food. Your taste for salt will sharpen as you reduce the amount you add to your food at the table.

Neglecting potassium and calcium in the diet

Diets high in potassium promote better health and may result in lower blood pressure.

Good sources of potassium are fruits such as cantaloupe, bananas, apricots, and oranges, as well as dairy products, lean meats, and dried legumes. Interestingly, salt substitutes often include potassium. So you can kill two birds with one stone when you're trying to improve your blood-pressure readings.

Just like potassium, calcium can help reduce your blood pressure. Key sources of calcium are dairy products — some experts would remind you to use low-fat dairy products such as skim milk or yogurt. You can also find calcium in sardines, certain grains and legumes, and even vegetables such as broccoli. Calcium helps maintain bone and muscle tissue — particularly important as you recover from stroke.

Alcohol: A little is good, a lot is bad

Those who have one drink of alcohol per day have a reduced risk of stroke and heart attack. That doesn't mean that if you don't drink you should start — it's never been shown in a clinical trial that *adding* one glass of alcohol per day will help those who drink *less*. But for those who enjoy alcohol in moderation, at least this is one pleasure in life that may not be bad for you.

Key word being *moderation*. More than two to three drinks of alcohol per day can *add* to your risk of high blood pressure. In addition, if you have a brain injured by stroke, you shouldn't be drinking that much, anyway. Alcohol can be much more intoxicating for those with injured brains. And, of course, alcohol is known to directly injure the brain when consumed in large quantities. If you are drinking too much now, after a stroke, look hard at whether you are depressed. Antidepressants work much better than alcohol and don't raise your blood pressure.

Would you believe bad kidneys?

Problems with your kidneys may raise your blood pressure. They play a major role in controlling your blood pressure by controlling the volume of blood and the amount of sodium and potassium in the blood. Any disease of the kidneys may affect blood pressure. It is particularly critical if you are young and have especially high blood pressure to check out your kidneys.

One cause of high blood pressure that may be treatable is narrowing of the artery that takes blood to one kidney or the other. The usual cause is a plaque of atherosclerosis in the main artery to one or both kidneys. If the blood flow through one of the kidneys is reduced too much, your blood pressure can go very high. Doctors can often open up the arteries with catheter tubes and small balloons inside your arteries. A metal stent is left in place to keep the artery open. If that doesn't work, surgery is possible.

Identifying other medical problems

Some cases of high blood pressure are caused by uncommon medical problems. You may want to have blood tests to see if you have any of the diseases listed here. The tests are expensive and odds are you probably don't have the diseases. If severe enough to cause high blood pressure, these conditions usually manifest in other symptoms as well.

Sleep apnea: Sign of high blood pressure

We are just beginning to learn about *sleep apnea,* a condition associated with loud snoring and gasping during sleep. In some individuals, the back of the throat collapses when they sleep, and blocks the air pathway to the lungs. The result is long periods of time between breaths. This condition is aggravated by excess weight.

Patients with sleep apnea often have high blood pressure. It's not known whether treatment will reduce blood pressure, but some people feel much better when they use a mask attached to pressure breathing machines at night. Some surgeons offer treatments for sleep apnea. Be especially diligent about seeking a wide range of second opinions before agreeing to such surgery — especially if you have already had a stroke.

Disease	Cause
Hyperthyroidism	Too much thyroid hormone
Pheochromocytoma	A small adrenal gland tumor
Hyperaldosteronism	An overactive adrenal gland
Cushing's syndrome	Too much steroid in your blood
Heart disease	Heart valve disease

One of these conditions, *pheochromocytoma,* can be very elusive and hard to diagnose. High blood pressure unresponsive to treatment may be the only symptom.

Drugs that may lead to high blood pressure

Many medications contain chemicals that can raise blood pressure. Here a few of the most common offenders:

- ✓ High doses of aspirin and similar drugs
- ✓ Decongestants
- ✓ Diet aids
- ✓ Steroids

You're wise to consider and list all medications — including diet supplements, diet aids, and vitamins — you take. Even the medicated salve that you rub on your sore muscles goes on the list. Birth-control pills, Viagra — the whole medicine cabinet. Then show the list to your doctor who is working with you to manage your stroke risk and every doctor who prescribes medication for you. It is important to have a complete list not only in relation to your high blood pressure, but because such supplements may interact in an undesirable way with other medications you may be prescribed.

Lowering Blood Pressure to Reduce Stroke

What are the benefits of treating blood pressure? For people who have never had a stroke, treating blood pressure cuts the risk of stroke nearly in half. In older patients, treating people with systolic high blood pressure reduces the chances of dementia (see Chapter 7) by half. If you've had a stroke, the chances you will have a second one are reduced by 30 percent if you treat your high blood pressure.

There isn't much good data on how *much* to lower the blood pressure. Most evidence shows that the lower, the better. However, in the majority of studies, the average reduction in blood pressure has been only about ten points.

If there isn't a treatable cause of high blood pressure (*hyperthyroidism,* for example), there are two basic ways to lower your blood pressure:

✔ Diet and exercise

✔ Medication

Because they don't treat the *cause* of the high blood pressure, these treatments have to be continued as long as you live — or until someone figures out a treatment that permanently fixes the problem. Regular and frequent monitoring of your blood pressure helps ensure that your treatment program is working. If you are taking medicine for blood pressure, you should still exercise and eat a healthy diet.

Control through diet and exercise

If you're overweight, consume an unhealthy menu of high-sodium and high-fat foods, *and* you avoid regular exercise, you may be able to lower your blood pressure by making some positive lifestyle changes. Even if you are recovering from a stroke, you can follow these recommendations:

- ✔ Exercise enough to make you breathe faster.

- ✔ Get your weight under control.

- ✔ Eat more fruits high in potassium (such as cantaloupe, bananas, apricots, and oranges).

- ✔ Restrict your sodium intake by cutting back on table salt.

- ✔ Consume low-fat dairy products to increase your calcium.

- ✔ Enjoy alcohol up to one or two drinks per day but avoid more.

- ✔ Avoid cold tablets and diet drugs that have warnings about high blood pressure.

Control with medication

Because I'm a doctor, you may think I am too quick to turn to drugs to lower blood pressure. The truth is, too many who suffer from high blood pressure are too slow to start treating it in the most successful manner possible. Although diet and exercise *may* help lower blood pressure, they alone are often not as effective as medication. This may be because people can't keep up the effort, or their lives don't really allow for them to — or because the underlying cause is not related to their diet.

But taking medication does require you to be responsible. You must take the prescription as directed and get needed testing on time to make sure the drug is working and not causing dangerous side effects. If your blood pressure is especially difficult to control — not uncommon — you may need to take two or more drugs to get your pressure below 140/90. If so, then you have to be aware of all the possible ways the two drugs can cause problems together that they wouldn't cause alone.

Lowering blood pressure too much

Drugs can reduce your blood pressure too far. As I go through the different types of drugs in the following sections, I won't repeat this warning for each different type. If your blood pressure is too low, then you will feel light headed or weak. When you stand up suddenly, your blood pressure may drop so low that you faint or almost faint. If you are having these symptoms, call your doctor. You'll probably be told to stop taking the medicine. This doesn't mean forever, though. This means you change the type of medicine or the dose before trying again to adjust the prescription to your system.

Don't stop taking blood-pressure medicine suddenly without checking with your doctor. Your blood pressure may "rebound" or shoot up higher than ever as the restraint of the drug is suddenly released — this can be dangerous.

A trial-and-error process

A lot of people are concerned about taking medicine. If you are one of them, don't overreact to failure by quitting. Getting your blood pressure under control is a trial-and-error process that may require a lot of telephone calls and visits to your doctor. Be sure you have a doctor you can work with and who is patient with your sensitivity. Make sure you have a clear channel of communication. You should be able to talk to either a doctor or nurse when you call to report a problem serious enough to make you think you should stop the drug.

For men only

A possible side effect with almost all blood-pressure medications is impotence. If you are an older man, especially if you have just had a stroke, problems getting and keeping an erection can already be an issue. Any preexisting problems may potentially get worse when you start blood-pressure medication. Usually, any problems can be resolved by either adjusting the dose or changing the drug — bring up the issue with your doctor.

Drugs for Lowering Blood Pressure

Most doctors will start treating high blood pressure with one of two inexpensive and effective drugs that have very few side effects and are well-tolerated by most people with high blood pressure. These drugs are the *diuretics* and *beta blockers*. But there are dozens of alternatives. Eventually you can find a drug or combination of drugs that works for you.

If you have just had a stroke or have other problems with your memory, you may need a system to be sure you don't miss a dose — or take a double dose. Even people with good memories can benefit from such a system. Those little plastic containers that allow you to set out your pills for a week at a time are very useful for this — you'll find them at any drugstore. Keeping written records works as well, especially when you are taking several medications several times a day. That way you can check the list before you take each set of pills.

Thiazide diuretics: Water pills

Thiazide diuretics are a class of drugs that decrease blood pressure by increasing the amount of salt excreted by the kidneys. The salt, eliminated through your urine, takes a lot of water with it. You will find yourself headed to the bathroom more frequently. To avoid dehydration and constipation, you will need to start drinking more water. You may be waking up in the middle of the night unless you take your dose in the morning. Of the many thiazides, *hydrochlorthiazide* is the most common. Doses of 12.5 milligrams to 25 milligrams are safest. If the dose gets higher, be sure you don't want to change to another drug. If 25 mg works well, ask your doctor if you can try 12.5 to see if you can get the same result.

You want to take the lowest effective dosage to minimize potential side effects. Thiazides may potentially do any of the following:

- **Deplete potassium:** Symptoms of low blood potassium are not anything special — something vaguely like the flu. Regular blood tests can catch this problem easily, but it is so uncommon at low doses that many doctors will only check if you already show symptoms. If you start thiazides and then find yourself feeling run down, tired, and weak, be sure to mention this to your doctor and ask if you need a blood test for potassium.

- **Aggravate diabetes:** This usually occurs only when higher doses are used. Checking your blood regularly can help detect these problems.

- **Raise cholesterol levels:** At higher doses, blood-pressure medications may increase cholesterol levels in the blood. Routine blood tests are important to monitor.

- **Constipation and dehydration:** Drink more water to avoid these common side effects.

- **Interact with other drugs:** Before beginning a thiazide prescription, be sure to let your doctor know if you are taking digitalis, coumadin, lithium, vitamin D, gout drugs, or drugs for diabetes. The doses of these drugs may have to be changed if you must take them when you are on thiazides.

Beta blockers: The anti-adrenalin

Beta blockers are drugs that work on your nervous system to lower blood pressure. They have the opposite effect of adrenalin, reducing the pulse rate and the forcefulness of heartbeats. Beta blockers have been shown to be particularly beneficial for patients who have had heart attacks and evidence of severe atherosclerosis.

Reducing blood pressure is a life-long commitment

A 54-year-old man went to his physician because his daughter had told him he should have a colonoscopy for early detection of colon cancer. During his exam, he mentioned he had had a spell a month or two earlier in which the left side of his face and left arm felt numb. He felt a little dizzy at the time and then the spell cleared up within minutes. The doctor checked his blood pressure: 155/102. The doctor asked him if he had tested for high blood pressure before. The man said he did years ago, but he had changed his diet and it had returned to almost normal. He didn't go back to see his doctor and had not had his blood pressure checked for several years. His business was very demanding and stressful and he just didn't have time. He was referred to a neurologist, who ordered an MRI scan. The scan showed several small strokes at the base of the brain and in its central core. His examination was normal and he had no recollection of any other spells. The neurologist listened to his neck and ordered an ultrasound test to see if there was narrowing of any major brain arteries. There was a thick plaque of atherosclerosis in his carotid artery but it was not thick enough to require surgery. He returned to his regular doctor.

He was started on thiazide diuretics, 25 milligrams per day, and advised to check his blood pressure every day for the next week before returning to his physician's office. His blood pressure declined over the ensuing week to 142/94. He continued the same dose for another two weeks. His blood pressure remained high at 144/92. His doctor then prescribed a low 40-milligram dose of propranolol twice per day. Two weeks later, his blood pressure was 138/86. His pulse rate was 66. The doctor increased his dose to 80 milligrams two times per day. Two weeks later his pulse rate was 60 and his blood pressure 130/80. He continued on this regimen. In the meantime, the doctor had found that he had elevated blood cholesterol and low HDL. He was started on statins and referred to a cardiologist for a full work-up.

The man became annoyed at all the time his medical care was taking. He felt his business needed him at the moment and that he would start taking better care of himself after the current crisis was over. He canceled his cardiologist appointments for several months and failed to renew his prescriptions. One morning while getting the newspaper, he started having unusual left-side chest pain. He went to the emergency room. No evidence of a heart attack was found, but his blood pressure was 162/108. He was referred back to his doctors to resume treatment of his blood pressure. This time he went to his appointments.

If you are a bundle of nerves living under constant stress and pushing yourself too hard, beta blockers, accompanied by an exercise program, may be the course for you. Although they are not sedatives or muscle relaxers, beta blockers blunt some of the physical aspects of anger and tension. You may find yourself more relaxed when giving speeches and more in control when tempers might otherwise flare. While on beta blockers, feelings of frustration, fear, or anger may not translate as readily into the physical signs of high pulse rate, red face, or dry mouth.

Beta blockers can have side effects, however. They can aggravate asthma, increasing the frequency and severity of attacks. They can interfere with the normal rhythm of the heart. Because they take some of the force out of your heartbeat, they can cause fatigue and limit your ability to exercise.

Rebound high blood pressure is a risk if you suddenly stop your beta-blocker medication. If the dose is too high or you accidentally take an extra tablet, your pulse rate may drop too low, a dangerous situation. The pulse rate shouldn't get too far below 60. Unfortunately, beta blockers can also blunt your body's normal reaction to low blood sugar — sweating and anxiety. This can be dangerous for you if you are a diabetic taking insulin because you may not be able to tell when your blood sugar is dangerously low.

ACE inhibitors: New kids on the block

Angiotensin converting enzyme (ACE) inhibitors are relatively new drugs. They are free of many of the side effects of thiazides and beta blockers, but clinical trials indicate they may be less effective than other drugs in lowering blood pressure. They have been shown to be particularly effective in the treatment of heart failure and can be a desirable alternative to beta blockers or thiazides — especially for diabetics and patients with kidney disease.

Be aware that there are some potentially serious side effects. ACE inhibitors can *raise* the level of potassium in your blood (opposite of thiazides, which lower the level). Having plenty of natural potassium in your diet is usually good, even when taking ACE inhibitors. Special potassium supplements and salt substitutes may not be such a good idea, though, when combined with ACE inhibitors. Check with your doctor.

Potassium in your diet does not usually raise your blood potassium levels because healthy kidneys keep it under control. But high potassium levels in your blood can be dangerous. This high-potassium reaction is more common in patients with kidney disease and heart failure. The best way to monitor it is to check blood levels of potassium after starting the drug. Other than slow, possibly irregular, pulse, there are no symptoms. ACE inhibitors have another unusual side effect: In a number of people, the drugs cause a chronic dry hacking cough. Some people hardly notice it; others can't stand it.

As with any blood-pressure medication, check your blood pressure frequently after starting the drug to be sure it's not too high or too low. ACE inhibitors can cause a rapid drop in blood pressure, particularly if you are dehydrated.

Calcium antagonists and other drugs

Calcium antagonists — or *calcium channel blockers* — were introduced after thiazides and beta blockers, but before ACE inhibitors, for the purpose of treating the most difficult cases of high blood pressure that seemed to remain resistant to other medications. They work by directly inhibiting the contraction of the muscles in the blood vessels. The result is blood vessels that have larger diameters and are easier for the blood to pass through. That means it takes less pressure to move the blood. Calcium channel blockers can cause headache and flushing. Occasionally they lead to mild swelling of the legs. Like ACE inhibitors, they work well for patients with diabetes or kidney disease.

If a case of high blood pressure is extremely resistant to treatment, other drugs may be prescribed. It's beyond the scope of this book to describe all the medications that can be used in these difficult cases. The more difficult the treatment, the more important it is for you to get regular blood tests and to check your blood pressure frequently.

High blood pressure may be called the silent killer — but its devastation is anything but quiet. When nearly a third of the adults in the United States have high blood pressure, and 40 percent of them are unaware of it, the potential damage this insidious villain can inflict is frightening. Whether you're recovering from a stroke — or you're just committed to preventing one — perhaps the most important and easiest step you can take to protect yourself is to keep tabs on your blood pressure. If it's high, follow a course of diet and medication to lower it to a healthy level — and eliminate that silent killer so that it is no longer a threat.

Chapter 9

Fat and Stroke Risk

Fat gets a bad rap in the press. True, it's not good to carry around an extra 20 pounds, nor should you indulge in a bacon cheeseburger and fries too often. Fact is, though, fat is an important part of our diet and an essential component of our bodies. We require some reserves of fat in our body and we need to keep that store supplied by calories taken in the form of fat.

But too much fat — in our diet and, subsequently, in our body and blood — leads to serious health consequences, not the least of which is stroke. In a nutshell, if the body's cholesterol level is too high, atherosclerosis develops (check out the glossary for more on this condition), which can lead to heart attack and stroke. A fat-heavy diet — too many pork chops and four-egg omelets — can certainly weigh down your blood with dangerously high levels of a fat called cholesterol. But in some people, the propensity for high blood cholesterol can't be controlled by diet, and drugs may be required to lower the cholesterol to a safe level.

What makes cholesterol such a villain? Is cholesterol all bad? How do we go from pizza to white stroke? What's fat got to do with blood clots in the brain? That's what this chapter's all about.

Fat and the Body

Researchers continue to explore the relationship between fat and atherosclerosis, heart disease, and stroke. Newspapers and magazines bombard us with information. Sometimes, small studies showing a possible trend, without definitive results, are widely published.

The result is that doctors and patients have jumped to conclusions that haven't been borne out in clinical trials. Some studies have showed that people who ate more cholesterol had more heart disease. It took a long time before trials were done to see what happened when people intentionally reduced the cholesterol in their diet compared to those who didn't. The trials didn't show a consistent difference. Now more trials are beginning to build a solid foundation that outlines the opportunities available to you as a stroke patient and someone at risk of atherosclerosis and heart disease.

What we have learned with a great deal of confidence is that *the amount and type of fat in your blood* is more important than the amount of fat that you eat. And the amount of fat you eat is less important than the *type* of fat you eat.

Fat: Slow-burning fuel

The way fat in your diet is turned into fuel for your daily energy needs is pretty interesting. And complicated. Basically, a carefully controlled, slow-burning fire from within combines oxygen with fuel to produce heat, water, and carbon dioxide.

We breathe in oxygen and breathe out carbon dioxide. We consume food and excrete the unusable "ashes" of our internal fires. The more complex sugars and starches in our diet are rapidly converted to *glucose* and similar simple sugars. These act as quick-burning, readily converted fuel throughout our systems — sort of like gasoline. Proteins burn more slowly, perhaps like coal, with many complex reactions.

The fats are the slowest-burning form of fuel. They are akin to petroleum oil, perhaps — highly concentrated, complex stores of energy. Pound for pound, fat contains twice the energy of sugar or protein. Fat's form of energy, however, isn't immediately available. Fats have to be refined and processed in your cells before their energy can be recovered and used.

So what happened to that salted butter that drenched your large popcorn at the movies last night? Or the egg-and-sausage biscuits you packed away for breakfast this morning? Or the pizza with extra cheese you grabbed for dinner? Here are the gruesome details.

Breaking down fat in the digestive system

Converting the fat we eat requires special digestive enzymes that are made in the liver and pancreas. The liver is essentially a large chemical processing unit that handles most of the complex reactions involved with the digestion of food and the removal of many toxins from the blood. The pancreas is also a digestive organ but is more specialized. It makes insulin to control blood glucose levels and also makes powerful digestive enzymes to dissolve and break down the fats that we eat.

The fat in our food doesn't dissolve very easily. Ever try to clean up grease spilled on the floor? As you attempt to wipe, it smears around. Water alone doesn't help. You have to add soap. The soap dissolves some of the fat and forms little globules with grease in the middle and soap around the outside in a protective shell that will dissolve in water. What you get is a slurry of water made cloudy with tiny spherical globules of soap-ringed grease.

Something similar happens in the lower part of the stomach as food leaves to enter the small intestine. The soap used by the body is called *bile.* The liver produces bile, which breaks the fat into small globules and works with the *lipase* from the pancreas to reduce the fat molecules to their constituent parts so that they can be absorbed by the small intestine. The small intestine churns the fat together with the bile and slowly absorbs the fat.

Fat begets fat. Special fat receptors in the stomach slow down the release of fatty food into the intestine — so that the intestines don't overload the bloodstream with large amounts of fat. Slowing the digestion in the stomach brings its own problems. Food left for hours ferments and irritates the stomach. Your grumbling stomach wants solace. You feel hungry (ever crave a few scoops of ice cream hours after you eat pizza?). Fat in your system is unique in that it encourages you to eat more.

The stomach churns the fat into small globules that can also be readily attacked by *lipases,* enzymes produced by the small intestines and the pancreas. Lipases take the large fat molecules in our bacon burgers and omelets and break them down into simpler fat molecules, which are smaller and can pass through the membranes of cells lining the intestines and then into the bloodstream to pass through the liver or directly to the heart. Along the way, tiny fat globules are coated with special proteins that work a little like soap to keep the fat dissolved in the blood. This system is highly efficient — about 95 percent of the fat you take in makes it into your bloodstream!

Getting to Know the Two Types of Fat: Cholesterol and Triglycerides

Before I go further into fat's journey through the bloodstream, allow me to introduce you to the two major forms of fat we find in the body and in the food we take into our body:

- Cholesterol
- Triglycerides

Cholesterol is waxy

Cholesterol is manufactured in our body — almost four-fifths of the cholesterol in your blood is homemade right in your liver. We also take in cholesterol when we eat meat, cheese and dairy products, and eggs.

Cholesterol is a waxy form of fat, quite firm and water-repellent. It is present in all cells as part of the outer cell membrane, with the highest concentration in the sheath that wraps around nerve fibers. This fat called cholesterol has some special functions: It forms the molecular backbone of several hormones, including estrogen and testosterone. And it is a fundamental component of vitamin D and the bile we need to emulsify fats when they are digested.

The processing of fats varies from person to person, depending on diet and genetics. Some individuals have unusually high levels of cholesterol in their blood despite consuming a cholesterol-free diet. This can usually be traced to an inherited abnormal enzyme or molecular abnormality.

The amount of cholesterol you should allow in your diet each day is a scant 300 milligrams, one-third of a gram. So it depends on what you eat: A boiled egg, for example, contains about 225 mg of cholesterol; a chicken breast, around 60 mg. As vital as it is to your cells, you can eat only a small amount of cholesterol before it becomes a threat to the health of your blood vessels.

Triglycerides are greasy or oily

Triglycerides are the most common type of fat in our diet and in our bodies. Think of vegetable oil, olive oil, and shortening. Salads are dressed with them, potatoes are fried in them, foccacio is dipped in them.

There are three classes of triglycerides:

- Saturated: Solids, such as shortening and butter
- Unsaturated: Liquid, such as vegetable and fish oils
- Trans: Begin as unsaturated, but hydrogen is added for processing and longer shelf life (such as hydrogenated vegetable oil in peanut butter)

Unsaturated fats are the most benign of the triglycerides. In fact, these fats can be downright good for you (more about that in the next section).

But watch out for saturated and trans fats. These forms of fat cause the body to produce more cholesterol, increasing the risk of atherosclerosis and, subsequently, heart disease and stroke.

Dieticians recommend that all the fats combined provide only 25 to 35 percent of the calories in our diet. This generally means we should eat no more than 60 to 100 grams — 4 to 8 tablespoons — of fat per day, depending on body size and how much food we consume. Candy bars, donuts, cookies, and hotdogs can, by themselves, contain a tablespoon or two of fat.

So, to summarize: Cholesterol, needed by the body in small amounts, is primarily produced by your body, though you can raise your cholesterol level by consuming more cholesterol — found in animal products. *Or* you can increase your cholesterol by eating some forms of triglycerides — specifically saturated and trans fats — which cause your body to produce more cholesterol. Now, how does all that fat get around your body?

Fat Transporters: HDL, LDL, and Others

The bloodstream is a highway-transport system that carries fats to their destination. But it's a water-based system, and water and fats just don't behave well when they get together. So to keep peace, special transport proteins serve as bodyguards, accompanying fats on their journey. Without these bodyguards, the fats and the water in the bloodstream would "mix it up," causing all sorts of traffic jams and congestion in your blood vessels.

To prevent that, here's what happens: After they are processed in the intestine and absorbed into the intestinal cells, fats are packaged in small droplets protected by the proteins. These fat-protein packages are called *lipoproteins.* There are four types of lipoproteins. Their long names are real tongue-twisters, but you may already be familiar with their nicknames.

HDL: The good

HDL, which stands for *high-density lipoprotein,* is recognized as the *good* fat transporter. HDL's smooth surfaces do not stick to the blood vessels — thus, no clogging of the thruways and risk of blood clots. Another favorable attribute is that HDL collects cholesterol from other tissues and brings it back to the liver for processing and excretion. This lipoprotein, then, not only reliably carries its passengers to their destinations, it finds the bad guys and turns them in for deportation.

The functions of lipoproteins circulating in the blood are very complex, and the relationship of blood vessel health, heart disease, and stroke is not completely understood. Study after study, however, supports the finding that people who have more HDL in their blood have less heart disease and stroke.

LDL: The bad

If HDL is good, then LDL — *low-density lipoprotein* — is recognized as the *bad* fat transporter. LDL has earned its reputation for a few reasons. It is the major carrier of cholesterol through the blood vessels. LDL doesn't hold tightly to the cholesterol or triglycerides that they carry, depositing them throughout the body's tissues. LDL's outer surfaces are coated with proteins that stick to blood vessels and attract a lot of mean friends, including white blood cells and platelets that get into the fray and invite their own friends. The result is a waxy plaque of atherosclerosis that begins to enlarge as more LDL collects at the site.

VLDL: The ugly

These *very-low-density lipoproteins* are fat trucks that contain little protein but are loaded with triglycerides delivered to fat and muscle cells for storage. VLDL particles are formed in the liver from excess fat or sugar in the diet. They have a triglyceride core with a thin layer of protein. VLDL breaks up easily, and the fragments of their wrecks expose blood vessels and other tissues to the toxic effects of their hard, fat cores.

Chylomicrons

Chylomicrons are fat and protein particles that transport both cholesterol and triglycerides from the intestine directly to the rest of the body. The source of HDL, LDL, and VLDL particles is the liver. The small intestine is the source of chylomicrons. Unlike most food you eat, fat carried by chylomicrons bypasses the liver and goes directly to the rest of your body where the oils and hard fats are removed for storage in fat or muscle cells.

Chylomicrons are largely triglyceride fats and, as such, not healthy. They increase your risk for heart disease, although the relationship to stroke is not as clear. They are controlled the same ways that LDL is. When LDL is elevated, the triglycerides are often elevated, too. The focus among doctors now is generally to focus on lowering the LDL cholesterol while keeping an eye on the chylomicrons/triglycerides to be sure they come down as well.

The stroke connection

So what does all this have to do with stroke? These fats and their bodyguard lipoproteins can irritate the sensitive lining of your blood vessels. This leads to atherosclerosis. Once irritated, the blood vessels can become increasingly inflamed, scarred, and overlaid with potholes and patches. Eventually, the atherosclerotic plaque ruptures and blocks the vessel entirely or becomes so rough that stroke-causing clots form there. Either way, white stroke can result.

Testing for Fat Trouble in Your Body

How do you know you're at risk for stroke because of high cholesterol? Not necessarily from the numbers on your bathroom scale — though if you're carrying a spare tire around your waist, that may be a bad sign. But getting a sense of the shape you're in is a starting point. Checking your blood for levels of cholesterol and its components is the next step.

Your weight is not always an accurate indicator of your cholesterol level. Thin people can have high cholesterol, and overweight individuals may have healthy cholesterol readings. That said, weight is often an indicator for heart disease, and a suggestion that cholesterol may need to be investigated.

Body mass index

The following Body Mass Index (BMI) table is a tool to help you assess your health risk due to your weight. Find your height on the left and scan across to find your weight. The figure at the top of your weight's row is your *body mass*. If your body mass is greater than 24, you are officially at higher risk of heart disease, diabetes, and stroke. (Desirable values are in gray. Values lower than 18 are unusual and may not be healthy for some people. Check with your doctor.)

Pears take heart

Shape may be another clue that the heart and brain are at risk because of weight. Studies indicate that "apples," individuals who carry weight at the waist or higher, may have a greater risk for heart attack, diabetes, and stroke than those who tend to put on weight around their hips.

"Pears" may fret about their bottom-heavy figures, but they're apt to be healthier than their "apple" counterparts. Even if your BMI is 24 or lower, you may be at higher risk if you are a man with a waist larger than 40 inches or a woman with a 35-inch or larger waist.

	19	20	21	22	23	24	25	26	27	28	29	30	31	32	33	34	35
4'10	91	96	100	105	110	115	119	124	129	134	138	143	148	153	158	162	167
4'11	94	99	104	109	114	119	124	128	133	138	143	148	153	158	163	168	173
5'0	97	102	107	112	118	123	128	133	138	143	148	153	158	163	168	174	179
5'1	100	106	111	116	122	127	132	137	143	148	153	158	164	169	174	180	185
5'2	104	109	115	120	126	131	136	142	147	153	158	164	169	175	180	186	191
5'3	107	113	118	124	130	135	141	146	152	158	163	169	175	180	186	191	197
5'4	110	116	122	128	134	140	145	151	157	163	169	174	180	186	192	197	204
5'5	114	120	126	132	138	144	150	156	162	168	174	180	186	192	198	204	210
5'6	118	124	130	136	142	148	155	161	167	173	179	186	192	198	204	210	216
5'7	121	127	134	140	146	153	159	166	172	178	185	191	198	204	211	217	223
5'8	125	131	138	144	151	158	164	171	177	184	190	197	203	210	216	223	230
5'9	128	135	142	149	155	162	169	176	182	189	196	203	209	216	223	230	236
5'10	132	139	146	153	160	167	174	181	188	195	202	209	216	222	229	236	243
5'11	136	143	150	157	165	172	179	186	193	200	208	215	222	229	236	243	250
6'0	140	147	154	162	169	177	184	191	199	206	213	221	228	235	242	250	258
6'1	144	151	159	166	174	182	189	197	204	212	219	227	235	242	250	257	265
6'2	148	155	163	171	179	186	194	202	210	218	225	233	241	249	256	264	272
6'3	152	160	168	176	184	192	200	208	216	224	232	240	248	256	264	272	279
6'4	156	164	172	180	189	197	205	213	221	230	238	246	254	263	271	279	287

Testing your blood for cholesterol

The most accurate way for determining your blood lipid levels is to have your blood tested under fasting conditions (see next section for more). Typically, a single blood sample can be used to measure cholesterol and triglycerides, as well as the three lipoproteins in your cholesterol. The results help you and your doctor estimate your cardiovascular risk.

Drugs that affect your blood test

Prior to a blood test for lipids, follow your physician's restrictions on diet, exercise, and medication use. Some substances can affect the accuracy of test results. Increased cholesterol levels may be reported if you take the following:

ACTH	anabolic steroids
beta-adrenergic blocking agents	corticosteroids
epinephrine	oral contraceptives
phenytoin	sulfonamides
thiazide diuretics	vitamin D

Lower values for cholesterol may result from taking the following:

Allopurinol	androgens
Captopril	chlorpropamide
Clofibrate	colchicine
Colestipol	erythromycin
Isoniazid	lovastatin
MAO inhibitors	neomycin
niacin (vitamin B3)	nitrates

Tell your doctor about all prescription and over-the-counter medications you are taking. By the same token, don't skip taking prescribed medicine the morning of your blood test without checking with your physician.

If your cholesterol or LDL levels continue to cause concern despite adequate treatment, further testing may be done. Although it's a more expensive and complicated test, *lipoprotein phenotyping* may be needed to determine exact levels of each of the four lipoproteins. The test can help identify inherited tendencies toward high cholesterol levels.

Although not related to lipid levels, two other tests for determining stroke risk are often done from the same blood sample: *homocysteine* and *C-reactive protein* tests. These two elements, when present at certain levels, predict increased risk of stroke. When blood vessels are injured or irritated, white blood cells, platelets, and other components of the blood signal a problem to the rest of the body. When the liver receives the signal, it produces C-reactive protein. You want your test results to show 10 or fewer *micromoles* per liter for homocysteine — and you don't want to see *any* measure of C-reactive protein in your blood.

Fasting before your blood test

All the interpretations of the blood lipid test results are based on the assumption that you eat nothing for 12 hours prior to the test. It is *not* the goal to analyze the fat content of your food, but to estimate the load of fat you carry in your blood between meals.

What fat food looks like in your bloodstream

If you eat a fat-heavy meal and then draw blood a few hours later, the blood will settle into three layers — a fat parfait, if you will: red cells at the bottom; a thin, faint-yellow layer of white blood cells in the middle; and, on top, a milky layer of serum cloudy with the fat from the meal.

Sometimes there can be so much fat that the top layer looks like whipped cream. It takes four to six hours to clear this fat out of your blood. This is one reason to fast before blood tests that measure cholesterol and other fats in the bloodstream.

You've read how almost every bit of fat in the diet gets into the bloodstream one way or another. And how fat in the stomach slows down the digestive process. It takes up to 10 hours to clear all the fat from your last meal out of your blood. If you forget and eat something, don't bother to have the tests done — you may as well throw the results away because only the HDL and total cholesterol levels will be close to accurate. You need the LDL values. Just in case you were thinking of really starving yourself to have a good test, you shouldn't wait more than 14 hours or the results may be changed by your body's response to the prolonged fasting.

Interpreting blood test results

Upon review of your blood test results, your doctor will take into account your unique set of circumstances to evaluate and offer an action plan. But "normal" ranges of blood lipids help provide guidelines for patients and professionals alike. Your treatment plan will depend on a great many factors including your age, your prior history of heart disease and stroke, whether or not you have diabetes, and other risk factors. There are guidelines but they are not simple to read, and they are updated as new information is gained from ongoing clinical trials.

Desirable values for cholesterol, triglycerides, and the lipoprotein breakdown are as follows:

Test	Desirable Value
Cholesterol, total	100–199 mg/dL (milligrams per deciliter)
Triglycerides	0–149 mg/dL
HDL	40–59 mg/dL
LDL	0–99 mg/dL
VLDL	5–40 mg/dL

Total cholesterol

When talking about blood lipids, people are no doubt most familiar with the target for total cholesterol, the sum of all the lipoprotein components. The desirable range is below 200 milligrams per deciliter. Levels greater than 240 predict a very high risk of stroke and heart disease. Until menopause, women tend to have lower levels of cholesterol than men the same age. Values for both men and women tend to increase with age. Pregnancy, when cholesterol levels tend to be high, is an exception.

Triglyceride levels

Normal levels are less than 150 mg/dL (milligrams per deciliter). Higher values mean higher risk for stroke and heart disease. Very high levels of triglycerides require treatment similar to that for high LDL.

HDL levels

Remember, HDL is the *good* fat transporter, so a higher range of this lipoprotein is positive news. An HDL reading above 40 is desirable; at 60 or above is even better. At this level, some think the HDL will start carrying excess cholesterol out of the body, reducing the likelihood of atherosclerosis inside your blood vessels. Some recommend that for women 45 and older, the target HDL should be 60.

LDL levels

A desirable level of LDL — the *bad* fat transporter — is 99 milligrams or lower. Whether this or another level of LDL is your treatment goal depends on the plan you work out with your doctor. An LDL level above 190 is a red-light condition for your heart and brain.

Cholesterol-to-HDL ratio

Some research indicates that the ratio of the cholesterol level to HDL level also predicts the occurrence of stroke and heart disease. Divide the cholesterol level by the HDL level. According to the American Heart Association, the level of total cholesterol should not be more than five times the level of HDL (a ratio of 5:1).

I don't hear this ratio used as much by physicians, who tend to look separately at the cholesterol and HDL levels. Using the ratio might let a few feel better about their high cholesterol over 200 if their HDL level was high.

Causes of high cholesterol

Diet	Kidney disease
Genetic factors	Uncontrolled diabetes
Liver disease or hepatitis caused by alcohol or infection	Bile-duct obstruction of the liver usually due to gall bladder problems
Hypothyroidism	Inflammation or infection of the pancreas

Diet and Cholesterol Control

Following a diet low in cholesterol and saturated and trans fats is a smart move. But it may not be enough to get your blood lipids to a safe level if you have an inherent predisposition to high cholesterol — or you simply have a hard time passing up the fried chicken and gravy.

Eating right versus eating less

Eating right and eating less are too different issues. Eating *right* to reduce your cholesterol levels and decrease stroke risk means changing the type and the amount of fat in your diet. It means replacing saturated and trans fats in your diet with unsaturated fat. It means checking your blood levels of HDL and LDL and making sure they are in or moving toward the healthy range.

These days, many people are appropriately concerned about their weight. Obesity by itself increases risk of stroke and heart disease. Obesity can cause and aggravate high blood pressure. Obesity also increases risk of diabetes, which injures blood vessels and accelerates the process of atherosclerosis, leading to stroke and heart attacks.

It's not a bad strategy to eat less *and* eat right. I suggest, however, trying to keep your weight down, but giving a priority to keeping the LDL and total cholesterol in your blood in the healthy range.

What's the right diet?

For anyone who wants to control their blood lipids, I recommend one of two courses: If you're diabetic, follow a diabetic diet that not only controls the fats in your diet but also controls the total number of calories, avoiding rapidly absorbed sugar (see the nutrition page at the American Diabetes Association Web site at www.diabetes.org). If you're not diabetic, follow the American Heart Association diet recommendations, which include limiting saturated and trans fats, substituting low-fat dairy products for their whole-milk counterparts, and eating a greater proportion of calories in fruits, vegetables, and grains. (For complete dietary guidelines, visit www.americanheart.org.)

Some scientists praise the Mediterranean diet, which focuses on vegetables, legumes, fruits, nuts, grains, and fats from olives and vegetable oils as well as a relatively high emphasis on fish. Studies show that following an eating plan traditional to many Mediterranean countries may result in lower cholesterol levels and reduced rate of heart disease. This makes sense: More unsaturated fat in the diet is consistently associated with lower LDL and higher HDL levels in the blood.

CASE STUDY

Cholesterol's the likely culprit

A 66-year-old woman was fixing breakfast for her husband one morning. She sat down with a cup of coffee as she waited for the eggs to boil. Her husband heard the crash of her cup dropping to the floor and came into the kitchen to find his wife dazed, her face contorted unnaturally. She had difficulty speaking, producing strangled sounds when she tried to talk. He couldn't tell if she understood him. She was not moving her right arm. He called 911 and tried to get her to lie down, but she was afraid to walk.

In the emergency department, she was diagnosed with a white stroke. After a CT scan showed no bleeding, she was treated with TPA. An hour later she seemed a little better. The next morning she could talk and understand her husband, but still had some weakness of the right hand. Tests were run to determine the cause of her stroke. She did not have diabetes, high blood pressure, or atrial fibrillation of the heart. She did have moderate atherosclerosis of the carotid artery to the brain. Her LDL cholesterol was high at 139 and her good HDL cholesterol was low at 36. Her body mass index was somewhat high at 28. She returned home three days later. Her doctors prescribed aspirin and the statin drug Atorvistatin, 10 milligrams per day. She was also advised to lose weight and was scheduled for follow-up blood tests and an office visit two weeks later.

I hesitate to mention the Atkins diet — you know: low-carb and lots of animal proteins. If you're on this bandwagon, I recommend that you test your blood cholesterol levels frequently. I also suggest discussing this with your doctor. I really don't know of any good clinical trial data supporting this diet, even though plenty of people have bought into it. But if periodic blood tests indicate that the diet is increasing your bad LDL cholesterol, I'd say the increased risk of heart disease and stroke far outweigh the benefit of whatever weight loss you've experienced.

Monitoring your efforts with blood tests

When you make changes to your diet with the goal of reducing cholesterol, regular blood tests are an important measure of your success. You wouldn't diet to lose weight without getting on the scale at regular intervals, would you?

Keeping Fats in Check with Statin Drugs

As I mentioned earlier, deciding whether you should take statins is a complicated process involving a detailed knowledge of your risk factors and the levels of the different lipids in your blood. Some doctors may be very conservative, and others very eager, to use statins. These drugs have already saved thousands of lives in the short time they have been available. But there are serious side effects in some individuals. You don't want to take statins if you don't need to. I can't write down a simple formula for you to figure it out on your own because it isn't simple if done right. See your doctor. This may be one situation where you want a second opinion about a medical opinion. The opportunity is there to discuss your plan with more than one expert.

Despite your best efforts, diet and exercise can only do so much to lower your cholesterol. If, after three months, you aren't making headway toward reducing cholesterol, and your body mass index isn't coming down, then don't delay seeking medical treatment to reduce cholesterol.

The skinny on statins

Drugs called *statins* can reduce your chances of having a white stroke. More than 26 clinical trials have tested the effect of different statin drugs. When taken together, all these trials estimate that statins could reduce your risk of stroke by 20 percent. If you've had a stroke, the reduction would probably be greater. There is also some indication, but no scientific proof, that statins may reduce the number of fatal strokes by approximately 9 percent.

These is also good clinical trial evidence that statins actually lead to a reduction in the thickness of some atherosclerotic plaques — these drugs seem to partially reverse atherosclerosis — pretty amazing. Here are some common statin drugs:

Commercial Name	*Generic Name*
Lipitor	Atorvastatin
Zocor	Simvastatin
Pravachol	Pravastatin
Lescol	Fluvastatin
Mevacor	Lovastatin

How statins work

Statins stop your liver from making cholesterol. They don't stop you from *eating* cholesterol, though. Diet and taking statins have to work together to some extent. Don't assume you can go back to bacon and eggs for breakfast the day you take your first pill. Continue to avoid trans and saturated fats while taking a statin drug.

In addition to lowering LDL cholesterol, evidence supports that statins may reduce inflammation that causes atherosclerosis, though this is still under study. It also appears that statins may reduce C-reactive protein levels in the blood of some people with serious heart disease and stroke. C-reactive protein is a marker of blood-vessel inflammation, and high levels in the blood predict heart attacks and stroke.

Statins, as with any major drug, stimulate a bit of controversy. Although we don't really know about their long-term effects yet, the benefits seen in the trials are pretty hard to dispute.

Side effects of statins

Nausea, diarrhea, constipation, and muscle ache are some of the more common side effects of statin drugs. There are two serious side effects, however.

Liver damage

This is usually seen by an elevation of substances in the blood that indicate liver injury. See why it's important to get your blood tested regularly? Six to twelve weeks after you start the drug and then every four to six months is recommended by some. A mild increase in these substances does not necessarily mean you have to stop taking the drug. Yet. It does mean you may have to lower the dose and check your blood more every couple of weeks for a while. If a serious liver problem does develop, or the liver tests remain elevated, stopping the statins usually reverses the problem.

If you are going to take statins, then you need to follow your doctor's instructions and get blood tests done when recommended. Otherwise, warning of serious side effects may be missed.

Other drugs that reduce cholesterol can make liver problems worse. One of these drugs is gemfibrozil (Lopid). In high doses, the B vitamin niacin does a pretty good job of lowering cholesterol, but beware adding it to statins. I haven't read anything to indicate that consuming daily or B-complex vitamins cause this effect.

Muscle injury

This is less usual than liver damage. It is common for statins to cause a vague muscle pain. However, if the pain gets worse and the muscles become tender, the muscle cells can start to die. This places a lot of breakdown products from the dying muscle into the bloodstream that in turn starts a potentially deadly problem, leading to kidney failure and death. The problem is worsened by the following drugs: gemfibrozil (Lopid), erythromycin, drugs to kill fungus infections, and nefazodone (Serzone), an antidepressant.

Do's and don'ts for taking statins

Here's a handy list of things to keep in mind about statins:

- ✔ **Eliminate grapefruit juice from your diet:** Grapefruit juice, and *only* grapefruit juice, has an unexplained effect on the metabolism of several drugs, statins included. Don't drink it: Grapefruit juice will cancel the effect of the drug.

- ✔ **Take statin drugs at night:** Your liver makes cholesterol at night. For maximum effect, take statin drugs late in the day.

- ✔ **Get your blood tested regularly:** You need to monitor the results of the statin drugs. Check blood lipids, liver function, and, if needed, muscle-breakdown products.

✔ **Avoid certain medications:** If you're on statins, you should not be taking certain medications, including drugs that kill fungal infections, the antibiotic erythromycin, gemfibrazol (Lopid), the antidepressant Serzone, or high doses of the B vitamin niacin.

✔ **Be alert to certain side effects:** If you notice unusual muscle aches and pains, report these to your physician at once.

Statins beat out most cholesterol-lowering drugs

There are other drugs used for lowering LDL and raising HDL. High doses of the B vitamin niacin, for example, can do a remarkable job of lowering cholesterol levels in your blood. Like statins, niacin can put stress on your liver. But statins have proven to be the most effective means of keeping cholesterol in check, and, thus, are most often recommended by physicians.

Among the many risk factors that predict stroke, high cholesterol levels in the blood is one of the easiest to address. If you've determined through blood tests that your lipid levels are not optimal, your course of action is fairly clear and easy to follow. By changing your diet to reduce the intake of high-cholesterol as well as saturated and trans fats and/or taking statin drugs, chances are your subsequent blood tests will show some improvement. And you can feel pleased that you've taken steps to reduce the risk of atherosclerosis and subsequent stroke in the future.

Chapter 10

Other Risk Factors and Prevention

*P*reventing stroke is working. Since 1972, your chances of dying from stroke have declined by 50 percent. A lot of people have seen the opportunities that come from making an effort to prevent stroke. The result has been longer and healthier lives. Since 1970, the treatment of heart disease and stroke has added an average of 6 years to the length of an average American's life. This chapter isn't an invitation to be a rugged lonely individualist. This chapter is an invitation to join a growing majority of people who are seeing the opportunities available to them.

There is a reason there are blood pressure machines in almost every pharmacy in the U.S. They weren't there in 1970. There is a reason McDonald's has made significant efforts to reduce the fat in the food it serves. There is a reason fewer people are smoking than ever before. The reason is that people realize that the benefits from taking advantage of the opportunities listed here are real and worthwhile.

I believe I'm doing better at protecting my health because, by writing this book, I am reminding myself every day that I don't want to end up with dementia or become otherwise disabled by something I could have prevented. I made it to 50. Maybe I can live into my 90s and still remember my kids' names. The possibility that I might *not* make it motivates me to do everything I can to ensure the health of my brain for the next 40-plus years.

In the previous two chapters, I covered two major stroke risks: high blood pressure and high cholesterol. I devoted entire chapters to these topics because treating them effectively — or better yet, preventing them — is so critical to preventing stroke. The risk factors discussed in this chapter are of no less concern, however. I offer advice on treating these conditions or avoiding them altogether, steps that will help you reduce your risk of stroke or suffering from further strokes.

This chapter concludes with a worksheet and action plan designed to help you launch a journey on the road to a stroke-free future. Are you reading this book because someone you love has had a stroke? The advice here is just as valuable to you. And it's pertinent whether you're 60 . . . or 30.

Prevention is the focus of this chapter. Prevention is something our healthcare system does not invest much in. Our society's approach to our health is to wait until something bad happens — and then act. This is a poor way to deal with stroke and heart disease because by the time something bad happens, damage to your blood vessels — and brain — has already occurred. Therefore, I charge you with taking an active role in taking care of yourself. No one else is going to do it. The opportunities are there, but they are not going to force themselves into your life.

Reviewing the Major Risks

Many of the risks for stroke are linked together — one condition aggravates or causes another, like dominoes in your vascular system. High blood pressure puts more wear and tear on blood vessels and seems to worsen atherosclerosis, probably because the plaque formation has something to do with the healing process that occurs when the lining of an artery is injured. Atherosclerosis is further aggravated by diabetes. High blood glucose levels seem to lead to injuries in the blood vessels. Diabetes also injures the heart muscles, resulting in more sources of clots to break loose and injure the brain.

Accepting what you can't change

Some risks factors you can't control. Factors such as family history, age, sex, and race — and whether you've had a previous stroke — are situations you simply must accept. Your family history, for example. Because of genetics, lightning does strike twice in the same family. You can't change the fact that your parents, grandparents, aunts, and uncles all have or had high cholesterol and that you're likely to be predisposed to the same, but you *can* take steps to watch your diet and treat your condition with medication.

- ✔ **Family history:** A family history of stroke increases the likelihood of stroke for an individual. The fact that many of the risk factors for stroke — hypertension and atherosclerosis, for example — are also hereditary makes family history an increased concern.

- ✔ **Age:** Your risk of stroke increases with age. At least 70 percent of strokes occur in people age 65 and older.

✔ **Gender:** Men are more likely to suffer from stroke than women. But women may increase their likelihood if they smoke and take estrogen or birth control pills. More women die from stroke than men, but this is partially related to the longer life span of women and the fact that they are older (and more likely to die) when they have their first stroke.

✔ **Race:** African Americans and Latino Americans have strokes at double the rate (or more) of whites of the same age and sex. This difference is not entirely explained by higher incidence of high blood pressure and diabetes. There is good evidence that the other risk factors are the same. This means that blacks and Hispanics have even more to gain from the effort to prevent stroke.

✔ **Previous stroke:** If you've had one stroke, your chances of experiencing another (about 5 percent per year — the first year may be higher) are about ten times higher than if you've never had a stroke (about 0.5% per year, depending on your age).

Zeroing in on what you can change

Other risks *are* treatable or preventable. Here's a quick overview of these factors before I examine them more closely and explore how to *eliminate, reduce,* or *treat* them.

✔ **Hypertension:** High blood pressure, the most important factor determining the likelihood that you will have a stroke, is examined in detail in Chapter 8.

✔ **High blood lipids and cholesterol:** This issue is so complicated, I've devoted an entire chapter (Chapter 9) to blood fat and cholesterol and how to combat its devastating effect on the blood vessels.

✔ **Heart and vascular disease:** The numbers tell the story. Studies support that individuals who have heart disease are twice as likely to suffer a stroke as those who don't. The conditions vary and can often be controlled through medication, as well as diet and lifestyle changes.

✔ **Smoking tobacco:** Smoking cigarettes increases your chances of stroke by a factor of four. Plus it increases your chances of heart attack and emphysema as well. This condition, however, has one of the most effective, if not most difficult, treatments: Simply stop doing it! Stopping smoking for a year returns you to the same stroke risk as a nonsmoker your own age.

✔ **Diabetes:** Unfortunately, diabetes can't be eliminated, but it can be controlled with medication. The accompanying conditions of high blood pressure and obesity can also be controlled in order to reduce risk.

✔ **Obesity:** Individuals who are obese are more likely to have hypertension, diabetes, high cholesterol, and heart disease. Control is achieved through diet and exercise.

✔ **Oral contraceptives and estrogen replacement:** Both these common drugs increase the tendency of blood to clot. Hence, the increased risk of white strokes caused by blood clots. Doctors were surprised when they learned that birth-control pills, especially when combined with cigarette smoking, also increased a woman's chance of red stroke from rupture of a subarachnoid hemorrhage.

✔ **Drug and alcohol abuse:** Heavy drinking increases your risk of heart disease and stroke. Light and moderate drinking are associated with a decreased rate of both stroke and heart disease. These facts have been known for years, but it hasn't been confirmed by a clinical trial that *adding* light or moderate drinking to a nondrinker's life will decrease stroke risk. Experts haven't really figured this one out. What's clear is that if you are already having a glass of wine with your dinner every night, there is no apparent reason to stop.

Tobacco and Stroke

How bad for you is smoking tobacco? Here's what the Surgeon General says: *Smoking is the biggest preventable cause of death in the United States.* In the U.S., roughly 440,000 people die each year from smoking-related illnesses. Treating the effects of smoking puts a chokehold on our nation's health costs — we're talking in the range of $70 billion per year. And yet each day nearly 4,000 young people under the age of 18 light up for the first time, according to some estimates.

Smoke and blood

Remember the old song, "Smoke gets in your eyes"? A sad little ballad. But what's even sadder is when smoke gets in your blood. In Chapter 1, I spelled out how smoking can lead to stroke: that thousands of damaging chemicals — including nicotine and carbon monoxide — travel from your lungs to your bloodstream and then do their damage throughout your system. These substances cause blood vessels to constrict (there goes your blood pressure!), reduce oxygen (forcing the heart to work harder), scrape the inside of the blood vessels (forming plaques), and make blood "stickier" (leading to more vessel damage and paving the way for atherosclerosis and clots).

Many large studies have compared smokers and nonsmokers. Those who smoke consistently have more strokes and die more often from them, consistently have more white strokes and red strokes caused by subarachnoid hemorrhage, and consistently have strokes when they are younger. One study of more than 300,000 people showed that those who smoked were more than twice as likely to have a stroke.

And what about all the small strokes no one notices or does anything about? Vascular dementia is increased in smokers (read more about this in Chapter 7). And who knows how bad the impact of smoking really is — it's likely that many smokers have brain injury that wasn't severe enough to be noticed or reported to the doctor.

And here's an alert to those who live with a smoker: You might as well consider yourself a light smoker. Your risk of having a stroke is about 30 percent more than a nonsmoker who doesn't inhale someone else's smoke.

Treatment plan: Quit today!

The plan of action to reduce stroke risk caused by smoking is: Stop! There are programs to help you stop smoking. There are approved drugs to help you get over your dependence on nicotine. If you smoke, then chances are very good that you've tried to stop. The pain of stopping is immediate and the benefits seem a little vague when you are in withdrawal. You need to find what is motivating you to smoke and tackle that.

They say most people start because of social pressure and advertising. Well, it might work the other way, too. Does pressure from other people motivate you? Do your children lose respect for you? Does smoking make it more difficult to get along with your spouse? Do you want to find out whether your kids ever do have any children of their own? Do you want white teeth? Do you have enough wrinkles? Are you more afraid of lung cancer than having a stroke? Or are you more practical? Do you want to be sure you don't burn the house down? Are you tired of always coughing and your kids always having runny noses and coughs? Do you want to save money?

There are quite a few approaches to stopping smoking, including structured programs that offer various tools for quitting, including medication, psychological support, group support, and behavior-modification techniques. Some can be expensive — but isn't your *life* worth it? The following are a number of strategies and tactics for your stop-smoking campaign. Use one, a few, or many — whatever it takes.

- **Drugs:** Some drugs help reduce the craving for tobacco. The drug that seems to double the success rate for smoking cessation is called Bupropion, also known as Zyban or Wellbutron. It is also used as an antidepressant. When combined with nicotine patches, it does a little better. There are significant relapse rates, but some people who have not been able to quit in any other way have succeeded with these prescription drugs. Because of the tendency toward depression after stroke, an antidepressant isn't a bad idea. If you have had seizures, then your doctor may not prescribe antidepressants, as Bupropion and other antidepressants increase the risk of seizures.

✔ **Patches and nicotine gum:** Nicotine patches and gum help you meet your craving for nicotine without all the associated habits of smoking. Just the habit of lighting up after a meal or during stressful times can be hard to break. Without the additional stress of nicotine craving, you may be more successful at getting yourself out of the behavioral rut you are in.

✔ **Behavior modification:** Whereas some attack their smoking habit by quitting cold-turkey, others sneak up on a smoke-free life one cigarette at a time by gradually reducing their consumption of cigarettes. One variation of the gradual slow-down is the increasing difficulty approach. You smoke fewer, but you concentrate on not buying cigarettes, delaying smoking by five minutes, then ten minutes, then longer and longer. The craving diminishes as you learn to control it for longer times. Other tactics in behavior modification include prohibiting yourself to smoke in certain places — your house, for example — or at certain times, such as after dinner.

✔ **Substitution:** You may succeed by using gum, toothpicks, and activities that use your hands. Then, of course, there is eating — not a good use of substitution. Eating instead of smoking is something that doctors hear a lot about. You can choose to eat or smoke — you can also choose to go walking and do neither.

✔ **Social-engineering approach:** Avoid others who smoke and the places where smokers congregate. This is getting easier and easier as cities, states, and nations put more limitations on smoking in public. Telling others you are stopping will also help you keep your commitment. Others may help you by not offering you cigarettes or by giving you suggestions about how to stop. You can really use the community approach by joining a group of people interested in not smoking.

✔ **Visualization:** It works for some. Imagining black ugly lungs, piles of cigarette butts, and wrinkled faces motivates the young and beautiful.

The good news for smokers

Tricked you! There is no good news about smoking cigarettes. But there *is* good news for smokers committed to quitting. Good evidence supports that stopping smoking will reduce your risk of stroke, even if you have been smoking for decades or have had one or more strokes. The benefits of breathing better, not coughing as much, and not getting as many infections are always immediate and increase your health and well-being.

I haven't ever smoked or stopped smoking myself, so it's not easy for me to understand the challenge for smokers. I do remember a lecture by a heart surgeon who stopped smoking years before. He said the desire to smoke never went away. Years after he had stopped, he once got off the elevator on the wrong floor and followed someone down the hall who was smoking a Camel cigarette. "It just smelled so good," he said.

Quitting cigarettes is hard. Some say it is the hardest thing they've ever dealt with. Most people have to try more than once before they succeed.

Of course, everyone stops smoking eventually.

Every cigarette you don't smoke is an improvement in your health. High blood pressure, diabetes, atherosclerosis, and your age are intrinsic parts of you that you may have been born with. You found cigarettes and brought them into your life. You can send them away. It isn't easy, but your lungs, your heart, and your brain will thank you. Good luck — I hope you succeed.

Heart and Vascular Disease

If you have had heart disease, you are more likely to have a stroke in the future. If you have had a stroke, you are more likely to have a heart attack in the future. Once again, we see how interrelated the heart and the brain are to each other. The reasons and level of risk vary based on the type of heart disease. Several heart diseases are connected to stroke because heart disease produces conditions that increase blood clotting, which results in stroke. Treatment almost always includes some medication to slow blood clotting.

Atrial fibrillation

This is a condition in which the contractions of the upper chambers of the heart (the *atria*) are irregular and result in inefficient pumping of blood. This leads to pooling of the blood in the heart chambers and elsewhere, which results in blood clots that can cause severe white (ischemic) strokes.

If you have atrial fibrillation, you should be treated for it. Aspirin or warfarin are the standard treatments, with warfarin usually preferred. The risk of stroke from atrial fibrillation adds up at about 5 percent per year. You can't let this go on very long before you are more likely to have a stroke than you are to win a coin toss.

Heart attack

If you have a stroke and you have had a heart attack in the past, then it is a good idea to look at the heart to see if it contains any blood clots that might break loose and cause further strokes. This can usually be done with ultrasound imaging. No invasive procedures are needed in most cases.

Having a stroke means you might also have a heart attack. A cardiologist (heart specialist) or other doctor can look for conditions you should treat to prevent a heart attack. For example, a stress test might show that one of the arteries to your heart is almost completely blocked. This might be treated with a stent to hold the artery open. Drugs that prevent stroke by slowing down clotting and reducing cholesterol in the blood also help prevent heart attacks.

Heart valve disease

If you have a mechanical (artificial) valve, your risk for stroke is significantly increased. If you do have a stroke, it is critical to communicate and coordinate your care between your heart specialist (cardiologist) and your stroke specialist. First, because you are undoubtedly on an anticlotting medication — possibly warfarin. But it may be at a different dosage than required for your stroke condition. Your clotting control will have to be reevaluated after the stroke, and your medication may need adjustment. Additionally, the valve itself must be checked.

Treating slow blood clotting

In terms of our concern about heart disease and the link to stroke, our main course of action is to treat for the prevention of the clotting caused by the condition. And I've already discussed that treatment in several chapters — the prescription of two types of blood-thinning drugs: antiplatelets and anticoagulants. Aspirin and drugs like aspirin thin blood by deactivating blood cells called *platelets* that stick together and plug leaks in blood vessels. Warfarin is a common drug often prescribed; its commercial name is Coumadin. Warfarin stops clotting by depleting your body of a key ingredient needed to make the glue that sticks a clot together.

In most types of heart disease and after white stroke, transient or permanent, aspirin or a drug like aspirin is the best choice for preventing blood clot formation. For atrial fibrillation and artificial heart valves, warfarin may be the best alternative.

Aspirin

Aspirin is the most commonly used drug to prolong the time it takes for a clot to form. Many physicians prescribe one 325 milligram full-size aspirin per day to prevent stroke. Others swear by the 81 milligram small-size aspirin.

If a patient can't tolerate the irritation to the stomach that aspirin often causes, the doctor may prescribe another antiplatelet drug. One of these drugs is clopidogrel (trade name is Plavix). Another is a combination of a low-dose aspirin and a drug called dypiramidole (Aggrenox). Trials have shown both of these drugs beating aspirin.

Warfarin

An aspirin every day is really simple and easy and works in most situations. Warfarin has been proven better than aspirin when it comes to preventing blood clots that form in the heart — for patients with atrial fibrillation or heart valves, for instance. Warfarin, also known as Coumadin, prevents clots by depriving the body of vitamin K, a substance in green leafy vegetables that helps blood clot. When prescribing warfarin instead of aspirin, your physician will take into consideration the risk factors you have for stroke and your age. If you have had a prior heart attack, high blood pressure, diabetes, or are age 75 or more, then you have more to gain from taking warfarin.

But warfarin does carry risk. Taking warfarin is a major undertaking. Done right, it can save your life. Done wrong, it can result in a major — possibly fatal — red stroke brain hemorrhage. Careful monitoring of the use of warfarin is critical to its success in reducing risk of white stroke.

Blood clotting

Two much clotting leads to heart attack, stroke, and the lung clot called a *pulmonary embolism*. All of these can kill you. But too *little* clotting can result in bleeding in the stomach or intestines, in the eye, or around your just-brushed teeth. If your blood is too thin and doesn't clot well, you could be at high risk for brain bleeding — red stroke.

Taking any blood-thinner can lead to easy bruising or bleeding gums. But taking too much warfarin can cause widespread severe bleeding. It is critical to monitor the dosage of warfarin carefully in order not to shift the balance from preventing the risk of white stroke to increasing the risk of red stroke.

The blood test that measures the time it takes for your blood to clot is called the *prothrombin time* or *protime* (PT). PT is the key to fitting your dose of warfarin to your needs. The results of the PT test are given as a ratio, which can be thought of as the relative time it takes the blood to clot. The technical term for the ratio is the International Normalized Ratio (INR). If the INR is three, then it takes, roughly, three times as long as normal for your blood to clot. If the INR is 1.5, then bleeding from a cut that normally would stop on its own in five minutes would take 7 or 8 minutes to stop.

Your doctor will set a target for your INR and adjust your dose of warfarin to reach and stay at that target amount. Reaching target is difficult because there is so much variation from person to person. Also, it takes two or three days for the dose of warfarin to take full effect. This means the INR from a blood test reflects the response to the warfarin you took two or three days ago. Fortunately, you don't have to worry too much about this. Your doctor has a lot of experience figuring out the best dose. You need to be patient because it can take a week or two.

What you can do to help warfarin do its job

You should be proactive in supporting a positive treatment experience. Here are some steps you can take to help your doctor achieve the optimal prescription for you:

- ✔ Take your medicine the same time every day and eat similar meals to the extent possible. The best time to take warfarin is before dinner.

- ✔ Consider how often and how consistently you eat leafy green vegetables. They are good for you, but they provide a lot of vitamin K, which counteracts the effect of warfarin. Eating a lot of leafy greens one day, then none for the next few days can make it hard to get consistent INR readings.

- ✔ Adhere to your dosage instructions. The usual dose of warfarin is between 2 and 5 milligrams once per day. Making a commitment to taking the drug requires diligence on your part. If you forget to take your meds or the right dosage, then warfarin is not for you. Better to take aspirin, which doesn't need to be monitored so carefully.

- ✔ Watch for signs of bleeding (check your gums after brushing your teeth) and bruising.

- ✔ Be sure to make your appointments for checking the PT time to keep your blood from getting "too thin." If you need a dosage adjustment, better to make it sooner rather than later.

Heart failure

When any disease involving the heart becomes so severe that the organ can't do its job, the result is heart failure. There are several causes of heart failure. One of the most common is a heart attack, which injures the heart and leaves it too weak to keep up with all the work it needs to do. Every time a healthy heart beats, it squeezes out about 55 percent of the blood in the largest chamber of the heart (the left ventricle). If you have heart failure, your heart only manages to get out 40 percent or less. When this happens, fluid can build up around the ankles and in the lungs, making it more difficult for you to walk and breathe. Other symptoms you might have are coughing, waking up at night short of breath, and chronic fatigue.

Causes of heart failure include atrial fibrillation, pneumonia and other infections, heart attack, anemia (low red blood cell count), heavy alcohol consumption that injures heart muscle, and poorly treated or untreated high blood pressure.

Heart failure is thought to promote clotting inside the heart and stroke similar to the way atrial fibrillation causes clotting and stroke. A lot of patients with heart failure have atrial fibrillation. Those who do should be on warfarin, usually. Other heart failure patients should be on aspirin or warfarin.

Heart failure leads to increased clotting and an increased risk for stroke. That risk increases depending on the level of heart failure. Every year about 2 percent of the hundreds of thousands of mild heart failure patients have a stroke. The percentage rises to 4 percent with severe heart failure.

Controlling Diabetes

In a nutshell, diabetes is a condition in which the body does not produce or use insulin properly. Diabetes can lead to cataracts in your eyes, decreased vision because of injuries to the retina, kidney disease, and nerve damage. And stroke.

Insulin reduces the amount of the sugar called *glucose* in your blood. Too much insulin, and your blood glucose drops so low that your brain stops working and you can lose consciousness and die. Too little insulin and your blood can be so filled with glucose that it injures cells. In diabetes, either your pancreas stops making enough insulin or your body stops responding to insulin. The result is the high levels of the glucose in your blood that are the hallmark of diabetes.

What does diabetes have to do with stroke? Diabetes makes blood vessels more prone to injury. It is as if diabetic arteries do not endure the wear and tear of life as well as nondiabetic arteries. The effects of major risk factors for stroke — atherosclerosis and high blood pressure — are increased in diabetics. See the domino effect here? A case of multiple-risk factors conspiring to set you on the path to stroke.

The doctors who treat diabetes have a large number of tools in their medical bags to find the perfect combination of treatments that work for you. Work closely with your doctor. The more you know about the different drugs and the principles of management, the better the two of you will be able to work to keep your blood glucose under control.

As with many drugs, antidiabetics cause interactions with other drugs. Simply changing doses may resolve any problems, but it's critical to communicate any and all prescriptions to the physician treating your diabetes. These drugs include aspirin, acetaminophen, ibuprofen, sulfa drugs, some antibiotics, warfarin and its cousins, a drug called probenecid given for gout, and beta blockers used to treat blood pressure and many other conditions. And then there are the vitamins and herbal supplements that you prescribe for yourself. Put these on your list of medications as well.

Diabetes increases your risk of stroke. The closer you keep your blood glucose to normal levels, the healthier your arteries will be. The more tightly you control your blood glucose, the more careful you will have to be in managing your diabetes. You will have to convince your doctor that you can pay attention and follow instructions precisely.

And don't get so focused on your diabetes that you forget other important risk factors. When you have diabetes, you have a lot to gain in terms of stroke prevention by treating high blood pressure and stopping smoking and getting your blood lipids in good shape. Diabetes makes virtually all other risk factors for stroke worse. Cerebrovascular dementia, in particular, is worse with diabetes and high blood pressure combined.

Fighting Obesity with Diet and Exercise

America is in the middle of a national obesity epidemic that is threatening recent progress in combating high blood pressure and atherosclerosis. And these lead to more heart attacks and strokes as we age.

The principle of weight gain

I can tell you the one basic principle that explains all the extra fat tissue you have on board. Here it is:

The amount of weight you gain is equal to the difference between the amount of energy you *consume* and the amount of energy you *expend*.

You lose weight by a combination of two strategies: First, you *exercise more* to build muscle mass and burn energy from fat reserves. The greater muscle mass is always burning glucose, even when you are resting. Just like your brain. Second, you *consume less energy.* Energy is measured in calories. Calories come from food. Need I say more?

Changing your eating habits

If you are overweight, it's likely an effort that took years to achieve. You have developed eating habits that help you sustain — and perhaps continue to add to — your extra pounds. I don't have to tell you about the miracle diets that pack the shelves in your local bookstore. There are all kinds of quick-fix cures that promise the pounds will melt away like ice cream in the Sahara. I'm not going to endorse, promote, or give space to one particular diet over another in this book.

I *am* going to urge those of you who need and want to lose weight to consider it a long-term commitment. Research the topic, give it some soul-searching, evaluate your lifestyle values, explore various eating plans, talk to your doctor or a nutritionist — and find an eating plan that you feel you can stick with and incorporate into your life. Eating is a lifelong activity. And *how* you eat is a habit you can change to promote healthy weight.

I mention diets in Chapter 9. Let me reiterate the importance of monitoring critical numbers when you are changing your diet. You don't want to lose weight at the cost of high cholesterol in your blood, smoking cigarettes, and raising your blood pressure with diet pills and loads of salt. Measure your weight, check your blood pressure frequently, and work with your doctor to get the cholesterol in your blood tested.

Seeing through the advertising hype

Let me offer this advice, too: *Turn off the TV and take a walk!* In a culture like America's, the average person confronts *immense* forces when he or she decides to eat less. Billions of dollars are spent to sell you food. These advertisers are smart. They don't just sell food — they sell love. They offer convenience, warm family gatherings, popularity, cost-savings, even health, beauty, and romance through food. Who wouldn't be persuaded to drive to the nearest chain restaurant after viewing happy, fit, attractive people downing huge quantities of fat-soaked food — at a special price? Obesity is sold every day by a huge gamut of corporations who want you to buy their products.

That isn't to say you and I aren't part of the problem. It's a lot easier to sell us fat, sugar, and salt than carrots, lettuce, and pinto beans. Campaigns to get folks to stop smoking have been relatively successful. Campaigns to reduce obesity are beginning to launch right now. We need them. But until they reach the same saturation as the restaurant and junk food advertisers, you'll have to rely on your own discriminating skills to control the advertisers' power over your purchases and eating habits.

Exercising as a life-long habit

The other strategy for weight loss is to expend more energy. In a word, exercise. Ugh! I walk to work about twice a year, but I probably think about it every day . . . at least at this one extra long stoplight. Treadmills and elliptical exercise machines? Extremely boring for me. I have been able to get some situated so I could watch a movie on a DVD player. That makes it easier.

You can probably tell that I am not one of those people who practically live in workout attire. My point in sharing my personal exercise aversions is that for most of us, exercise *is* an effort. Our jobs and lives don't require much physical exertion, so we have to incorporate such activity into our routines. And for many of us, it's not something we look forward to.

My advice, as it was for eating less, is to explore exercise seriously. Read up, talk to your doctor, meet with a personal trainer. Consider the spectrum of physical activities — from pilates to power-walking, from handball to horseback riding — and find something you can incorporate into your routine as a life-long habit. Something you can enjoy.

Exercise doesn't have to be complicated — you don't have to buy expensive machinery, join a pricey fitness center, or take classes to learn a new sport. Your route to weight loss can be as simple as walking for 45 minutes a day in your neighborhood. The great benefit of walking is that you can take it anywhere. If you're traveling, you don't have to worry about packing extra equipment. If it's raining, you can find a mall to walk in. And it's as easy to do alone as it is in the company of a friend.

Making a Plan for Reducing Stroke Risk

Now that I've reviewed the various risks that may result in stroke, I want to pull everything together into a manageable action plan. I suggest a two-part strategy for tackling the situation. First, take steps to address medical problems that offer the greatest threat — with the result that the treatment offers the greatest benefit:

- Stop smoking.
- Get treatment for high blood pressure.
- Take medication for slowing blood clotting.
- Control your blood cholesterol.

The second part is to act *before* things get bad. If you wait to treat your blood pressure until you have a heart attack or a stroke, that's too late. Blood-pressure tests and cholesterol screenings are routine parts of exams. Even if you are a young adult reading this book out of concern for a parent or grandparent who has suffered a stroke, you are getting information about your blood pressure and blood lipid levels that you could put to good use *now*.

At your last check-up, you may have learned that your blood pressure or your cholesterol levels were on the high side of normal. Your doctor may have said something like, "Well, it's a little high, but we don't need to consider medication at this point. Just watch out for it."

I say this *is* the time to take action! You are already very late in starting to prevent heart attack and stroke if you hear things like the remark in the preceding paragraph. You don't have to let your arteries harden until you have blood pressure so high it requires medication. Today you eat pizza, chocolate shakes, and French fries; tomorrow you take blood-pressure pills and spend hours in doctor's offices. Work with your doctor *now* to learn everything you can to prevent high blood pressure, atherosclerosis, diabetes, and other risk factors from ever getting out of control. It's possible. This is an opportunity for you to do something now that is guaranteed to pay off for you in the future.

Collecting the evidence

It's a great idea to establish a relationship with a physician that allows you to work together to anticipate health problems and start treating them early. If you've already had a stroke, you may already have a file drawer full of medical information. Certain data is important — whether or not you've had a stroke — in order for you to effectively monitor your condition.

- **Blood-pressure tracking:** Know your blood pressure and keep track of your readings. You don't have to visit the doctor every day to keep tabs on this critical bit of information. This detective work can be done at a free machine in a drug store. Or buy your own machine. Best things about getting your own machine: portable, private, easy to use, and available for daily use in a convenient place.

  Blood pressure is usually measured once a day, yet you live with it 24 hours a day. It is usually higher in the morning and lowest during sleep. Your blood pressure may not go down as much at night as it should. It may be wise to track it several times a day for a period of time — your own machine makes this affordable and practical.

- **EKG reading:** EKG stands for *electrocardiogram*. This test indicates irregular heart rhythm or heart disease. It also tells whether you have had a (silent) heart attack or if your heart is enlarged due to a failing heart.

- **Cholesterol level:** This one requires drawing a bit of blood. A *lipid panel* will tell you about the different types of cholesterol, and whether yours is normal or high. A lot of emphasis is placed on LDL and HDL cholesterol, the bad and the good, respectively. Let your doctor tell you the best levels for you — right now the recommendations vary considerably depending on your medical condition. Be sure you know the numbers and have agreed on a target level to reach with your doctor.

- **Diabetes testing:** A blood sugar test screens for early diabetes. Don't forget to stop eating 12 hours before the morning of the test. This usually means nothing after dinner the night before and only water in the morning — without water, you may be dehydrated the morning of your test. Get instructions from your doctor about which of your morning pills you should take. This is especially important if you are diabetic.

- **Other tests:** You may also want to get tests of liver and thyroid function and indicators of muscle injury to determine possible drug side effects.

- **Ultrasound for atherosclerosis:** Atherosclerosis of the carotid artery is an important risk for stroke. The ultrasound tests pose little risk of injury. You'll learn whether one or both of the carotid arteries are blocked with plaque and find out more about your heart. An arteriogram might give more complete information, but that involves punching holes in you, which increases risk of stroke and of injury to your blood vessels.

If you have a carotid or transcranial ultrasound test, be sure someone else outside the laboratory evaluates the results. Some labs are pretty much referral centers for a particular surgeon or group of surgeons. This is somewhat like taking your car to the dealer to change the oil and being told you need $500 in repairs. Get a second opinion before you go ahead with any procedures to fix your arteries.

✔ **Chest X-ray:** This test can give more evidence about your heart.

✔ **CT or MRI scan:** If you've already had a CT or MRI scan of your brain, then collect the reports so that you have a record of your brain's condition.

Stroke prevention checklist

Now that you've gathered the important information about your health, the next step is to consolidate it in a way that allows you easy access. Doing this can help you better monitor your condition and work to prevent future stroke. A fairly comprehensive checklist is in the next section. I have put it in a format that allows you to use the form in this book (if you have a really sharp pencil). Or you can photocopy it and mark on the copy for practice. The following checklist is the foundation of your "prevention file," something to which you will attach a lot of papers that will monitor your efforts. Take it with you to check-ups to keep track of progress in your stroke prevention status.

Setting your prevention goals

Your stroke prevention checklist may be a work in progress, but it will help launch your prevention plan immediately. Add a conversation with your physician to identify what further information is needed and to determine what the evidence is telling you so far — and you're ready to begin. Here are some tips for mapping out a successful plan:

✔ **Write it down:** Complex form or a simple list. The point is to commit your goals to paper, whether it's a single item or lengthier.

✔ **Establish a timeline:** If you list "Lose 30 pounds" as one of your goals, determine a deadline goal for achieving that goal. Be realistic.

✔ **Break it down into steps:** If you jot down "Stop smoking in six weeks" but stop there, chances are you'll still be stubbing out cigarettes two months from now. But if you break it down into manageable steps, it's easier. Your breakdown may include steps such as, "Week One: Get a patch," "Substitute a walk for a cig break at work immediately," "Week Two: Reduce per-day cigarette consumption by half," and so forth.

✔ **Keep your list close at hand:** Tape it to the refrigerator. Post it on your bulletin board. Reduce it, laminate it, and stick it in the driver's-license slot of your wallet. The point is to keep your goals in front of you.

Personal history	
Atrial fibrillation	Yes No Year:
Heart attack	Yes No Year:
Heart failure	Yes No Year:
Other heart disease	Yes No Year:
Family history (parents, grandparents, aunts, uncles, brothers, sisters)	Circle:
Heart attack	F M GF GM A U B S
High cholesterol	F M GF GM A U B S
Stroke	F M GF GM A U B S
Diabetes	F M GF GM A U B S
High blood pressure	F M GF GM A U B S
Your own blood tests	Record value and date
Cholesterol	
Total	
HDL	
LDL	
Complete blood count	
Hemoglobin	
Hematocrit	
Sedimentation rate	
White blood count	
Platelet count	
Electrolytes	
Sodium	
Potassium	
BUN	
Glucose (fasting)	
Chemistry panel	
Creatinine	
Liver function tests	
Thyroid function tests	
Prothrombin time	
Partial thromboplastin time	
C-reactive protein	
Homocysteine	
If diabetic	
Hemoglobin A1C	
C peptide	
Electrocardiogram	
Standard	Date
24 hour monitoring	Date
Blood pressure	
Last date measured.	
Most recent blood pressure	/
24 hour blood pressure monitoring	Date
Weight	
Weight in pounds	
Computed body mass index	
Abdominal girth	
Amount of exercise in minutes per day	
Alcohol consumption	
Number of drinks per week	
Tobacco consumption	
Number of cigarettes per day	
Carotid ultrasound	
Presence of stenosis	Yes No Date:
Percentage occlusion of carotid artery, if any.	
Carotid intimal plaque thickness, if available.	
Cardiac testing	Dates
Cardiac ultrasound	
Stress testing	
Brain imaging	Dates
CT scans	
MR scans	
Chest x-ray	Dates
Medications. Name of medication and name of prescribing doctor	Doses

Working toward a stroke-free future

Sometimes, for those at high risk for stroke, the prospects for a healthy future may seem bleak — especially when considering risks that you have no control over. If you've had a stroke, you can't rewrite history after all. Your family history, your age, your gender: These factors you can't change.

But here's the good news: Some of the most significant risk factors — high blood pressure, high cholesterol, and use of tobacco, among others — can be controlled through effective treatment or change in lifestyle. You *can* reduce your risk of stroke by taking proactive steps to prevent or treat the related risks. But it does take your active involvement and ongoing commitment.

Part IV
Treating Stroke

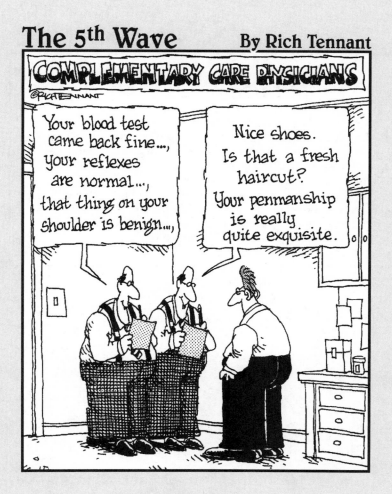

In this part . . .

Stroke is a major emergency, so the first thing to do is call 911 and get to the hospital emergency room. Once there, doctors will scramble to find out which type of stroke has occurred, because different strokes call for different treatments. This part is full of advice for the stroke victim and family members struggling with medical treatment options. I cover the different tests that are likely to be done, the drugs and surgeries available, and the rehabilitation process to help speed recovery.

Chapter 11

Get Thee to an Emergency Room

*R*apid recognition of what's happening and getting treatment as quickly as possible are the best chances you have for recovery from stroke. The problem is, sometimes it's not so easy to tell that you're having a stroke. For example, you could be having a stroke if suddenly

✔ Your arm begins to feel numb, and you have a hard time controlling your fingers.

✔ You can't understand what others are saying to you.

✔ You have difficulty recalling or saying words.

Even though you may not feel any pain, the situation is very serious, and permanent disability is a real possibility. Some treatments that are effective in reducing disability following a stroke aren't as effective unless they are given soon after the onset of stroke. One of the most effective treatments can't be started more than three hours after a stroke starts.

Once a stroke starts, part of your brain is dying. You have to get to a doctor as soon as possible to prevent or limit permanent damage. You are not the only one who has to rush. Doctors and nurses in the emergency room need to act quickly to be sure you get the best treatment.

The truth is that many people are frightened or confused by their stroke symptoms. Waiting to see if the paralysis goes away is a common response. Many patients don't make it to an emergency room for several hours. Some come the next day because they don't want to make a lot of fuss about what may be nothing.

Others defer action because they're worried about the expense of what may turn out to be an unnecessary hospital visit. Quite a few people take the time to call a family member or a physician's office first before calling an emergency number. All of these are natural reactions, but stroke symptoms are serious and warrant swifter action.

If you suspect that you or your loved one is having a stroke, *don't wait.* Get thee to the emergency room immediately!

In this chapter, I take you through the process of responding to the emergency of acute stroke — and stroke is *always* an emergency. I've broken the process down into logical steps, from recognizing stroke symptoms to being a proactive patient in the hospital and afterward.

At the end of the chapter, I present some practical pointers so you don't feel as helpless in the hospital system as you might otherwise feel. If your hospital and community are among the thousands that are prepared to treat stroke rapidly, so much the better — but you can do things that may be even more important.

Recognizing Stroke: Sudden Loss of Brain Power

The word *stroke* means a sudden or swift action — a golf stroke, a stroke of luck, the stroke of a pen. *Stroke,* the disease, is also sudden — and requires a swift response. When you have a stroke, you suffer a sudden loss of part of your brain function. You're normal one moment and suddenly very different only a minute or two later.

Usually there is no pain associated with a stroke. Now, that's not true 100 percent of the time. Sharp neck pain or very severe headache may be present with a few strokes. But specific symptoms indicate that something is suddenly and clearly amiss with the brain. The key concepts bound together by the word *stroke* are

✔ The suddenness of the onset, within minutes.

✔ The brain as the source of the problem.

✔ The emphasis on loss of brain function.

Symptoms that say "stroke"

The Brain Attack Coalition, a group of national organizations to treat stroke, has agreed on the following as the best description of the symptoms of stroke:

✔ Sudden numbness or weakness of face, arm, or leg, especially on one side of the body

✔ Sudden confusion or trouble speaking or understanding speech

✔ Sudden trouble seeing in one or both eyes

✔ Sudden trouble walking, with dizziness, or loss of balance or coordination

✔ Sudden severe headache with no known cause

Stroke is defined by a *loss* of brain function. Symptoms such as nervousness, trembling, and shaking are signs of *increased* brain activity — they are not present in stroke.

What if you are incapacitated?

Of course, there's often a catch-22 with regard to responding swiftly to stroke. If you are the victim, the very symptoms that signal the stroke may also prevent you from taking action. If you experience loss of feeling or paralysis or cannot speak or find yourself in a state of confusion, you may not be able to seek help. You may have to rely on family members, friends, or even strangers to call for emergency help.

If you've suffered from stroke previously or suspect you are a candidate for stroke, share important information about symptoms and discuss emergency action plans with those near to you. You may want to share this chapter — or the entire book, for that matter — with loved ones or friends.

What to do if someone is having a stroke

When someone is having a stroke, you will notice some peculiar behavior immediately: The mouth may droop on one side of the face, as if the face is slack on that side. This droop is often accompanied by slurred speech. Talking becomes a struggle — often the sufferer can only get out a word or two and then becomes mute.

If you only remember only one thing about stroke, make it this: Pay attention to language. No one symptom occurs in all strokes, but speech problems are among the most common telltale signs.

Bystanders may have to ask the person questions to get the full picture of what's happening: "Can you lift your arm? Can you make a fist? Do you know what day it is?" If someone has any problem at all with these tasks, then he or she may be suffering from stroke.

All strokes are not the same

A stroke usually does not affect the entire brain; typically, about 5 to 30 percent is affected. And different strokes can affect different areas. This means that one stroke doesn't always look like another, and different symptoms can appear in different combinations for each stroke. The brain is organized in such a way that different capabilities are located in separate places. For example, movement of the right arm is controlled from an area of the brain just beneath the skull above the left ear — likewise, the left arm is controlled from a similar spot above the right ear.

Because stroke affects any one of hundreds of blood vessels that supply blood with oxygen and glucose to all the different parts of the brain, the symptoms of a stroke can vary depending on which blood vessels are affected.

Consider 600 stroke patients whose stroke was caused by a blood clot blocking a brain artery. They were seen right after the onset of their stroke, and a systematic examination was done.

81 percent had difficulty speaking clearly.

68 percent lost feeling on one side.

65 percent had weakness of the face, arm, or leg on one side.

58 percent had decreased vision on one side.

58 percent had trouble paying attention to one side of their body.

52 percent had trouble using language.

52 percent had difficulty looking to the right or left.

31 percent were drowsy or lacked alertness.

7 percent had difficulty with balance.

There are two lessons from this list that I would like to emphasize: (1) Pay attention to language. (2) There is no symptom of stroke that occurs in all strokes.

The stroke victim may try to downplay the situation, assure concerned bystanders that he or she is not in pain, or try to persuade everyone to wait awhile before calling for help. In that situation, if you are the bystander, keep calm and collected, but don't delay. *Take charge and take action.* You are dealing with a person who has an injured brain. Call 911. It's the right thing to do even if it is embarrassing, expensive, or turns out to have been unnecessary.

Here are the responsibilities of the stroke bystander:

- Know the signs of stroke and recognize them quickly.
- Call 911 or a similar emergency system.
- Note and remember the exact time when the stroke started.
- Go to the emergency room with the stroke victim or get someone else to go who knows the patient and knows what happened. It's as helpful to ER personnel to be able to talk to someone who saw the stroke happen as it is to talk to a family member.

Timing is everything

Bystanders or family members can be critically important in determining the timing of the stroke. If you were not with the victim at the stroke's onset, remember when you first noticed the symptoms. If the person who had the stroke can't say when it started, try to find someone who can verify the last time that he or she was normal.

As with heart attacks, most strokes start in the morning or early afternoon. If a family member appears to have a stroke soon after waking up, the stroke may have occurred during sleep. It can make the difference between getting treated or not if you can show that someone was normal, if only for a few minutes, after waking up. For example, consider an individual who gets up and goes to the bathroom at 6 a.m., returns to bed, and is found paralyzed in the right leg at 7 a.m. If you know that the individual went to the bathroom, then you know that the earliest the stroke could have occurred was 6 a.m. If you don't know or don't remember that the patient was okay at 6 a.m., then you might think that the stroke started the night before — the last time that you saw the person being normal. For treating white stroke, to be safe, the doctor has to assume a stroke started that last time the patient was known to be normal.

If you are present when a person has a stroke, or soon after, look at a clock. To be given treatment in the emergency room, it may be necessary to know when the stroke started. Ask the individual what he was doing when the stroke started. "What show was on television? Did you wake up with the stroke? When was the last time you felt normal?" If he or she can't talk, ask for a nod yes or no. The individual may be more willing to answer questions from you than from unknown medical personnel.

Getting to the Hospital: The EMT Scoop and Run

Time flies when the brain is starving for glucose and oxygen (see Chapter 2). If the heart stops, the brain can't last more than five or ten minutes before extensive injury destroys most of its functions. That's why Cardio Pulmonary Rescue (CPR) mouth-to-mouth resuscitation and chest compression are performed when the heart stops.

With stroke, the heart is not affected and continues beating. Partial blood flow continues, and the brain can survive longer — but every minute still counts. That's why it's critical to call 911 immediately as soon as you suspect a stroke is occurring.

A typical stroke scenario

A 76-year-old woman calls 911 and says, "Something is wrong." As she continues to talk, the dispatcher can clearly hear the words she speaks, but they are disorganized and make little sense. He suspects stroke and dispatches an ambulance to the woman's home. On arrival, the EMTs find that her doors are locked. A supervisor approves breaking a window, and the woman is found on the floor of her living room by the telephone. The television is on.

She speaks to the EMTs, but her words don't make sense. She is bright and cheerful, but when asked if she can stand up, she shakes her head no. The EMTs notice that her right arm seems weak. When asked when the stroke started, she keeps repeating that she was watching a particular television show. "I thought . . . maybe strange . . . strike . . . stroke, yes, stroke, maybe stroke," she manages to say. Apparently she had crawled from her chair to the telephone to call 911. She is taken without delay to an emergency department.

She arrives 45 minutes after the onset of her stroke. Nearly 25 minutes later, after blood tests, evaluation by a team of stroke experts, and a CT scan of her brain that shows her stroke was probably caused by a blood clot, she is given the drug TPA, a drug used to dissolve the clot that caused the stroke. If her arrival at the emergency department had been delayed, she would not have had the opportunity of being treated with TPA.

Several hours later, she has improved somewhat, but still has difficulty understanding language and speaking. Four days later, she is discharged to a rehabilitation center, walking with a limp and still having difficulty with communication. (See Chapter 13 for more about rehabilitation.)

Some delay is inevitable in getting help for stroke. You may take a few minutes to recognize a stroke before taking action. The 911 call can take two to five minutes to report critical information, including symptoms and a call-back number. The arrival of Emergency Medical Technicians (EMTs) on the scene varies with distance. So, even in the best circumstances, the patient may not be in the care of medical personnel for 15 minutes or longer after the stroke is recognized.

With this time loss in mind, many EMTs employ a *scoop and run* approach toward stroke emergencies, with the goal of spending minimal time at the scene and getting crucial care as quickly as possible. In the ideal situation, the EMTs at the scene conduct a brief neurological examination (checking out the basics of how the brain and the nerves that control movement are working). They ask questions, take blood pressure, and count the pulse rate. They may start oxygen, measure serum glucose (sugar content of your blood), or perform a more detailed assessment of brain function. Then they get the patient on a stretcher and into an ambulance. Minimal time on the scene can be as little as 10 minutes, but 20 minutes is more realistic, even with the most efficient emergency medical system (EMS) people who are trained to respond to stroke.

Unnecessary time may be spent filling out forms and preparing the patient for travel unless some routine procedures are skipped. Special *stroke protocols* (rules of procedure) allow EMTs to spend minimal time at the scene and encourage them to get the patient in the ambulance and moving toward the hospital as soon as possible. In addition, the EMTs may communicate with an emergency physician or a hospital stroke team member while on the way to the hospital. This communication helps the hospital prepare for the rush of activity needed to evaluate stroke in the ER.

Deciding on a Hospital

As the EMTs close the ambulance door, the next critical decision is where to go — the nearest hospital? Or a hospital offering special services for stroke patients, even if it's farther away? Does the ambulance driver have standard instructions regarding where to take stroke patients? What are the criteria for a good stroke care center?

Of course, you don't want to be asking these questions while racing the clock. That's why the more you can arm yourself with information about your community's stroke resources ahead of time, the better off you'll be in a stroke emergency.

Determining stroke severity by number

Doctors, nurses, and EMTs use a simple scale, the National Institute of Health Stroke Scale (NIHSS), to measure how severe a stroke is. It is not foolproof, but it's accurate for most cases and helps medical personnel plan hospital care, and it provides a good predictor of how well the patient will recover. Shorter versions are available for EMTs if they need it to save time.

If you have had a stroke, you may overhear hospital staff talking about your condition in terms of numbers: "The NIHSS was 16 at the time of admission, but it improved to 5 overnight." This scale starts at 0 for someone who is normal, and ends at 42 for a person with the worst possible stroke. A score from 1 to 9 is a mild stroke; from 10 to 19 indicates a moderate stroke; and 20 or above is a severe stroke (scores above 25 are unusual).

The NIHSS measures 15 different factors, ranging from whether you are awake and alert to whether you have good strength in your hands. For instance, if you can't say what month it is, or your age, then that costs you a point for each missed question. If you are drowsy and keep drifting off to sleep, that adds a point or two. (You won't be the first one to look in the mirror one morning and realize that your NIHSS might already be 1 or 2.) If your face droops on one side and has reduced movement, a point or two will be added depending on how weak the face muscles are.

The big points come from paralysis of the arms and legs. If your leg falls to the bed after being lifted by the tester, then that adds 3 points — 4 if you can't move the limb at all. Lesser degrees of weakness are more common. Speech problems can add up to 3 points. You get the idea.

A book cannot address this issue definitively because every response is influenced by local resources, geography, and politics. For example, the EMS services in your community may follow certain procedures in terms of which hospital they deliver stroke victims to. Your town may have a hospital that is well known for its stroke care. But following are some considerations for selecting a hospital.

Several national groups have started to establish guidelines (not standards, which are established locally) for determining which hospitals are qualified to claim status as a *primary stroke center. Primary* in this case means "the first place to go." Each hospital can read the published guidelines and decide whether it wants to do what is necessary to meet the guideline criteria. Not every community has such a center, and some have several.

Guideline requirements for primary stroke centers have been kept as simple as possible in order to maximize the number of qualified stroke centers. To deliver the best possible care, the first hospital you are taken to should be able to rapidly evaluate and treat stroke within 60 minutes of your arrival at the emergency room door.

The most widely known stroke guidelines are those published by the Brain Attack Coalition. Its guidelines make suggestions regarding resources and organization of a primary stroke center. To be a stroke center, a hospital must have

- Good EMS services that can communicate with the hospital when a stroke patient is *en route*
- An emergency department
- Laboratory testing capabilities
- A CT scan

The good news is that these resources are generally available in at least one area hospital.

Unfortunately, you don't have time to start comparing hospitals after your stroke symptoms start. Before your next stroke, you may want to call around and check at various hospitals in your community to determine which has a capable stroke center. Remember, time is important. A competent center ten minutes from your house may do you more good that a nationally known center two hours away. If you have time, you should also look for other criteria, which may be less common. A good stroke center should also

- Have a special stroke response team, adding specially trained personnel to the resources already available for stroke patients in the emergency department.

✔ Require administrative and financial backing of the institution. Call the hospital administrator's office and ask how the hospital supports its stroke team.

✔ Support its stroke personnel with ongoing training.

In addition to these factors, ongoing monitoring of quality is important for a good stroke center. For example, hospital administrators might monitor to ensure an acceptable response time from admission to treatment; 60 minutes is considered a widely attainable goal, but most centers with an experienced stroke team aspire to a quicker response. However, with changes in personnel and the passage of months and years, the average time to treatment may slow down rather than speed up. Periodic quality control reviews help sustain high levels of stroke care performance.

Advocating for the Stroke Patient in the ER

If you've ever taken a child or family member to the emergency room, then you've probably experienced a long wait, with the few minutes you actually spend with medical personnel spread out over several hours. The roughly 4,000 emergency rooms in the United States are increasingly crowded — emergency physicians can afford to spend only a small amount of time with each patient. For major emergencies — such as major trauma, heart attack, and stroke — other physicians are needed to back up the emergency physician.

Stroke is a major emergency. It's the brain! Because the stroke patient may not be in a position to speak up, it may be up to the family member or friend to make sure the individual is given the attention he or she needs.

If you are accompanying a stroke victim in the ER, don't be shy. He or she needs you to serve as advocate. *Don't* leave the person unattended while you fill out forms or explain insurance. Your first duty is to be sure the stroke patient is in the hands of someone who understands the severity of the situation.

If you are confident that the stroke started less than three hours before, your role is even more critical. Your responsibilities are to

✔ Report accurately what happened.

✔ Describe the patient's previous condition and any medications being taken.

> ✔ Determine whether the hospital has a stroke team and whether that team has been activated.
>
> ✔ Ask if personnel can treat the stroke with drugs to dissolve a blood clot.

If the hospital personnel will not treat the patient with drugs, the facility may not have the stroke expertise or the CT scan to determine whether rapid treatment is needed for the patient. Or there may be other reasons. In any case, you, as the patient's advocate, might suggest that the patient be transferred elsewhere.

The bottom line is that the person you are with is likely to be better off if a team of stroke physicians or an expert in stroke has been contacted and is managing the care.

If you're with a stroke patient in the hospital ER for more than five minutes without attention, something is wrong. If it has been less than two hours since the stroke started, then something is really wrong. Ask someone to see the patient and determine what kind of stroke the patient has and whether there is any treatment. Ask if the patient can receive the clot-busting drug (TPA), and, if not, why not. Two hours is important because TPA can't be started more than three hours after the stroke started, and it may take up to an hour to get the patient evaluated before starting treatment.

Understanding ER Stroke Strategy

For the stroke victim, the race against time continues in the emergency department. The next hour is called the "golden hour" because during that time the opportunity is greatest to prevent or limit permanent damage. Don't expect the doctors to stop and spend 20 minutes talking to the family. This is not the time. Brain is dying and the stroke response team must focus every minute on determining the cause of the stroke to treat as quickly as possible.

This is the challenge for the doctors: No treatment can save brain that is already permanently damaged — and after three hours of stroke onset, most of the damage is done. This is why it is critical to begin treatment immediately.

But there are four major types of stroke, and each type must be treated accordingly. In some cases, the *wrong* treatment could be fatal.

Therefore, the strategy for treating the stroke patient in the ER is this:

1. The doctors must *quickly* have some tests done to help decide what type of stroke the patient is suffering from.

2. They must treat the patient appropriately according to the type of stroke to keep the stroke from causing further irreparable damage.

Name that stroke

The doctors' observations and test results indicate which of the four main types of stroke the patient is experiencing. Detailed information is in Chapters 3 through 7, but the following is a brief recap:

- **Acute ischemic stroke.** Also known as *cerebrovascular accident* or CVA. This type of stroke is one of two types of white stroke caused by a blood clot plugging one of the brain arteries. Part of the brain isn't getting enough blood and, in time, it could be permanently injured. Nearly 80 percent of all strokes are this type.

- **Transient ischemic stroke.** Also known as a *transient ischemic attack* or TIA. This is another type of white stroke, also caused by a blood clot. But in this case the clot dissolves and the symptoms clear up a few minutes after they start. Although danger isn't as immediate, transient ischemic strokes are often followed by the permanent type — sometimes within hours, other times within a day or two.

- **Intracerebral hemorrhage.** Also known as ICH. This type of red stroke involves bleeding into the brain from a broken artery. This is the second most common type of stroke.

- **Subarachnoid hemorrhage.** Also known as SAH. This type is also known as a red stroke, but unlike the ICH, the bleeding is *around* the brain instead of *in* the brain. SAH is caused when a weak spot — also called an *aneurysm* — in the large blood vessel outside the brain begins escaping at high pressure.

Performing basic tests

Some clues help doctors determine which kind of stroke the patient is experiencing. For example, a severe headache with stiff neck is evidence of a subarachnoid hemorrhage. If all the symptoms have cleared up, then the doctors may conclude that the patient suffered from a transient ischemic attack. The team will run several tests, however, to confirm the type of stroke and to determine the best course of treatment.

Here are the basic tests and procedures that emergency department doctors perform for all strokes:

- Measure blood pressure, breathing rate, and temperature.

- Start an *intravenous* (IV) line for giving fluids and drugs into a vein.

- Draw blood for tests. This will help determine whether the patient has any conditions that would preclude certain treatments.

✔ Perform an *electrocardiogram* (EKG) to determine if the heart is okay. This test can quickly detect many common heart problems, which might have caused the stroke.

✔ Perform a CT scan to detect bleeding in or around the outside of the brain. A CT scan can determine whether the stroke is red or white. CT scans are computer-controlled X-rays that allow you to see the brain within the skull. For reasons only a radiologist could explain, a CT scan is also called a *cat scan* in the ER. It has nothing to do with cats and everything to do with making a rapid decision about whether bleeding is the cause of stroke.

It isn't always clear whether a stroke has occurred until other tests are done. Sometimes an MRI scan is helpful in determining what is causing the stroke symptoms.

In the case that a patient has complained of a severe headache with stiff neck — but the CT scan does not show any bleeding to support evidence of a subarachnoid hemorrhage — the doctors may decide to perform another test called a *lumbar puncture,* or *spinal tap.* The doctors concern here is not to mistake a small warning bleed for a migraine headache. If the spinal tap is negative, then there is much less likelihood of a brain aneurysm. The patient can be sent home with a possible migraine. Although this is not a common situation — less than 1 percent of stroke cases — it's important to make sure this is not a small bleed from an aneurysm that warns of an impending major rupture and subarachnoid hemorrhage (see Chapter 6 for more details).

Table 11-1 summarizes the tests done for stroke patients in the ER.

Table 11-1	Tests Done for Stroke Patients in the ER
All Patients	
Brain CT scan to see if the stroke is caused by bleeding	
Electrocardiogram (ECG, EKG) to check the condition of the heart	
Blood tests for other medical conditions that could affect treatment	
Some Patients	
Chest X-ray to see if lung disease is present	
Spinal tap (lumbar puncture) if subarachnoid hemorrhage is suspected but not found on CT scan	
MRI if CT scan does not clearly show cause of stroke	

This is a spinal tap

Although it sounds scary and has a bad reputation (not helped by its namesake faux rock band or their mockumentary), a spinal tap is a very safe — and relatively painless — procedure (occasionally a spinal tap will give you a headache, but usually not). A needle is placed in the middle of the back just above the hips. The same cerebrospinal fluid (CSF) that circulates around the brain also goes down through the spine surrounding the spinal cord and nerves. The fluid is normally as clear as water. A tablespoon or two of this fluid is removed through the needle and tested for the presence of any blood. If a subarachnoid hemorrhage has occurred, the fluid is pink or red with blood. Sometimes the blood can be pink due to inadvertent bleeding caused by the needle puncture, but there are tests to determine if the blood is fresh or several hours old.

Treating White Strokes

Remember, there are two types of white strokes (the blood-clotting kind): the acute ischemic stroke and the transient ischemic stroke. With the first kind, the doctors want to re-open the plugged vessel by dissolving the blood clot and restoring blood flow quickly before the brain is permanently injured.

The treatment that does that job is *tissue plasminogen activator,* better known as TPA — the only FDA-approved treatment for white strokes.

But . . . there are some *buts* regarding the use of TPA. If you find yourself diagnosed with a white stroke and you are *not* given TPA as a course of treatment in the ER, it could be because of one or more of these reasons:

✔ **There are risks associated with TPA:** It can cause serious, even fatal, brain bleeding (turning a white stroke into a red stroke) in about 6 percent of patients who receive it — most often people older than 75 who suffer a severe stroke.

✔ **Three or more hours have passed since the onset of the stroke:** Because the damage to the brain has already been done, the risks of TPA use may outweigh any potential benefit.

✔ **Your medical history or condition puts you at higher risk:** For example, you may have had surgery in the past two weeks. Or your blood may not clot normally.

✔ **The hospital can't do it:** Your particular hospital may not have a specially trained stroke response team or be equipped to administer TPA and monitor it carefully.

So, not everybody can take TPA. The following are some of the characteristics of patients who *can* benefit from TPA:

- ✔ The stroke causes significant disability and is not considered a minor stroke.
- ✔ The stroke is not rapidly improving.
- ✔ The symptoms of stroke should not be suggestive of bleeding from a ruptured aneurysm (SAH stroke).
- ✔ The stroke onset is less than three hours before beginning treatment.
- ✔ No major head injury or prior stroke in previous three months.
- ✔ No heart attack in previous three months.
- ✔ No bleeding from the stomach, bowels, kidneys, or bladder in the previous 21 days.
- ✔ No major surgery in previous 14 days.
- ✔ No history of previous intracranial hemorrhage.
- ✔ Blood pressure not elevated (systolic should be less than 185, diastolic less than 110).
- ✔ No evidence of active bleeding or recent injury causing a fracture.
- ✔ The blood should clot normally.
- ✔ Blood glucose concentration must not be excessively elevated.

TPA can be dangerous and requires fairly intense patient monitoring after it is given. Not all hospitals are equipped to do this. It is not unusual for physicians at one hospital to call a nearby major stroke center to seek advice or to transfer a patient there.

In the U.S., only about one-tenth of the patients who get to the ER in time to receive TPA actually do receive it. If TPA can't be given, doctors can take other measures to ensure the best possible outcome for a patient. Stroke patients tend to be older and, therefore, have other medical conditions such as diabetes and high blood pressure. Careful treatment of conditions such as these immediately after a stroke can improve the recovery from stroke.

Now, the second type of white stroke — transient ischemic stroke (also known as transient ischemic attack or TIA) — is a stroke of a different color, although it is also caused by a blood clot. TPA is not an appropriate treatment for TIA because the symptoms clear up so quickly, and the immediate brain risk is not as great.

A drug to reduce the chances of further blood clot formation may be started right away. This may be something as simple as a tablet of aspirin. Even though the patient has returned to normal, it's important to see what caused the blood clot. This can be determined during a stay in the hospital, or in some cases, as an outpatient.

If your stroke symptoms go away after a few minutes, you have likely suffered a TIA, which poses no *immediate* danger. You can feel lucky — but the danger is not gone. In fact, you can consider your TIA a valuable early warning sign. Get to the doctor — even to the emergency room, if necessary — for immediate evaluation. Many patients with transient stroke are back with a permanent stroke within hours or days. You should be tested as soon as possible. Surgical procedures and medical treatments are available that can reduce the risk of further stroke (see Chapter 4).

Treating Red Strokes

With a red stroke (see Chapters 5 and 6), patients are either admitted to an intensive care unit (ICU) or a special stroke unit for care. They usually leave the ER as soon as a hospital bed can be found for them.

Remember, the red stroke known as intracerebral hemorrhage — or ICH — is caused by bleeding within the brain. ICH is a very deadly form of stroke. Severe brain bleeding stops the patient from breathing and requires that tough decisions be made. The patient may need to be put on a ventilator to breathe in the ER. If the patient needs a ventilator, the chances of survival are very slim. At that point, the presence of someone who knows the patient's wishes about taking extreme measures to prolong life can be very important.

The goal of treatment is to stop the bleeding as soon as possible. Unfortunately, very little can be done other than lowering excessively high blood pressure, which has to be performed very carefully. Actions can be taken to help reduce brain swelling if that is a problem. A neurosurgeon may be called to evaluate the patient. Sometimes the blood inside the brain can be removed, and the patient does well, but the general rule is that surgery doesn't make that much difference. You have to trust the surgeon's judgment on this tough decision.

The other type of red stroke — subarachnoid hemorrhage or SAH — is brought on by bleeding *outside* the brain. Fifty percent of patients with this type of stroke don't even live to get to the hospital. For those who survive, the treatment — surgery to patch the aneurysm and stop the bleeding — is not started until the patient is in a hospital bed, often in a special ICU. Not all hospitals have neurosurgeons who can treat SAH strokes. In that case, the patient is usually transferred to another hospital, either from the ER or the next day from the hospital.

What you should know about your community's stroke center

If you suddenly find that one side of your body is paralyzed, it is clearly too late to research your community's emergency response. If you find yourself unable to find words or communicate, it is not the time to be asking around about the best hospital for stroke care. But if you're reading this book, you no doubt have concerns about the likelihood that you or someone close to you may experience stroke.

In that case, the news is good. You have time to learn more about the services your community offers for stroke victims. Now is the time to call your Emergency Medical Service (EMS) — using the non-emergency line — and ask about how they respond to stroke. Call your favorite hospital to see if it is a designated stroke center.

Here are some questions you should ask:

✔ Do EMS personnel receive special training to respond to stroke?

✔ Do they follow special EMS stroke protocols?

✔ Do EMS personnel communicate with the destination hospital when a stroke patient is on the way?

✔ Are hospitals that do not have stroke response teams bypassed?

✔ Are any hospitals in the area designated as primary stroke centers?

✔ Is there a designated stroke team at the hospital of your choice? If so, who are they and how often do they meet to evaluate their performance?

✔ Does the emergency department have special protocols for stroke?

✔ Does the hospital have a stroke unit with specially trained nurses?

✔ Does the hospital meet or intend to meet standards being set by Joint Commission on Accreditation of Healthcare Organizations?

If you want to bore down into the details, I suggest looking at the Web site of the Joint Commission on Accreditation of Healthcare Organizations. It describes primary stroke center standards and lists certified hospitals. Like many Web sites, the JCAHO site is not that well organized. I suggest going right to the Search option at the top of the page and searching for *stroke*. The page that describes the "Primary Stroke Center" program takes you to a list of Disease-Specific Certified Organizations.

One major concern with SAH is that the bleeding will start again. A second hemorrhage is often fatal. Surgeons or radiologists can repair the weak spot where the vessel ruptured. Usually, the sooner this is done the better, often within the first day or two, and there are some drugs that prevent the blood around the brain from causing further injury. These drugs are usually started during the first day in the hospital rather than in the ER (see Chapter 5).

There are several diseases that can cause symptoms that look like stroke and feel like stroke but are not stroke. Some migraine headaches have fooled doctors and patients alike. Likewise, diabetes and occasionally epileptic seizures have been confused with stroke. Sometimes during an illness like pneumonia or a bladder infection, the brain *decompensates*. The symptoms of an old stroke may return even if there is no new brain injury. It's as if the stress of the new problem causes the brain to forget what it learned to compensate for the disabilities of the old stroke. There are tests that can usually detect one of these other causes of stroke symptoms that are not really strokes:

- If the patient has other illnesses or has had one or more prior strokes, the situation may be unclear in the ER. About 30 percent of patients who come to the ER with stroke symptoms are found to have an old prior stroke. This can make it difficult to figure out what is going on.

- If the stroke symptoms are thought to be caused by an imbalance in blood chemicals such as blood sugar, then these imbalances can be corrected.

- If another cause is suspected, such as a migraine headache that can cause paralysis, then the migraine can be treated in the ER.

- If the symptoms continue to cause paralysis or another, new disability, then the patient is usually admitted for observation and further testing.

Chapter 12

Treating Stroke in the Hospital

*Y*ou've heard the expression, "We're not out of the woods yet." When you find yourself in a hospital bed after stroke, this familiar saying couldn't be more apt. You made it through the initial stroke trauma, surviving the trip to the emergency room. The immediate threat to your life may have been contained and your condition stabilized. But whether you suffered a white (ischemic) stroke, intracerebral stroke, or subarachnoid hemorrhage, you're not out of the woods yet. One-fifth of all stroke patients do not survive their initial hospitalization. Although death may not occur in the first hour or day after stroke, brain swelling and other threats often kill patients within a few days of their stroke onset.

The news isn't all grim, however. Modern hospitals offer wonderful resources for stroke victims. In hospitals of 20 and 30 years ago, you might have stayed for weeks after stroke. Today, treatments are intense and expensive — and more effective than in the past. You are out of the hospital usually in days instead of weeks. Good evidence indicates that the result is better survival from stroke and fewer second strokes.

This rapid and intense approach may present challenges to the patient and family, who need time to adjust and to gather critical information before they must return home to confront life after stroke on their own. In the few days available, it is important to learn everything possible so you can take care of yourself when you get home. You must absorb a tremendous amount of information and prepare for profound changes.

were in the emergency room, the overall goal was ensuring your
..om stroke. In that process, emergency physicians attempted to
... what type of stroke you had so they could begin treatment as
...ossible and stabilize your condition. Now you're ready for the next
... your hospital stay.

... many of the medical problems are the same for each type of stroke,
...pter is written for *all* types of strokes. After the emergency room,
most ᴏf the problems encountered in the hospital are those shared by all
injured brains. A range of challenges might develop during the first few days
after a stroke — some directly connected to the injured brain (brain swelling,
for example), and others leading to a related outcome such as swallowing difficulties or blood clots in the leg. In the hospital, however, you are under the
care of experts who have the diagnostic and treatment resources to deal with
these issues and do their very best to see you out of the woods.

Preventing Further Strokes

Having had one stroke, you are vulnerable to more. The goal of your doctors
becomes preventing another stroke from causing more brain injury while you
are in the hospital.

By the time you reach your hospital bed, your doctors will probably know
what type of stroke you had. However, further testing is needed to gain more
information about exactly what caused the stroke, how it should be treated,
and what can be done to prevent future strokes. Depending on what the tests
show, you may need surgery or drugs to keep you safe from another stroke.

Testing to determine the cause of stroke

In the emergency room, the physicians test to find out what sort of stroke —
white, subarachnoid, or intracerebral — you had so they can take steps to
stop the damage and protect your brain. After that, your doctors test to
better understand what caused the stroke — whatever the type — in the first
place. Several tests help determine the cause of stroke.

Finding narrowed arteries with carotid ultrasound

If you were diagnosed with a white (ischemic) stroke, your doctors may give
you a *carotid ultrasound* to determine whether you have narrowing of either
carotid artery. In this test, sound waves are bounced off the moving blood in
the carotid artery to see if the artery has any obstruction. This involves covering your neck with a wet jelly and sliding a wand over the area.

The results are usually given as a percentage of blockage in the artery. Although standard measurements have been established, they vary and hospitals don't seem to consistently follow the same ones. You would be surprised at how much the readings can vary from one hospital to another. Overall, though, you can count on the test to identify blockage and tell you roughly how serious it might be.

The more obstructed your carotid artery, the more you stand to benefit from surgery to remove the atherosclerosis blocking your artery. (Read more about atherosclerosis in Chapter 9.) If you've had a white stroke and have more than 70-percent obstruction on the same side as the injured brain (the opposite side of the weak face, arm, or leg), strong clinical-trial evidence suggests that you have much to gain from surgery.

This all depends on whether the surgeon has a good track record for performing this surgery without complication. Often, any surgery on the carotid artery is delayed until you've substantially recovered from your stroke. But with a transient or mild stroke, surgery may be done right away.

Looking for atherosclerosis with a cerebral angiogram

Some surgeons prefer an *angiogram* (or *arteriogram*) before proceeding with *carotid endarterectomy*. This procedure is uncomfortable and carries a small risk of causing another stroke. A long, thin, plastic tube is inserted into a large artery in your groin area and pushed upstream to the mouth of the carotid artery in your chest where it branches off to head into your neck and on to the brain. At that point the tube is manipulated into the carotid artery and dye is injected under pressure while a series of X-rays is taken. You are typically awake for this procedure, but sedated to reduce your anxiety. Some people say the dye going into the brain is very uncomfortable.

A brain angiogram is not needed for every patient. They are most commonly done in patients who have SAH to look for an aneurysm. They are also done in patients with white stroke if ultrasound or magnetic resonance tests (MR angiogram) show atherosclerosis blocking flow in an artery.

Tracking down plaque with a transcranial doppler ultrasound

The *transcranial doppler* test looks for atherosclerotic plaques in the larger brain arteries inside your skull. *Transcranial* means "through the skull." This test uses a special high-intensity sound wave to "see" through the bone of your skull. Otherwise, it is similar in principle to the carotid ultrasound test.

Although the test often determines that plaque is partially blocking an artery in the brain and is indeed the cause of the stroke, unfortunately, there is no surgical treatment to re-open the artery like carotid endarterectomy (see above). This narrow area is called a *stenosis* of the artery. Some experts recommend opening up these narrowed areas from inside. As yet, there isn't much data to support the benefits of this procedure. Aspirin probably works as well or better than warfarin to prevent future stroke when there is narrowing of a brain artery inside the skull. (Aspirin is better than warfarin in almost all cases except with a blood clot in the heart or atrial fibrillation.)

The transcranial doppler test is also used when you have a red stroke due to SAH. The doppler can tell if vessels are going into spasm in reaction to all the bleeding, and immediate treatment can be given.

Reducing the risk of another white stroke

Four critical steps can help prevent a second white stroke:

1. Take a drug to slow down your blood clotting.

2. Have carotid endarterectomy to check for blockage.

3. Learn the signs and symptoms of stroke so you can get to the emergency department faster in the future.

4. Control your high blood pressure better, get your cholesterol down, stop smoking, and control diabetes.

Checking your heart

If you've had a white (ischemic) stroke (or a red — intracerebral — stroke, for that matter), you don't *just* have high risk of another stroke. You also have high risk of heart disease. An exam by a cardiologist during your hospital stay is critical in determining the status of your heart and blood vessels. An electrocardiogram (EKG) is an easy and virtually pain-free test. The suction cups some doctors still use on your chest wall may leave bruises, but besides that, the test is just another small event in the complex day of the recovering stroke patient.

Your doctor might schedule a stress test of your heart, which consists of a fast walk on a treadmill. This can be a bit of hard work if you haven't been doing regular aerobic exercise. Obviously, any disability from your stroke will have to be taken into account. If you have a paralyzed arm or leg, you can't take the test without some special help and equipment.

Checking your cholesterol level

Blood tests tell you and your doctor whether you need any cholesterol-lowering drugs. If your cholesterol level is high, reducing the amount of fat in your blood — through drugs and diet — can help prevent stroke. What is defined as "high" cholesterol has been a changing number in recent years. Your doctor will help you figure out what to do in your individual situation. For example, it is thought to be more worthwhile to treat cholesterol aggressively with drugs if you have other risk factors such as diabetes and high blood pressure.

Considerations for diabetics

Are you diabetic? This might be a good time for evaluation by an endocrinologist who specializes in diabetes. Controlling your glucose can have a lot of benefits for your health. Clinical trials have not proven that managing glucose levels better will reduce your chances of stroke, but uncontrolled diabetes makes all the other risk factors worse for you. There are many other benefits of good control of your glucose: for your eyes, kidneys, and presumably many other parts of yourself.

Preventing future ICH red strokes

High blood pressure is the most common cause of intracerebral (ICH) red strokes — those that bleed within the brain. If you are over 50 or 55 and have high blood pressure, the cause of your stroke is usually just that. If you are especially young and do not have high blood pressure or another reason that explains your red stroke, then further tests may be conducted. A *cerebral angiogram* is a likely procedure to be scheduled. MRI scans might pick up the presence of *arteriovenous malformations* (AVMs) and some other abnormalities of blood vessels.

After your intracerebral stroke, you may have had surgery to remove part of the clot. If that's the case, you'll receive some very specific instructions before you are discharged from the hospital. You can also count on making office visits to your neurosurgeon for at least a few months after the surgery.

Avoiding further SAH red strokes

You prevent the recurrence of bleeding from brain aneurysms by either clipping them off from outside through the skull (a big deal) or by coiling them off from the inside (still a big deal, but perhaps a little safer). Before such surgery, doctors are likely to run a series of MRI studies and an angiogram to accurately locate the aneurysm. Sometimes it's hard to tell which aneurysm actually did the bleeding when two or more are found.

During your time in the hospital, your doctors will likely talk about some important steps to take at home: treating your blood pressure, for instance. Those who have suffered a subarachnoid hemorrhage will undoubtedly be reminded of the high risks of smoking. For women, the increased risk of subarachnoid hemorrhage from the use of estrogen will probably also be discussed. You may be instructed to avoid birth-control pills or estrogen.

For female readers: If you are *not* on birth-control pills or hormone-replacement therapy (estrogen) when you are admitted to the hospital with your stroke, your doctors may neglect to explain the risks of estrogen related to red stroke. But the risk remains whether you take estrogen currently or start up after your stroke. You'll want to share the information about your stroke history to all your doctors — including your gynecologist.

Asking for a second opinion

A 33-year-old woman jogging in the park was seen staggering, stopping, and putting her hand on the back of her head before falling to the ground. She was taken by ambulance to a nearby emergency room, where she remained unconscious. Within 30 minutes, a CT scan was completed. The emergency physician told the woman's husband that he believed she may have had a brain hemorrhage based on seeing blood filling the subarachnoid space around the base of the brain. He explained that final diagnosis depended on a radiologist and neurosurgeon.

The neurosurgeon and the radiologist concurred with the emergency physician and diagnosed a subarachnoid hemorrhage. The neurosurgeon advised that the woman be sent to a large hospital in a major nearby city for treatment of the probable aneurysm that had ruptured. The woman was delivered to and admitted to the neuro-surgical intensive care unit. Her blood pressure was monitored overnight, her headache pain was controlled, and she was given drugs to prevent her arteries from closing shut (this closing is called *vasospasm*). Her husband spent the night researching subarachnoid hemorrhage on his laptop in his hotel room.

The neurosurgeon met with the husband immediately and advised an angiogram first thing to determine whether blood clots were present in his wife's brain. The doctor explained that the procedure, which involved injecting dye into her arteries, had some risks, but that the diagnosis was critical. The husband agreed and was comforted that his wife opened her eyes and looked at him in the ICU during his short visit. After the angiogram, he found her sleeping peacefully. She had a big bandage on the crease where her left leg met her torso at the site where the radiologist inserted the plastic tubes for the angiogram.

An hour later, the neurosurgeon told the husband that the test showed a brain aneurysm that bled and that it should be closed off soon. The surgeon recommended that it be done with a small clip. The husband listened and said, "Tell me again what could go wrong." The surgeon repeated the risks: another stroke, infection, death. Concerned about these possibilities, the husband asked if there were other options.

Three more doctors diagnosed the patient: another surgeon, a neurointerventionist, and a neurologist. After assessing the options, the husband finally decided on a different procedure — in which the neurointerventionist would try to close the aneurysm with coils placed from the inside during another angiogram-like procedure. The husband preferred the uncertainty of how long the coil would last over the risk of the surgical complications with the clip. If the coiling effort failed, then surgery would be considered. The neurointerventionist performed the procedure that afternoon without any incident.

Several days later, the woman began to get drowsy and her right-hand weakness and speech problems suggested a white stroke. Another emergency angiogram showed that some of her brain arteries were in spasm and much narrower than usual. Treatment for the vasospasm was begun. Three weeks later, the woman was discharged from the hospital. She was still a little clumsy with her right hand and had some difficulty finding words from time to time. She was considered to have a moderate disability at the time.

Monitoring for Brain Swelling

Brain swelling is a very serious complication of stroke and can occur for a number of reasons. If you have a white stroke, the brain area injured by a lack of blood will begin to swell. In red stroke, the brain swells because of the extra blood from the bleeding. In addition, the blood can block the flow of fluid in the ventricles and the backed-up fluid expands the brain. Finally, any blood inside the substance of the brain causes inflammation and swelling.

Regardless of the cause, the swelling presses the brain against the inside of the skull. This increased intracranial pressure makes a person drowsy and can even put someone in a coma. Doctors can measure the pressure by drilling a hole in the skull and putting in tubes or other devices. Placing a tube in one of the fluid cavities of the brain can relieve the pressure if the outflow of fluid is blocked. Other treatment measures include raising the head higher than the body, using a ventilator to cause rapid breathing, controlling blood pressure, and giving drugs. None of these treatments works very well or for very long.

Brain swelling from white stroke

A 63-year-old man was sitting at home watching television when he noticed that he couldn't move his left arm. In fact, the left arm looked funny to him, like it was someone else's. He checked it a little while later. By the time the show ended it seemed a little better. He walked upstairs to bed and realized that his arm hung straight down and his hand wouldn't grip the banister. While getting ready for bed, his symptoms cleared, and he went to sleep relieved. His wife woke beside him at 5 o'clock in the morning to find him breathing noisily. When she tried to wake him up, she noticed his eyes were looking to one side and he didn't move his left arm or leg. He could speak but seemed dazed and confused.

In the emergency room, a CT scan showed a massive white stroke on the right side of the brain with evidence of brain swelling. He was admitted to an intensive care unit. Later that day he was more responsive, but completely paralyzed on his left side. The next morning, he was worse and

breathing irregularly. A new CT scan showed that the swelling of the brain had increased.

Doctors explained to the family that the brain swelling could kill him; that treatments often did not work and that if they did, he might be left with a major disability. The family authorized the doctors to treat the man, as there was a reasonable chance he could speak if he survived. The doctors started drugs and procedures to minimize the swelling. The next day his condition worsened. A CT scan showed that there had been bleeding in the area of the white stroke infarction. He died the same day.

There is no way to be sure that this fatal stroke could have been avoided if he had come to the emergency department the night before, but chances are pretty good that the severity of the situation might have been recognized. If he had been hospitalized and observed carefully, he might have been a candidate for treatment to open up the blood vessels to the brain.

Doctors often can't control the rise of pressure inside the skull. The result is that the brain first shifts to one side and then begins to press down against sharp edges in the skull at the base of the brain. These sharp edges cut into critical areas of the brain that keep you alive. Brain swelling and subsequent damage is one of the most common causes of death in white or red strokes.

Responding to Seizures

During the trauma of stroke, the lack of oxygen and injury to the brain puts its protective systems out of balance. The result can be a seizure. A very small percentage of stroke patients (1 or 2 percent) may have a seizure while in the hospital. The shaking often starts in an arm or leg and then rapidly spreads to include the whole body.

Seizures are usually treatable and typically do not happen again if anti-seizure medications are started. Several medications are available, including ophenytoin (Dilantin) and carbamazepine (Tegretol). If you have a seizure in the hospital, your family should call for help. In the meantime, they can turn you on one side or the other to prevent you from inhaling into your lungs any saliva or vomitus in your mouth. You have heard of putting a stick or spoon in the mouth of someone who is seizing. Don't do it unless you know exactly what you're doing. Someone sticking anything in your mouth while you are having a seizure is a risk to your teeth and their fingers. Sometimes, just an arm or some other part of you will be shaking from a small partial seizure. You may even be awake and alert. You still need to call someone to see what's going on. A major seizure could be starting soon.

Of course, if you have had seizures before your stroke, this increases your odds of having seizures *after* a stroke.

Other Problems in the Hospital

A lot of other troubles and complications can occur while a patient is hospitalized. This section outlines some of these.

Blood clots in the legs

You've probably read about "coach class syndrome," a condition that strikes passengers of long airline flights. Sitting in a cramped position with their legs pressed down into the seats for long periods of time puts flyers at risk of developing blood clots in the veins of the legs. This same situation — sitting or lying in a bed for days — puts hospital patients at risk for clots in the legs, a situation that can prove fatal.

How leg clots are a risk

The blood in your leg veins is moved along slowly toward the heart in part by the gentle squeezing whenever you contract the leg muscles. The veins have tough but thin walls that are easily squeezed by muscles. They are likewise easily distended by blood seeping into them from the tiny capillaries that connect to arteries. Because the legs are typically in a position lower than your head, blood is more likely to collect there — and clot — when you are inactive. Once a clot begins to form in the leg veins, it stimulates the formation of more clots. Large clots as thick as one of your fingers can form inside the largest veins deep in the thighs and calves.

These large clots are a danger in a few different ways. First, they can attach themselves to the sides of the vein and become painfully inflamed. This condition is called *thrombophlebitis.*

Or the clot can break off and travel through the veins toward the heart. Like tiny streams meeting in the plain to form a small river, veins converge and become larger as they travel toward the heart. Once a clot breaks loose in a vein, it is bound to reach the heart where it can either block the heart and kill you immediately or go through the heart into the lungs. Think back to high school, when you learned that the right side of the heart takes blue blood without oxygen from the veins and pumps it through the lungs, where it turns red as it picks up oxygen and goes into the left side of the heart where it is pumped out into the body.

Pulmonary embolism: When clots hit the lungs

If the clot is small enough to pass through the right side of the heart without causing damage, its next stop, as it transfers to the outgoing transportation system — the arteries — is the lungs. Small clots block only small bits of lung, and blood flows through alternate pathways.

But intermediate or large clots headed to the lungs can completely block off blood flow. The whole blood-pumping mechanism can shut down with disastrous results — often sudden death. The name for this whole process is *pulmonary embolism. Pulmonary* refers to lungs. The *embolus* is the clot flying from the heart and slamming into the lung's smaller vessels.

If your doctors don't treat you to prevent these clots, and you are bedridden, chances are 25 to 50 percent that clots will form. You know now that the clot is inevitably going to reach the heart, where it typically moves through without damage but can then move on to the lung and result in a pulmonary embolism. Death is a real possibility.

Treatments for preventing blood clots in the legs

Obviously, the best thing to do is to keep the clots from forming in the veins in the first place. Shifting your position stirs the blood and moves it toward the heart, keeping it from forming blood clots. So get moving! The last thing you may feel like doing — after all you've been through — is to get up and take a walk down the hospital corridor. Or, if you're unable to do that, do simple leg exercises from your bed every hour or so. But I hope you'll understand after my explanation here that the floor nurse is not really a heartless drill sergeant intent on making your stay as unpleasant as possible — he or she is, in reality, looking out for your welfare when he or she insists on getting you to "shake a leg."

Doctors can also do the following to prevent leg clots:

✔ Treat you with drugs, such as heparin, to make your blood less likely to clot. These medications can be administered orally or as injections under the skin or in a vein.

✔ Place elastic stockings that squeeze the veins and move the blood.

✔ Insist that you regularly work your legs against that annoying board at the end of the bed, designed to keep you flexing and extending your ankles and keep the blood moving and your calf muscles stretched out.

Struggling with difficulty swallowing

After a stroke, it's not unusual to have some difficulty swallowing. Stroke can cause weakness of the muscles of your mouth and throat, just as it can make an arm or leg weak. Manifestations include drooling, a newly hoarse and gurgly sound to your voice, difficulty with coughing, getting food trapped in your mouth, trouble with chewing, and difficulty swallowing anything. In fact, 30 percent of stroke patients experience these problems.

Choking, lung infection, and other dangers

With all these challenges, what often happens is food or liquid passes into the airway rather than the esophagus and stomach. In short, liquid or solids end up in your lungs. This is not good. In fact, it can kill you. Better hope that someone is there and the Heimlich maneuver works for you if this happens.

Fortunately, death due to choking isn't the most common problem caused by difficulties with swallowing. Malnutrition gets that dubious honor. For a while, you feel like you're trimming down, but then when you begin to see emaciation in the mirror, you recognize you're not eating enough. Poor nutrition makes you weak and limits your ability to recover from stroke.

Another common result from swallowing difficulties is lung infection or pneumonia. All that food and liquid in your airway carries bacteria into your lung, which can lead to a serious chest infection. Get ready for a lot of chest X-rays and antibiotics. Even with all the best efforts of modern medicine, pneumonia still kills about one-third of all patients who die from stroke in the first year. Most of these deaths occur after people leave the hospital and are bedridden in their home or a nursing home.

Testing for swallowing problems

While you are in the hospital, your doctors are likely to test you for swallowing problems right away — before starting you on a regular diet. If you choke while drinking water, then it is likely that you will have problems with food and other liquids as well. If you can't swallow properly, you still have to eat. Many swallowing difficulties go away in a few days. Because you have to eat in the meantime, you may have a tube put through your nose and down the back of your throat into the esophagus and stomach. Not very comfortable at first, but more comfortable than pneumonia or not eating or drinking anything. You will gag and cough as the tube is passed into the back of your throat through your nose, but then think of the convenience of not having to chew your food.

If your swallowing problem is not too severe, a speech therapist can show you ways to swallow without choking. You may need a special swallowing test to diagnose exactly which muscles are weak and to help guide the therapy. You want to know its name? *Video fluorography* and/or *barium swallow*. Read more about swallowing difficulties in Chapter 16.

Monitoring your heart

Your heart needs your brain to keep going. When the brain is injured, the heart can't really be trusted to keep things under control by itself. It can lose track of its rhythm and that can literally stop you dead in your tracks. You are also more prone to have a heart attack just after you have had a stroke. Chances are good that you've already been checked for that in the emergency department once you got to the hospital.

For severe strokes or those that affect the brainstem or deeper portions of the brain that control the heart, doctors may continue to monitor heart rhythm during your stay. If an abnormal rhythm starts, they may administer drugs to get it beating normally. Dangerous rhythms are most common during the first 24 to 48 hours after a stroke. They are particularly common after a red stroke.

Blood pressure is usually controlled by the brain. Given a brain injured by stroke, blood pressure can be unstable, especially when the patient starts getting active again after the first few days in bed. Getting up to get to the bathroom or on your feet in physical therapy, blood pressure can drop. You can count on doctors and medical personnel keeping a close and frequent eye on your blood pressure while you are in the hospital. The worse your brain injury, the more frequently your blood pressure will be measured.

Bleeding stomach ulcers

A small percentage of stroke patients bleed from stomach ulcers. A stay in the hospital isn't a day at the beach for your stomach, and I'm not talking about hospital food. Plenty of treatments and procedures give the stomach a hard time. For example, a stomach tube can cause the stomach to bleed. Certain drugs — heparin, aspirin, or steroids — can result in bleeding. In fact, just the stress of being in a hospital can cause an ulcer that bleeds. If you have a history of stomach ulcers or pain, your doctors may give you drugs to reduce the injury to the stomach while you are in the hospital.

Avoiding pressure sores

Pressure sores aren't that common anymore. Also known as bed sores, these painful skin ulcers result when patients who are unable to move themselves are left lying in the same position for long periods of time. Hospital staff are well aware of the importance of keeping patients moving, not just to avoid bed sores but to reduce the risk of blood clots in the legs. That said, a few guidelines will help ensure that you avoid skin irritations from lying in bed.

- Don't lie on your weak or numb side — the side of your body affected by the stroke.
- Avoid being moved by shoving, dragging, or pulling on your weak side.
- If family members or friends are attempting to assist you, great — but they may need some training from the floor nurse or attendant.

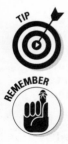

If you are a family member, take this time to learn how to lift, support, or assist your loved one in getting around. Watch what the nurses do and learn to do it yourself. You'll be doing it at home, unless you hire a full-time nurse.

Small injuries can rapidly become major sores. If splints are applied to your arms or legs, leave them there. Cooperate with nurses to be sure you move around and reposition yourself. And assist by eating and keeping hydrated by taking in adequate fluids. This will keep your skin healthy and able to heal. Once they develop, pressure sores are not easy to treat. Severe sores can require plastic surgery. It they get infected, you'll require antibiotics — possibly intravenously, possibly prolonging your time in the hospital.

Preparing for Life After Stroke

While you are in the hospital recovering from stroke, you and your family have a short time to absorb and tap into valuable information and resources that will aid in your adjustment to living with stroke after your discharge.

This comes at a time when all you want to do is rest and recover from the shock of stroke. But if you're going to get the most out of your hospital time, you need to become a good listener and note-taker.

Getting the most out of your hospital stay

These steps will help you optimize your hospital experience:

- **Take advantage:** The hospital staff is there to help you plan for after you leave the hospital. They have a lot of experience with stroke patients — welcome their input and seek out their advice and knowledge.

- **Work hard:** I've said it in earlier chapters, but the sooner you start therapy, the better your odds for recovery. Cooperate with the hospital therapists to develop a post-hospital plan and learn as much as you can about becoming as independent as possible.

- **Observe:** Watch how the nurses take care of you. You and your caretaker can start practicing some of what you learn — whether it's tips for getting out of bed into a chair or strategies for bathing.

- **Gather — and give — information:** Keep a list of tests done and their results, drugs prescribed, and all the medical issues that have arisen. Be sure that the physicians caring for you know your prestroke medical history. Doctors often don't have access to all your old records, and even if they did, may not take time to dig through them.

- **Plan with your family:** Anticipate the daily and weekly schedule after you return home. Talk about the help you'll need and how you'll get it. Set up a schedule. Make arrangements. You have much to gain by launching a strong plan for dealing with the challenges of the future.

Getting hold of your discharge summary

Ensuring that you have thorough, accurate, and up-to-date discharge information is critical to transitioning to life after stroke. You'll need this detail for yourself and your follow-up physicians and therapists. Preparing the document called the *discharge summary* is the responsibility of the primary discharging doctor. Hospitals can usually prove that they handed the discharge instructions to the patient or caregiver as they left the hospital. But for whatever reason, these important instructions often get lost.

Don't leave as if escaping from jail. If the nurses are in a hurry, ask them to please sit and talk with you. Insist on getting all the information and instructions written down. Have a family member or friend take notes. Get a phone number. No matter how obvious, write it down. Be sure you have all the pills you need to take or a prescription. Following these instructions can have a significant and positive impact on your future health. Accurate discharge info is of *extreme importance*. Just imagine if the following errors or omissions resulted from poorly executed papers:

✔ You had a white stroke and aspirin or an equivalent is not on the list.

✔ Blood-pressure medications have been changed or deleted.

✔ A medication that you have taken for years is not on the list.

✔ Warfarin is on the list, but the need for blood tests is not mentioned.

✔ There are no medications listed to lower your cholesterol.

✔ No follow-up appointments are mentioned.

A hospital stay is extremely important to help you recover and adjust to your circumstances. Take the care to collect information, tap into the expertise that surrounds you, make contacts, ask questions, and observe during this time.

Chapter 13

Rehabilitation

. . . .

In This Chapter

▶ Determining who will benefit from rehab

▶ Understanding the rehab strategy

▶ Meeting the rehab faculty

▶ Boning up on the curriculum

▶ Paying for rehabilitation therapy

▶ Graduating from rehab and starting your new life

. . . .

*W*hen it's time for the stroke patient to be discharged from the hospital, the doctors may recommend one of three courses of action:

✔ Patients who have mild or little damage may be able to return home immediately.

✔ Those suffering from severe damage with little hope of recovery of their independence may be referred to a nursing home.

✔ Individuals likely to benefit from rehabilitation therapy — and that's as many as 20 to 30 percent — will probably be directed to a rehabilitation center.

Approximately 50 percent of stroke patients need some kind of rehabilitation. Those who don't get it in a rehab center have to arrange for it at home or in a nursing home.

The term *rehab* may conjure up images of celebrities escaping to luxurious private facilities where they lounge around landscaped grounds, wear designer robes, and dine on gourmet fare prepared by famous chefs. In truth, a rehabilitation center is not a place where the stroke survivor is pampered and waited on hand and foot. Instead of spa resort, think back-to-school. Yes, the rehabilitation center is more of an educational institution offering a crash course in skills that will help the stroke victim regain independence and lead a fuller life.

In many cases, the rehabilitation center is a boarding school — the "students" eat, sleep, and learn there during the course of treatment. Though the average term of stay is short, from one to four weeks depending on stroke severity, the program is intense and requires active participation and commitment, not just from the stroke victim but from family members or caregivers, too.

In this chapter, I offer the "course outline" for the rehabilitation process. I discuss who might make a good candidate for therapy, explain the strategy behind rehabilitation, introduce the rehab team, outline a typical daily schedule, and offer information on Medicare, Medicaid, and insurance coverage of rehab.

Who Should Go to Rehab

If you want a clear answer about who should and should not go to a rehabilitation program, you will search in vain. The answer depends on many different factors: doctor recommendation, severity of stroke and the damage incurred, level of care that can be provided in the home, and, no less important, the attitude and openness of the stroke patient and the family toward the rehab experience.

Home, sweet home?

After a stroke, most patients are anxious to leave the hospital and return home to familiar surroundings and routine — it's a natural inclination to get back to normal as quickly as possible. But in their haste to get out of the hospital, many stroke patients may find themselves struggling to adjust to new limitations, and their caretakers may be ill-equipped to help. A wife may suddenly find herself struggling to help her husband get in and out of bed, take a bath, and use the toilet. A husband might need to take time off work to attend to his wife's needs, including feeding and clothing her. Out of loyalty, family members may fail to express their doubts about their ability to handle a person with brain injury. Or they may simply be unaware of how changed a family member can be after a stroke.

I strongly encourage stroke patients and their families to be open to rehabilitation therapy if that is what the doctors recommend. Although you may intend to refuse anything but the shortest possible route home, you really should first consider the recommendations and the potential benefits of time in a rehab program.

"Why can't I have rehab in my own home?" you may ask. Of course, with unlimited resources, you can turn your home into a rehabilitation center and have the appropriate specialists come to you. However, this turns out to be very difficult. Scheduling difficulties, space limitations, and lack of equipment may be a few challenges. Even more critical, you'd miss out on the interaction with other patients and families in the same predicament.

If I've successfully persuaded you to accept a doctor's recommendation for rehab, then my next goal is to convince you that it's equally important for family members — particularly a close partner such as a husband or wife — to be involved in every step of the program, too.

What the doctor looks for

The rehabilitation doctor considers several factors when recommending a stroke victim for a rehabilitation program. Three factors favor your going to rehab:

- Stroke severe enough to limit independence, but not severe enough to make it unlikely you can improve
- Physical strength to endure three or more hours of physical therapy every day
- Capability to learn and benefit from the rehab experience

The doctor is more likely to suggest a nursing home rather than a rehabilitation center if the patient

- Has had a prior stroke
- Is very frail from other medical problems
- Can't make it to the bathroom without help
- Has serious problems with memory or thinking
- Is unable to understand or cooperate with therapists
- Requires constant medical monitoring
- Is unlikely to be able to return home after maximum rehabilitation

How much rehabilitation is needed?

Most stroke patients who go into a rehab center stay for weeks — not months. (Though many have told me later that they wished they could have stayed longer.) But each stroke patient is unique and, consequently, will follow different programs with different time requirements.

For example, patients with mild deficits may need only one or two weeks at the rehabilitation center. On the other hand, if the patient is paralyzed on the right side and has difficulty speaking and understanding language, he or she may require three weeks of rehabilitation before returning home. If the weakness is on the left side, the patient may not have speech difficulties, but may have trouble paying attention long enough to accomplish anything. Also, this patient may be more likely to fall, because the brain doesn't take notice of the fact that the left arm or leg isn't working. In this case, a longer stay — perhaps four weeks — in rehabilitation may be needed (if appropriate). An experienced doctor can usually make a good guess about the time that will be needed in rehab. However, the initial plan can be changed based on how things actually work out, which may vary from original predictions.

The Rehab Strategy

As I said earlier, the goal of rehabilitation is to help the patient adjust to life after stroke as much as possible — regaining function as capacity allows, adapting to limitations by developing new skills, and learning to use tools to help compensate — all with the purpose of helping the stroke survivor return home and lead an independent life.

Keeping muscles ready for recovery

When your left or right side is paralyzed by a stroke, the inactivity of the muscles on the affected side can cause serious problems — without use, paralyzed limbs draw up tightly into awkward positions that become permanent as muscles form tight, unstretchable bands called *muscle contractures*.

To keep muscles ready for action as the brain recovers, the muscles must be kept flexible and strong. Daily stretching and strengthening exercises keep muscles fit and supple. This is preventive maintenance for future recovery. Even if no function returns, it is still important.

Making do with what's left: Substitution

Most time in rehab is spent learning to use what you *have* in order to replace what you've *lost*.

This involves instruction and practice, but it may also require specially fitted braces and simple tools to help with some tasks. The recovering brain can't shut down and wait to heal before resuming its work. It has to keep things running the best it can. First comes survival, and for this the parts of the brain distant from and not connected to the injured area have to take on new activities previously managed by the injured part of the brain. Think of this as _substitution_.

Here are some examples of how the stroke survivor substitutes:

- ✔ Your right hand is partially paralyzed, and you cannot yet hold a pen. You try writing with the left hand; it is clumsy but it gets the job done.

- ✔ Your left leg is too weak to support you. By using your right arm and leg for strength, you learn to get out of bed and into a wheelchair. Not as good as walking, but it gets you where you need to go.

- ✔ Your right foot points down when you take a step. You wear a foot brace that keeps your foot at 90 degrees from your leg. This makes it easier to walk and keeps a contracture from happening to your calf muscle. The brace substitutes for your calf in raising up your foot when you walk.

- ✔ Your right hand is weak and can't hold a spoon or fork effectively. You use special utensils to make it easier to get the food into your mouth.

Brain recovery: Use it or lose it

During the days and weeks following stroke, the brain does actually generate a few new cells. And some injured brain cells may learn to activate new connections that bypass the injured neurons and begin functioning again. In this process, some lost abilities may return. Most of this biological recovery seems to be finished after three months, although there may be some ongoing recovery for a year or more.

But here's the exciting news: Some evidence indicates that exercising these injured cells may increase the speed and extent of recovery. Here's how it works: First, the injury from stroke is variable and patchy, depending on the way the blood flows and the access of blood supply near the injured tissue. True, stroke completely destroys some brain cells. But those that are only partially injured can partially recover. Growth of new blood vessels may be stimulated; formation of new connections to other brain cells may be fostered.

And what is it that stimulates these new, healthy connections? _Using those brain cells._ Exercising the arm or leg weakened by stroke or repeatedly grasping a pen in a weakened hand. Physical activity appears to be important in stimulating those injured cells to recover, especially during the first few months after the stroke — although significant improvement has been observed in a small percentage of patients 6 and even 12 months after a stroke. Such early effort also has the effect of increasing muscle strength and reducing the possibility of contractures, which is the first rehab tactic. Sometimes the improvement is small — but even small changes in hand strength can have a large impact on your ability to gain independence.

A rehab success story

A man in his 50s, a computer programmer, had a right arm and leg stroke that spared his comprehension of speech but limited his ability to speak clearly. After his hospital treatment was completed, he was admitted to a rehabilitation center. His rehabilitation nurse explained that she was there to encourage him to reach his maximum potential. He diligently followed his program, a unique plan designed to deal with his particular stroke symptoms.

The first days on the unit, he was moved in a wheelchair, but he quickly graduated to a walker. He worked hard in the facility's gym. Each day he received three hours of therapy directed at the practical issues of living, such as eating, brushing his teeth, buttoning shirts, and, eventually, typing. In addition, he participated in programs to help reconnect him to people. He was taken on trips into the community, including restaurants, department stores, and grocery stores. His nurses urged him to be as independent as he could.

At the same time, a social worker began to make arrangements for his return home. These arrangements included continuation of the physical therapy and actual modifications to the layout of the furniture in the home and moving in special equipment to help improve his independence. After one month in the rehabilitation center, he was able to return to both his home and his job. His recovery was attributed to his ability to understand language, his eagerness to cooperate with his therapists, and his high spirits.

In previous decades, the major goal for rehabilitation was to focus on substitution while avoiding intense therapy that might put too much stress on the recovering brain. These days, most experts agree that physical activity promotes brain reorganization and enhances recovery.

Preventing additional strokes

Another critical rehab goal is to prevent future strokes. Those who have already suffered a stroke are the likeliest to have a stroke. It's critical to do everything possible to avoid another one. See Chapter 10 for a list of preventive steps. Your medical care and evaluation needs to continue after you leave the hospital for rehab. This includes taking medications, continuing tests to determine the cause of your stroke, adjusting your blood-pressure medications, getting your cholesterol under control, and more. Stroke prevention should not wait for you to "settle down" after your stroke. A second stroke is more likely in the weeks immediately after a first stroke. If you let down your guard, you miss the opportunity to prevent stroke.

CASE STUDY

Things may get worse before they get better

A 78-year-old man experienced the sudden onset of numbness, weakness, and slurring of speech. His wife recognized the symptoms and called 911. While in the hospital, he then had a second stroke. After eight days, he was transferred to a rehabilitation unit. Upon admission, he was unable to walk because his right leg would not support his weight, and his ability to move his right arm and hand was limited. His speech had improved to the extent that he could participate in a short conversation.

After three weeks, physical therapy enabled him to move from chair to bed and to walk with the help of one person and a walker; the occupational therapy helped him dress himself. With plans to continue rehabilitation one day a week, he was discharged. He and his wife were both eager for his return home.

But things did not go well: Shortly, he gave up using the walker and returned to a wheelchair. His wife started helping him wash and dress. He began spending more time in one room, lying on a couch. Other than a weekly outing with a friend, he refused to leave home, feeling he was too much of a burden to his wife.

He continued to go for weekly physical therapy but didn't use what he learned there at home. He was now afraid of falling and no longer felt comfortable and secure in his home. After two months, his hand movement still did not improve, yet he learned a way to play cards using a holder rigged up by a friend. This improved his motivation to begin dealing with the other impairments caused by his stroke. When his wife was sick, his daughter had to move in with him to care for him until his wife recovered.

Everyone has to adjust to the consequences of stroke in his own way. Working through the depression and discouragement is not easy for anyone. Renegotiating relationships and dependencies takes time and patience on everyone's part. Setting expectations at a reasonable level is as difficult for the patient as it is for the family. Eventually, almost all patients and families come to terms with stroke disabilities and are able to get on with their lives. The message of this book is not that you *should* recover completely from your stroke or that you *should* do this or that. The message is more that there are a lot of opportunities to help you recover, however you choose to do it. Success is usually wrought out of multiple hard knocks and failures.

The rehab curriculum

Enrolling in a rehabilitation center is a full-time commitment — you are "in school" 24 hours every day. Rehabilitation nurses oversee patient care around the clock and work closely with patients to encourage self-care and attention to personal hygiene.

Although all stroke rehab patients are encouraged to follow a similar level of commitment and diligence, each patient receives a custom "curriculum" based on unique needs, deficits, and goals. Specific sessions with various specialists are scheduled in most units. A typical day's schedule might be as follows:

6:00 – 7:00 a.m.	Morning dressing in your room
7:00 – 8:00 a.m.	Breakfast in a dining room with others
9:00 a.m. – noon	Sessions with therapists
Noon – 1:00 p.m.	Lunch in a dining room with a group
1:00 – 4:00 p.m.	Sessions with therapists
5:00 – 6:00 p.m.	Dinner in a dining room with a group

Some centers run on five-day schedules, others on six-day schedules. Patients may be encouraged to wear their own loose-fitting clothes for exercising, a sweater or jacket, pajamas, and comfortable shoes. Depending on individual limitations, patients may be encouraged to get themselves around in the unit to the various activities and meals. This is a good place to really push hard to see how much you can do on your own. It is safe, and the people about can suggest ways to work around difficulties.

Furthermore, there is good evidence that the harder and sooner you push, the better the brain may recover lost capabilities. Pushing your limits stimulates your brain to recover. The more you try, even if you don't succeed, the better you will do in the long run.

Meet the Rehab Faculty

Rehabilitation is a team effort. The players include the stroke survivor, family members or caretaker, and the trained experts who work with the rehab program. A physician — either a *physiatriast* (a specialist in rehabilitation medicine) or a neurologist (a specialist in the nervous system and its diseases) — usually heads up the team. The rest of the team focuses on various therapies, physical needs, and transition from rehab to the real world. Let's meet some of the key players.

Physical therapists: Helping with mobility

When most of us think of rehabilitation, we think of physical therapy. And, indeed, the physical therapist plays a crucial role in the recovery of a stroke patient, working with a patient to increase general strength, condition muscles, develop endurance, and help the patient regain as much function and independence as possible through enhanced mobility.

In an intense program, you may spend three hours six days a week with a physical therapist. An hour every weekday is more usual. Not everyone has the strength and endurance to tolerate even an hour. The exercises depend on the disability and come in three parts: teaching, practicing, and home-work. If the difficulty is with walking, for instance, you will be re-taught how to walk, you will practice what you are taught with a therapist present, and, if useful, you will be given suggestions about how to practice and keep new skills when you are back in your room on your own.

After stroke, some patients neglect and ignore the parts of their body dam-aged or paralyzed by stroke, making it difficult to eat, dress, wash, or move. The physical therapist addresses the mobility aspects of this neglect and assists the patient with exercises that involve walking, standing, transferring from chair to bed, and using a wheelchair or walker. The physical therapist also identifies needs for braces and other special equipment.

Occupational therapists: Everyday skills

You might think an *occupational therapist* has something to do with employ-ment. Actually, occupational therapists teach stroke patients ways to perform the simple tasks of everyday living — cooking, eating, dressing — through individually designed exercises and the use of special tools. The occupational therapist is familiar with the patient's impairments and teaches the patient how to dress, eat, bathe, groom, use the toilet, and perform other routine tasks. It's surprising how hard these simple tasks can be when you have only one good hand or if you are sitting in a wheelchair.

The occupational therapist not only helps the stroke patient with therapeutic exercises that strengthen and increase range of motion, but also teaches the patient new ways of approaching tasks and suggests special tools or equip-ment to help achieve success. An hour with an occupational therapist can be very tiring. Listening and learning take a lot of effort. Practicing new skills can fatigue your brain. Practicing on your own after you have rested really locks in what you have learned and speeds your progress remarkably.

If there is anything that is good about stroke, it is that stroke usually leaves one side or the other normal. Occupational therapists are magicians at teaching you how to do with one hand what usually takes two hands. Long-handled tools can pick up items dropped on the floor, special spoons are easily gripped without spilling, zipper pullers, and slight of hand tricks will handle buttons on shirts. Where there is a will, there is a way. The occupa-tional therapist is your opportunity to learn how to get everyday tasks done once you decide to do them.

Speech therapists: Bridging gaps

Speech therapists (also called *speech language pathologists*) focus on speech, but also address other communication-related problems, including swallowing and breathing, understanding, hearing, and vision (reading). They may evaluate the patient's risk of choking or inhaling food while eating by running tests to determine whether the throat muscles are working properly. They might work with patients to improve the clarity of their speech and teach them methods to overcome problems with memory and thinking.

Speech therapists also address problems related to *aphasia* (ay FAY zha), the inability to understand language, which is common among stroke patients. The word *aphasia* is thrown around quite a bit, and you will surely hear it if you or a family member suffer stroke-related language problems. It does not refer to grammar or a stutter or slurred speech, but to problems that arise when part of the brain that spent years learning a language is not functioning. Hence, someone in your own family can sound as if he or she is speaking a foreign language. Or a patient may be able to understand spoken language fairly well, but *written* words are unrecognizable or have no meaning. The speech therapist helps the patient find a communication method that works until the language understanding improves (as it often does).

An hour with a speech therapist is spent learning the components of processes most of us have never thought much about. How does your tongue move when you are saying the word *liquid*? How do your lips move when you say *baseball*? What exercises would be helpful if you wanted to learn to speak more clearly? Relearning speech is made more difficult because practicing speaking involves another person. You have to show your disability to others and face their reactions as well as cope with relearning to speak. Often you find yourself preferring one person or another to practice with. You are lucky if you can find one who will wait while you struggle to get words out right.

Working around aphasia is like finding secret passages in an old house. Stroke patients with aphasia often seem to know what they want to say, but only communicate the frustration of not being able to say it. Eventually, though, the brain begins to figure out how to get messages out, and the pathway is often unusual. Sometimes words come out in other languages that you know, or through writing. Showing someone pictures may bring out a word unavailable from memory. Solving language comprehension problems and learning to express yourself with limited language skills is daunting.

Nurses: Medical management

While in the rehabilitation unit, medical management of the patient's stroke continues. Rehab nurses monitor blood pressure and other vital signs and administer medication. They also participate in the rehabilitation program — sometimes in ways that may surprise you. For instance, they may expect you to do more for yourself than their counterparts in the hospital did. Instead of bringing dinner bedside and feeding you, the rehab nurse may encourage you to go to the dining room, even if it means struggling out of bed and using a walker to get there. This is part of the program.

Social workers: Making sense of it all

Social workers facilitate the transition from rehab to the real world, helping families plan for services they'll need upon the patient's return home — or transfer to a nursing home. They have the difficult job of trying to make the whole medical-care system work for the patient. They help you understand what help you can expect from your insurance and your community, including your employer, if you have one. Their goal is to get you out of the hospital and into a situation where you can be as independent as possible and still maintain your health. Often they face a significant challenge as needs frequently outstrip the resources available.

A social worker might arrange for special equipment to be used in the home, schedule outpatient nursing and rehabilitation home visits, and connect you to support groups. Social workers are also concerned with the social process of reintegrating the patient with family and community after rehabilitation.

Other specialists involved in the rehab program may include the following:

- Neuropsychologists measure changes in your cognitive abilities and your personality. They can suggest ways to deal with many cognitive problems, including difficulty with memory.

- Vocational rehabilitation counselors work with you and your current employer to get you back to work, either at your old job or a new one.

- Dieticians help work around medical problems related to diet. This can range from counseling a diabetic to helping someone with difficulty swallowing.

- Orthotists fit braces and other assist devices.

Family and other caregivers

Family members and caregivers can learn important information and skills from taking part in the rehab experience. Skills include knowing how to help you move from a wheelchair to and from a car and to assist with range-of-movement exercises and bathing — and knowing what they are expected to attempt on their own and what they should be letting you do. The experts on the rehab team can do a much better job of making things work out for you when you return home if they know who will be available to help.

It is also important that the stroke experience not have adverse effects on the health of family members or caregivers. By participating in group discussions and interacting with the staff, loved ones have an opportunity to address doubts and uncertainties about their ability to provide the emotional and physical support required by the patient — before they find themselves in a difficult or impossible situation that makes them depressed or ill.

Paying for Rehabilitation

Just as private schools and universities carry a high price tag, most rehabilitation centers charge fees that all but the most affluent might find staggering. Some rehabilitation units are run as profit-making businesses, and although they may provide excellent care and services, you have to be sure you can afford the care. You may want to consult with other family members and physicians to see if there are alternatives that could attain the same goals with lower out-of-pocket costs. Fortunately, most stroke victims can seek financial support through government programs or private insurance.

Medicare and Medicaid

Medicare is the federal health-insurance program for U.S. citizens 65 years or older *and* for certain Americans with disabilities. Medicare has two parts:

- **Hospital insurance (known as Part A):** Helps pay for home health care, hospice care, inpatient hospital care, and inpatient care in a skilled nursing facility.

- **Supplementary medical insurance (known as Part B):** Helps pay for doctors' services, outpatient hospital services, durable medical equipment, and other services and supplies not covered by Part A.

Social Security Administration offices across the country take applications for Medicare and provide general information about the program.

In some cases, Medicare helps pay for outpatient services from a Medicare-participating comprehensive outpatient rehabilitation facility. Covered services include the following: physicians' services; physical, speech, occupational, and respiratory therapies; counseling; and other related services. A physician must certify that skilled rehabilitation services are needed and must refer a stroke patient. This ensures that an expert in the care of stroke patients thinks the effort and time are worthwhile.

Medicaid is a federal program operated by the states. The states determine eligibility and scope of health services offered and provide healthcare coverage for some low-income people who cannot afford it. Others who might be eligible are older, blind, or disabled individuals, or individuals in families with young children.

Medical insurance

You pick your insurance company before you have a stroke, not after. Now you have to figure out what you bought. There are a slew of private medical and health-insurance products, as well as health maintenance organizations (HMOs). They all handle coverage for stroke rehabilitation in their own way and vary to some extent, depending on the level of insurance and the particular benefits of the individual companies offering the insurance.

What care you get may depend to some extent on what is offered by your particular plan. While some plans provide for in-hospital rehabilitation, others emphasize in-home or outpatient programs. Talk with your care provider and your insurance company to determine what is best for you.

All insurance programs have limits, and some stop paying as soon as the patient stops making progress. Often, the hospital's social service department can answer questions about insurance coverage. Some decisions are based on opinion. If you feel the wrong decision has been made, there are often ways you can get the decision changed by communicating directly with the insurance company and your doctors. Be a squeaky wheel.

Graduating: Life After Stroke

Congratulations! It's graduation day — and you're ready to leave the rehabilitation center. Stroke survivors and family caregivers alike have looked forward to this day when home life can resume — if not "just like before," at least with the knowledge that they've gained new skills in order to adapt to life after stroke.

Like any educational program, the time you invest in rehab is worth only what you take home with you. For that reason, whether you're the stroke survivor or the caregiver, be sure you clearly understand what you must do to continue the efforts you've started. It is part of the procedure in rehab units to meet with the patient and family and discuss a follow-up plan. This is important stuff. Often, with the excitement of going home or the rush to get moving before the car gets towed from the front of the hospital, papers get lost and important advice is not heard.

The following checklist covers most of the critical issues that should be discussed as you prepare to leave the rehab facility. Use it as a "crib sheet" for your final meeting with the rehab doctor. Try to get detailed answers to each of the questions and then share this list with all family members — not just your spouse or caretaker. It is important for *everyone* involved to know what is expected of them. The family shares responsibilities for monitoring the success of the transition home and the stress on the patient and the caregiver.

- ✔ List of all known medical problems
- ✔ List of all medications and purpose of each, with accurate descriptions of the doses
- ✔ Name of a rehabilitation person who can be called if there are problems
- ✔ Schedule of outpatient and in-home visits clearly written out in one place
- ✔ List of equipment expected to be supplied at home and a telephone contact
- ✔ Schedule for family members not in the home to check in with caretaker and patient
- ✔ Name and phone number of a doctor to call for medical problems
- ✔ Instructions to call 911 if there is a second stroke

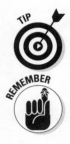

Make copies of the preceding list and distribute to all family members and caregivers.

The goal of the rehab unit team is not to take care of you. It is to train you to take care of yourself and to make the best use of your support system. With the intention of helping you, the team may have presented you with some tough challenges and difficult situations. But as you're ready to return to your community — home, social world, and work — you've gained an education that will help you not just survive but thrive as a survivor of stroke.

Part V
Living with Stroke

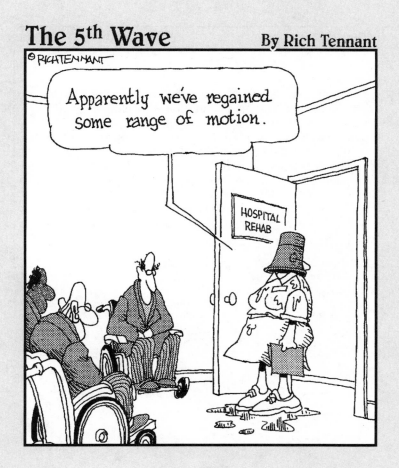

In this part . . .

*L*ife after stroke involves learning new ways of living and coping. There are limitations and challenges to be surmounted, and changes to familiar routines and plans have to be considered. These chapters cover returning home after the hospital, thinking about residential placement, dealing with the financial stresses, and confronting the hard choices and issues families have to face. It's important to not try to do everything yourself — be willing to ask for help. There is a lot of help to be had out there, and accepting it can help ease the pain for everyone.

Chapter 14

Returning Home: Adapting to a New Life

. . . .

In This Chapter
▶ What to expect the first year after stroke
▶ Committing to ongoing medical therapy
▶ Seeing your physician
▶ Continuing rehabilitation therapy at home
▶ Returning to work
▶ Getting organized and motivated

. . . .

*I*n this chapter, I address many of the issues you face after you return home and begin to adjust to life after stroke. During this transition time, you are confronted with a number of new challenges and responsibilities. One of those demands is to continue therapy either at home or at an outpatient facility. Another is to assess your capabilities. As you continue to improve and to know better what you can and can't do, you can begin to plan for the long-term.

An important part of the planning is to have some sort of estimate of how different your condition will be in six months to a year from the onset of stroke. By now you may have asked this many times of physicians, therapists, and other stroke patients. They really don't know an exact answer, and each person you talk to may offer different descriptions of your future. I offer you some information so you can form your own estimate of how you will do. This may allow you to do a better job of planning your approach to your new life after stroke.

The good news is that unless you have a second stroke, or another medical condition intervenes, you can be reasonably certain that your stroke symptoms will lessen gradually with time. How much depends on

✔ The severity of injury due to the stroke

✔ Your health in general and whether you suffer from conditions such as heart disease, cancer, or dementia

✔ Your efforts to prevent a second stroke

✔ What rehabilitation efforts you make to protect and enhance your recovery

Avoid the Three-Stroke Rule

It's a good idea to do everything you can to prevent a second stroke. The rule is: Three strokes and you're out. In a study of 150 or so stroke survivors in one town, 80 to 90 percent had had only one stroke; 10 percent had two strokes; and a few had three strokes. None had more than three strokes. Presumably, those that did were dead.

As to the type of stroke among those who survived a year or more, 90 percent experienced the white type, and 10 percent suffered from red strokes. About half of the stroke survivors had some kind or residual paralysis, close to 20 percent had some sort of language problem, and 10 percent had both paralysis and language problems. Another 15 percent had difficulty speaking, while 15 percent had lost part of their vision to one side, and 25 percent had loss of sensation on one side.

By the way, I have to repeat the obvious: If you do have another stroke, however small it is, call 911 and get to an emergency room right away. Don't call a family member. Don't call your physician. Call 911. *It's your brain.*

Recovering Slowly but Surely

Another study reflects the *positive* outlook for stroke recovery: The patients left the hospital at approximately seven to ten days after their stroke. When they were examined three months later, almost all showed some improvement.

Consider language recovery: More than half of the patients with language problems showed some degree of improvement by three months, and 25 percent of those had improved their language abilities to normal levels. This is the good news. On the downside, 1 out of 20 of those who left the hospital with no language problems became worse and developed language problems in the next three months due almost entirely to subsequent strokes.

Approximately 70 percent of patients leaving the hospital had no weakness in their right arms. Three months later, that had increased to 75 percent. And of the 30 percent who did have some degree of right-arm weakness, half or more showed some degree of improvement. More good news: 25 percent of those with some degree of right-arm weakness had no weakness three months after leaving the hospital. However, as with language, a few patients, 1 or 2 percent of them, got worse — possibly because of a second stroke, failure to maintain strength by exercising, or because they developed pain or stiffness.

In general, patients who continue to improve greatly outnumber those who lose ground during the three months after leaving the hospital. Typically, this holds true for face and leg weakness, although slight weakness in the face is sometimes more noticeable than slight weakness in the arms or legs. In general, if you maintain your muscle tone and flexibility, you can look forward to a slow but steady improvement in the strength of your weak arm or leg following your return home.

It is fortunate that the most severe stroke impairments — living in a nursing home or becoming dependent on a caregiver for mobility or normal everyday maintenance — are the least common outcome from stroke. There is no difference in recovery rates between men and women.

Rewiring the Brain

What is your brain doing to help out? Here's good news that may be surprising to people who thought the brain stopped growing at age 20: After an injury such as stroke, the brain reorganizes itself to adjust for deficits caused by the injury. Special brain-imaging studies show that after an injury, the brain can rewire itself and form new connections between brain cells, transferring the work of the injured area to some other, usually nearby, part of the brain.

Research shows that the brain forms more new connections if the patient is more active. For example, if you work six hours a day to move your weak hand, you will get more return of function than if you work three hours a day. This is not because the muscles are stronger, but because the brain makes new connections and regains the control that was lost due to the stroke. More good news: The more effort you make to "exercise" your brain, the better your brain will respond by rewiring its connections.

This is why rehabilitative efforts are so critical in the first few months after stroke — to help speed up and increase the extent of brain recovery from stroke. (See Chapter 13 for more information about this amazing brain function.)

New Disabilities Will Affect How You Live

So far I have been talking about specific brain functions that are changed by stroke. Let's look at how stroke can affect *how you live*. The following table shows the percentages of stroke patients who exhibit various limitations common to stroke. The numbers refer to the percentage of all stroke patients who develop a new disability that was not already present before their stroke.

Decreased ability to do household tasks	36%
Decreased socialization outside the home	31
Decreased ability to use outside transportation	31
Decreased vocational function	27
Decreased interest in hobbies and other pursuits	27
Dependency in the activities of daily living	23
Dependent in mobility	16
Decreased socialization at home	15
Move to a nursing home	13

Stroke changes your personality

You may notice something about the disabilities listed in the preceding table. Some of them have no direct relationship to the physical impairments caused by stroke. Decreased interests and reduced socialization, for example, are common problems after stroke. This could be a side-effect of problems with language and difficulty with transportation. But the data illustrate an important lesson for the stroke survivor and family: Stroke causes social impairments as well as physical limitations.

It may come as no surprise that caregivers and spouses often report that it's no picnic to live with a loved one after he or she suffers a stroke. More than 60 percent of those who've experienced taking care of a stroke survivor describe the loved one as less patient, for example. The following table lists the percentage of patients who lose some good personality traits.

Less patient	63%
Less capable	60

Less active	60
Less in control	57
Less independent	57
Less energetic	54
Less confident	43
Less easygoing	37
Less stable	37

From caregiver reports, it seems that about half of stroke survivors appear to be more bored, unhappy, worried, and frustrated than they were prior to their stroke. Further, but to a lesser extent, caregivers describe stroke survivors as exhibiting more dissatisfaction, irritability, and unreasonableness after their stroke than before.

The long and the short of it is that emotional and behavioral changes put more stress on the people living with the stroke victim than the physical impairments do. These changes can also slow and diminish recovery from stroke.

Stroke survivors may not be sensitive to the fact that their frustrations and impatience may manifest in behaviors that negatively affect loved ones. Think about it: You used to be able to brush your teeth with your right hand. Now, when you try, the toothpaste gets all over the sink. You get impatient and frustrated. You may yell, cry, throw things. Then you begin to notice that everyone in your family seems to be avoiding you — or tip-toeing around you during these times. For help for the caregiver, see the "Taking care of the spouse or caregiver" section later in this chapter.

It's hard to become more patient or easygoing. However, part of adjusting to life after a stroke is learning to live with your new limitations. Hopefully the information provided in this chapter will help you develop some realistic expectations for the future. I can't say the predictions made here will be any better than the weatherman's are at telling you whether it is going to rain on a particular day, but at least it's a start. If I accurately conveyed the data to you, you should think that the future is mostly sunny or at worst partly cloudy with only a 20- to 30-percent chance of rain.

In more than 90 percent of strokes, the weather in three months will be better than it is today.

Part of the improvement that is possible after stroke comes from learning new ways to do things, part comes from the brain rewiring itself, and part depends on your accepting the changes and getting on with the rest of your life.

Don't mess with depression

Depression. Suspect it is there. Hunt it down. Treat it before it wastes more of your time.

Depression, from moderate to severe, affects nearly half of stroke patients who return home. The depression usually doesn't last longer than seven or eight months, but if untreated, it can slow the recovery process dramatically.

You might already be thinking, "Who wouldn't be depressed after a stroke?" To some extent, depression after stroke is due to the unhappy situation and is a normal reaction. However, that doesn't fully explain it. Fortunately, depression is now treatable. The only difficulty is facing up to its presence, having the temerity to talk about it with a physician, and then getting it treated, sometimes by taking anti-depressant medication. As with blood pressure, a number of affordable, generic drugs treat depression.

"I take enough pills," you may think. "Besides, life is hard — I can't expect to be happy all the time. I should tough this out, struggle through." This attitude is all well and good when you're talking about confronting physical limitations and facing post-stroke difficulties. However, by neglecting to address depression, you may be holding yourself back from successfully adjusting to your new life — and you may even deprive your brain of the opportunity to restore some function. (Review the "Rewiring the Brain" section earlier in this chapter.)

Depression is more than unhappiness. People who are not depressed can be unhappy. Depression is a state of mind — a state of brain, you might say — involving a general decline in energy. The symptoms can be fatigue, lack of interest, social withdrawal, and irritability. Do these sound familiar? They are the very symptoms that make people who live with you unhappy and frustrated. They are the same symptoms that lead to canceling therapy appointments, not trying as hard as you can, and forgetting to do your range-of-motion exercises three times per day. Treating depression can be a key to moving forward in your recovery from stroke.

How do you find out if you are depressed? You can start by asking the people you spend time with — family members, caregivers, therapists. Many nurses are particularly good at picking up on depression. Be aware, though, that some individuals may not be frank with you. This is particularly true among those who have an emotional or social connection to you. Even a spouse — *especially* a spouse — may fear a confirmation of depression may make you even further depressed.

Approach the issue of depression with a spouse or loved one when you have time to delve deeper and explain that it is important to know whether you seem depressed. Under such circumstances, you are more likely to get honest and objective feedback. But even if your loved one conveys that you don't "seem" depressed, yet you feel unhappy inside, anxious, or empty, then it is critical to consult a physician.

Likewise, caregivers or family members should pursue a conversation with a stroke survivor if they suspect depression is an issue. This may be difficult — as I discussed earlier, stroke sufferers are often impatient and angry as they adjust to their condition. Initiate a conversation during a "neutral" moment — not when the individual has just shoved his or her walker to the floor in frustration. If you are unable to communicate successfully, share your concerns with your loved one's physician.

You may ask, "Isn't it the physician's job to diagnose depression?" Certainly if a doctor suspects depression, he or she will explore the possibility with the patient. But to diagnose a condition, the physician must have the critical information. A doctor could not, for example, be expected to diagnose high cholesterol without the appropriate blood tests. No blood test, urinalysis, or X-rays currently exist that detect depression. Although a physician may be able to recognize signs of depression in a brief follow-up exam, often these appointments are rushed and focus on more immediate *physical* concerns.

I would like to believe that most physicians look for signs of depression in their stroke patients — but to ensure that any issues of depression are addressed, it is critical that either the stroke patient or family member raise such concerns with the doctor.

Taking care of the spouse or caregiver

A stroke can have a big impact on the spouse or caregiver. Those close to the stroke survivor are also extremely vulnerable to depression and emotional problems resulting from dramatic changes in their loved one — and from the impact on their own lives. Stroke survivors should certainly be encouraged to be aware that family members suffer from the stroke, too. But they may not be in a position to ease the burdens of their caregivers. To some extent, caregivers have to learn that looking out for their own psychological well-being has benefits for both themselves and the person they are caring for. Someone who is depressed isn't likely to do a good job taking care of someone who is disabled.

If you are a spouse or primary caregiver to a stroke victim, be sure that you are taking care of yourself. You, too, have suffered a traumatic, life-altering experience and must be alert to its impact on you. Although there's nothing you can do to change the facts or the limitations and demands stroke places on your loved one and yourself, you must take measures to protect your health and emotional well-being.

Stroke support groups are outstanding resources for caregivers. By gathering with other caregivers and family members of stroke victims, you benefit from talking about your problems and getting reassurance from the experiences of others. These support-group meetings may also alert you to valuable information or concerns you may not have been aware of.

Enlist the help of others, either in your household or beyond. Adult children and even teenagers need to know how important it is for them to spend time helping the stroke survivor — and thereby giving you a needed break. And don't neglect your social life! Most stroke patients tend to be less outgoing during the transition period. This can also isolate the caregiver from previous friends and limit opportunities to socialize. You need to consider your own needs in your daily schedule.

Taking care of a stroke victim full-time may be too much for even the most loving spouse. Asking for professional help may be in the best interests of all. But that doesn't have to mean a nursing home. Daytime care centers may offer services to the stroke patient while the family member runs necessary errands, gets out for a lunch with friends, or spends time with children or grandchildren.

Ongoing Medical Therapy

You've had one stroke. You certainly don't want another. Yet the risk that you will have a stroke or a heart problem is very high. Second strokes are far more likely to happen in the first few days and weeks after the first stroke. Doctors know a lot about preventing stroke — many clinical trials have shown that available drugs and other treatments really work. You need to do everything *you* can to prevent stroke, too. This requires taking your prescribed medications and pursuing ongoing medical follow-up with stroke experts.

Starting meds: Time is of the essence

The transition from hospital to home can be a particularly critical time. It is essential to continue the treatment started in the hospital. If you have just arrived home from the hospital, you should have a list of recommended medications and corresponding prescriptions. If you don't, track down this information immediately. Call the hospital and speak to your doctor or nurse. Enlist a social worker, a family member, or a pharmacist to help you obtain this information.

Except in unusual cases, the staff at your doctor's office does not understand the urgency of immediate medication. They may suggest you schedule an appointment and ask you to come back in a week or two. *That won't do.* If your doctor is busy and not an expert in stroke, the importance of continuing to take your medication may be lost.

It is also important to watch for side effects of new drugs after you get home. Any new symptoms or discomforts that you experience may be due to medication side effects rather than your stroke. Read package labels so you have some idea what to look for.

Often, your first medical appointment after returning home may be several weeks away. I repeat my caution in the previous paragraph because I have heard so many times the same excuse for not taking medicine. Don't wait till later to start taking medications recommended in the hospital. You should fill prescriptions from the hospital the very first day and not miss a single dose.

The chances are very slim that you *don't* need to be taking any medication. Except in rare circumstances, most stroke patients require some preventive therapy to reduce the risk of a second stroke. You should probably be taking medications to control blood pressure and possibly *serum lipid* levels. You may need medication to control your diabetes if you have it. Aspirin, warfarin, or other drugs are usually necessary to help keep your blood from clotting too much.

You and your family are pretty much on your own now. You will need to look out for yourself. A nurse is not going to walk into your bedroom and hand out medicine three times a day. *You* must take a proactive role to ensure that you have the best possible recovery from stroke.

Birth-control pills and stroke risk

Female stroke sufferers who've been taking birth-control pills or other prescriptions with estrogen should discuss discontinuing this medication with their doctors. Estrogen, also common in hormone replacement therapies for menopause, increases the risk of all types of stroke.

Monitoring blood pressure changes

If you are taking drugs for blood pressure, now would be a good time to get one of those blood pressure machines. After you return home from the hospital, the change in your activity and diet may affect your blood pressure. Your stroke may also make it harder for you to stop by your drug store to test your blood pressure. Blood pressure machines — the ones that display the blood pressure on a digital readout — are affordable these days.

Take your blood pressure and pulse rate every morning and evening at the same time and in the same place. The reading should stay relatively constant. You can call your doctor's office to have the results evaluated. If you get light-headed when you stand up, the pressure may be too low. Check with a physician. Keep the records and take them with you to your next appointment.

Watching out for dehydration

For a variety of reasons, stroke sufferers often don't eat or drink enough. Perhaps it's physically difficult for you to hold a fork or raise a glass. Maybe you're experiencing loss of appetite due to depression.

But with stroke, dehydration becomes an even greater concern. Here's why: The lack of activity following stroke puts you at risk of forming blood clots in your legs. Most strokes are caused by blood clots. Without enough fluids in your system, your blood is likely to become thicker and more prone to clotting, not to mention making you more susceptible to infection and other disease.

Even if you suffer from a poor appetite, be sure to drink plenty of water!

Even if it sends you to the bathroom more than you want, drink two to three full glasses of water every day between meals.

How can you tell if you're drinking enough water? Your urine will be a light yellow or straw color, rather than dark yellow. This rule works well unless you are taking vitamins that turn the urine dark.

And don't skip meals, especially breakfast. It is not known why, but morning is the most common time for a stroke to start. Why take chances? Drink a full glass of water when you take your medication before breakfast. And beware: The coffee or tea you drink with breakfast not only increases your blood pressure a little, it may actually dehydrate you, as well.

Did you smoke before your stroke?

A lot of smokers who were not permitted to smoke in the hospital are eager to celebrate the return home with a cigarette. First thing they do after arriving home — if they haven't already done so on the drive home — is light up. Don't start smoking again. You really don't want another stroke. And there is no doubt that using tobacco in any form at least doubles your chances of stroke. Stopping smoking rapidly reduces your chances of a second stroke. Within a year of stopping smoking, your chances of stroke are equal to a nonsmoker. You stopped smoking while you were in the hospital. The hardest part is done. Now just keep on *not* smoking. One of the first things you should consider doing is removing everything smoking-related — cigarettes, matches, lighters, and ashtrays — from your home.

Seeing Your Physician

Did you know that a lot of people stop taking their blood pressure medicine when they find out the medicine has brought it down to normal? I guess they don't realize that they have to keep on taking it for the pressure to *stay* down. I know of a Fulbright scholar who stopped taking his statin drug after he was told that his cholesterol levels had returned to normal. He had a heart attack and was found to have extremely high levels of fat in his blood several years later.

I don't know whether seeing a physician would prevent you from making mistakes like these. I do think that having a stroke is a sign that your health is more precarious, at least for a period of time. I also know that recovery from stroke can take a year or more. Therefore, monitoring your medical condition during this time is key to avoiding setbacks and ensuring that you are making satisfactory progress in your recovery.

Be sure you've scheduled an appointment with your doctor soon after your return from the hospital. And be prepared to schedule visits more frequently than you would under normal, "nonstroke" conditions. After a stroke, you should have your risk factors evaluated more often.

You may want to see a stroke specialist in addition to your regular doctor — especially if your doctor has expressed that he or she is not familiar or comfortable with treating stroke symptoms. From the medical system point of view, it's a good idea to stick to a doctor who manages and integrates all of your care. You can be referred to see a stroke specialist once or twice a year.

The quality of the office staff can be as important as the quality of the physician. If the staff is brusque, uninterested, makes clerical errors, and doesn't return phone calls, try another physician's office. Often, physicians may have nurses that help with telephone calls. If you can't reach a physician, ask to speak to a nurse. If you still think you are getting the runaround, then one last resort might be to talk to the office manager. Sometimes it helps if a family member calls for you.

Checking up on your stroke

Here's another important reason to schedule that doctor's appointment soon after your return home: Critical testing to determine the cause of your stroke may still be needed if it wasn't done in the hospital. You may need to check whether fat deposits called *atherosclerosis* are slowing blood flow to your brain. You may need a CT scan or an MRI scan to see how much brain damage occurred during your stroke. It also may be helpful to know exactly where the damage is. Your doctor may advise an electrocardiogram (EKG) to determine whether you have an intermittently irregular heart rhythm — called *atrial fibrillation* — that is an elusive cause of stroke.

In addition to testing for cause of stroke, your physician will monitor your recovery progress and review other medical conditions that may affect your risk. Checking blood pressure, drug levels and side effects, surgery scars, and rehabilitation progress are all part of the doctor's job. If you need more therapy or different kinds of therapy, the doctor may make recommendations and arrangements. The physician may even arrange for your driving ability to be tested.

Bringing up other problems

Although you may be inclined to disregard other health issues not related to stroke, don't hesitate to discuss all medical concerns with your doctor. First, they may indeed *be* related to your stroke, even if in some indirect way. And, secondly, if not taken care of, they may have an impact on your stroke.

Are you having problems with sex or incontinence? Mention them. These conditions can usually be successfully treated. Many of the drugs for blood pressure can cause impotence in men, and anti-depressants can decrease interest in sex for men and women. The same drugs and others can affect urination and bowel movements.

If you're uncomfortable talking about these issues in front of a nurse or spouse, ask to speak to the doctor alone. But don't neglect the problem. It's just not necessary for you to suffer if help is available.

Loss of hearing is also another seemingly unrelated problem that could have a detrimental impact on your stroke condition — if only because you may miss out on hearing important information or advice from your doctor. If you suspect you have some hearing loss, ask to have your hearing tested.

The patient's role in doctor appointments

What is the patient's responsibility in the doctor-patient dynamic? Keeping appointments with physicians is a good start! Additionally, be sure to take all necessary information — including medical records — with you when you go. Many medical offices simply do not do a good job of this.

Here is a checklist of some of the records and information you might bring to your appointment:

- ✔ Brain scan reports
- ✔ Electrocardiogram
- ✔ Hospital discharge summary
- ✔ Laboratory results
- ✔ Blood pressure record
- ✔ Accurate, up-to-date list of medications — better yet, the bottles themselves
- ✔ List of unusual symptoms you may have had

As you undergo further testing, continue to keep track of lab reports and keep copies of MRI and CT scans, as well as X-rays. If you go to the hospital for a different reason, keep records of that. You may want to remind any therapists you have seen that you have an appointment and encourage them to contact your physician with their questions and reports.

Continuing Rehabilitation Therapy at Home

Don't wait to start recommended physical therapy, speech therapy, and occupational therapy. You may feel like you deserve a rest, but don't take a week or two off from your exercises, thinking you will start later.

The more you do, and the earlier you do it, the better your recovery from stroke.

You need the therapy recommended to start *right away*. Chances are, you already began rehabilitation while in the hospital. Don't lose momentum! You may actually be stronger when you come home from the hospital than you will be after you slack off for a few days and lose the conditioning you got at the hospital.

You should be taking some kind of therapy if

✔ You have difficulty speaking or understanding language.

✔ You have clumsiness or weakness in a hand or arm.

✔ You have difficulty walking or keeping your balance.

Rehabilitation is so important that it is paid for by most insurance policies or through Medicare, at least for the first few weeks after stroke. It's not fun, and arranging for therapy after returning home may be difficult, but the fact is *it is critical*. Your rehab also presents an opportunity for someone else to check up on your progress.

Rehabilitation's Catch-22

You will likely be scheduled to return to an outpatient facility for therapy. Some people don't go. You can imagine the reasons. For one thing, just getting in the car and driving to an appointment is now a major challenge. Maybe you shouldn't even be driving. But here's the Catch-22: The more you need therapy, the harder it is to get to it — because your mobility is limited, because it requires a strong helper to get you in the car, or because your wheelchair doesn't fit in the trunk.

Trust me: You'll be faced with times and circumstances that will discourage you so much you'll want to throw in the towel. This is exactly the time when it's essential to *double* your effort! And if you simply can't do it, then call for help and make some changes. Rehabilitation gives you more than just the therapy you need — it gives you the same skills that get you out into the community as you rebuild your life. It presents you with the tools you need to travel away from your home and out into your world.

In-home therapy is an option

If you're not able to find help in getting to your therapy sessions, you may need to make arrangements for the therapist to come to you — at least for the first few visits. However, in-home sessions pose problems of expense and

Range-of-motion therapy

If you have a weak arm or leg, then you've already been taught about the importance of range-of-motion therapy to avoid *contracture*. The muscles in the weak arm or leg will gradually shorten and tighten if you don't stretch them out fully several times (at least three times) per day. This is the absolute least you should demand of yourself every day. If you can't stretch every weak muscle out, then someone living with you needs to do it for you. If that's not possible, then you should probably be in a nursing home. Failure to do these range-of-motion exercises can result in a deformed arm or leg and decreased ability to walk or use the hand.

efficiency. The therapist's time is not well used when he or she is commuting to and from your home — and you may find you'll spend a lot of time coordinating, scheduling, and rescheduling appointments.

The important point is that you should not be coming home with the idea that you are just going to rest and recover. It will slow down your recovery if you don't start the treatment you need right away. Continue your therapy, either at an outpatient facility or in your own home.

Returning to Work

If your stroke was serious enough to put you in the hospital, then it's probably a bad idea to go from the hospital one day and back to your job the next. You may do it with no problem. On the other hand, your stroke can change you in ways you are not yet aware of, and you probably don't want to find that out in front of your boss or co-worker. The psychological and physical changes after a stroke are often not as apparent to the person with the stroke as they are to others. Test yourself. Spend some time with your family, make sure you can read as well as you used to, go up and down the stairs, and remember phone numbers or names of all the people at work.

Testing the waters slowly

Don't get me wrong. It is a good idea to get back to work. The movement, socialization, and discipline of old habits on the job are good for the recovering brain. But it's *better* to test how deep and warm the water is before diving in. Stick a toe in first — or you may find yourself drowning in a flood of work. You probably don't want to start too much and then have to back off.

Even if you have or soon will fully recover from your stroke, you may fatigue easily for the first few weeks or months after a brain injury. Consider returning to work on a limited schedule. You may try half days for a week, for example. Many patients are surprised how exhausted and tired they become after the first full day back on the job.

If you are limited in some ways, then you will have to negotiate some changes at work, either with special furniture or equipment or by a reassignment of duties. Some employers react differently than others and may be more or less able to accommodate your needs.

How well others accept your limitations will to a large extent depend on how well you accept them yourself. What little homily does this bring to mind? How about "Smile and the whole world smiles with you"?

Accepting job limitations

If the return to work is not going smoothly, you may need to evaluate changing your job duties and responsibilities. Most employers are willing to meet someone halfway if they are willing to make the extra effort to change or learn new skills. A lot of people define who they are by their job. This makes job change difficult. Employment counselors can work with you and your employer to adjust to these changes and create a work environment that's beneficial to all.

It's hard for me to say this, but depending on your age, this may be a good time to retire, especially if you were thinking about retiring before your stroke. If you had plans for travel — something you really wanted to do after you retired — then the time to do it may be now, while you can still get around and have the resources. If it makes you angry to read that, then I apologize. But if you would really rather be somewhere else while you are working, then you need to look into this.

You may have to work to survive, but you are different after your stroke and may be happier in a different type of job. Most people who were employed before their stroke are not employed a year after their stroke. To a large extent, this is because most people who have a stroke are older than 60. You may be set to retire, but have apprehension about giving up the security of a job. Take a breath and listen to your family and their concerns. Listen to those you live with. And watch yourself to be sure you are doing what you should to take care of your stroke. Again, are you taking your medicine every day? Are you getting to the rehabilitation center if that is recommended? (You aren't smoking again are you?) Are you sleeping well and making scheduled visits to your physician? Are you getting some exercise? If you are not doing the things you should, then your job may be getting in the way of your brain's recovery from stroke.

Driving

If you were used to driving yourself around before you had your stroke, you have to face the reality that you might be a risk to yourself and others. Another reality is that you may not be the best one to decide whether you should drive. In fact, you may have no doubts that you can drive and do it well. This could be the truth — in which a formal test should be no problem. Or it could be a result of the stroke that you don't recognize your own limitations. This is quite common. Whether you give them the opportunity or not, your family has a responsibility to you and others to keep you off the road if you might be dangerous.

I suggest that you not drive until you can pass a professional driving evaluation. Some states provide this through the state licensing agency. In others, you have to make your own arrangements.

Not driving can isolate you. You will have to depend on your caregiver or make adjustments to maintain your connections. It's a lot easier than dealing with the results of a bad automobile accident that you caused.

Get Organized and Motivated

I asked a nationally known expert in stroke rehabilitation what was important to make the best possible recovery from stroke. She had one piece of advice for a successful effort: "Get organized."

A psychologist I know once worked at a university. It fell to him to teach a course in study skills for students who had low grades. After a few sessions with them, it dawned on him that he should test them to see how much they already knew. He gave them a test and found out that almost all of the bad students knew what it took to be good students. It wasn't that they didn't know how to be good students. They just didn't do it.

Finding new ways to get organized

I don't know how to tell you the way to get yourself organized and to persist on the rehabilitation effort it will take to get the maximum recovery from your stroke. But I would guess that you already know how to do it. Writing down goals and making lists works for some people. Being competitive works for others. I suppose some people actually enjoy doing things the right way and doing what is recommended — you know, the people who read the directions on the soup can.

On the other hand, stroke can change your personality in subtle ways. You need to take stock of your new self and find a different approach toward getting the work of rehabilitation done. For starters, get inspired: Read some of the stories in the Part of Tens at the end of this book. George Frederik Handel moved to Germany from England and wrote his masterpiece "Messiah" while he was recovering from his stroke. I don't know how he found the strength to do this, but he did. And I'm glad he did.

Minding the basics

Did you take all your medication yesterday? Did you eat all your meals? Did you drink water between meals? If you have a weak arm or leg, did you do range-of-motion exercises yesterday? Did you make it to all your scheduled therapy sessions this week?

If you are having trouble keeping on target, I suggest you go back to the basics. I apologize for reminding you of what my psychologist friend would guess you already know. However, it may be worthwhile to jog your memory.

Rehabilitation works like any human enterprise. You are going to be much more successful if you have goals and lists and schedules of activities that will help you accomplish these goals. Will this be the time that you get a calendar, a pencil, a notebook, and a few sheets of paper and decide that you are going to be the good student? After all, this is not a class in geography or something else you doubt you will ever use. This is your brain. You can't give up on your brain.

 Write down what you want to accomplish in the rest of your life and what you need to do to get it done. Having a little more trouble remembering things? List your medications, the dosage, and how often you take them. Fill out schedules of doctors' visits and therapy sessions. Plan your day in the morning and follow the plan. A stroke may give you the opportunity to simplify your life in ways that you have thought about but postponed for years. And, of course, it helps to talk about these things with the people who live with you or help you.

Forming new habits: Give it 40 days

Hate lists? Hate schedules? Here's another approach you might take to give your brain a chance. *Not* doing things is actually a habit. How about changing that habit? I'm told you can form a habit of doing things in about 40 days. Some say more, some say fewer, but 40 days is a good estimate. If you can do something every day for 40 days, then it becomes a habit, and you don't need a list or a schedule or someone to remind you. It's just something you do. So pick a thing or two and start to form a habit. I suggest taking pills or doing range-of-motion exercises, because they are really important from the first day you return home. The more your stroke has changed you, the more new habits you will need.

Truth is, you will probably do some of the things, but it will be tough to do all of them every time. The more you do, the better your physical recovery will be, the easier you will adapt to your remaining limitations, the better your relationships with family and friends will be, and the quicker you will adjust to a fulfilling life after stroke.

Ready-made daily checklist

- ✔ Medications morning, noon, night
- ✔ Three square meals
- ✔ Three glasses of water
- ✔ Range of movement morning, noon, night
- ✔ Doctor appointments
- ✔ Laboratory test appointments
- ✔ Socialize outside the home
- ✔ Telephone calls
- ✔ Make a family connection
- ✔ Take a walk or get some exercise

Checklist for doctor's visit

- ✔ Check all your prescriptions. See if you need any renewals. Take list and pill bottles with you.
- ✔ Before the visit, make sure the doctor has the hospital reports and records from your stroke.
- ✔ Take any reports of tests or visits to specialists since your last visit to this doctor.
- ✔ Make a list of questions you have for your doctor.
- ✔ Ask about depression and other tough or embarrassing problems.
- ✔ Take a notepad and pencil and use it to remember what you are told.

Chapter 15

When You Can't Go Home Again

Some strokes are so severe that the patient can't return home. In these cases, the stroke victim isn't likely to be in a position to investigate alternatives, evaluate nursing homes, or even *make* the decision that a nursing home or assisted-living facility is the best choice. So in this chapter especially, the "you" I am speaking to includes the caretaker or loved one — an individual who has also suffered from the devastation of stroke.

When a stroke first happens, the medical care system steps in to help. As the hospitalization reaches the second or third day, that same system applies pressure to get the stroke patient *out* of the hospital — whether to an inpatient rehab facility, home, or nursing home or assisted living facility. Perhaps well before you have adjusted to this unexpected and traumatic event, you will be *encouraged* (to put it generously) to find another place for the stroke victim in short order — whether or not your family is emotionally or financially ready.

This encouragement is well meant. You will almost always find the hospital personnel to be concerned for your welfare. They know, however, that few families are ready to deal with a serious stroke disability. Without some gentle pressure, most families would delay or postpone making important decisions.

Whether through the recommendations of the doctors who are attending to the stroke patient or through the realization that you are ill-equipped to provide the necessary care at home, a nursing home or assisted living facility is an option that *must* be considered whenever a stroke causes significant disability.

In this chapter, I aim to guide you through the difficult process of deciding whether a care facility is the right choice, gathering the resources to fund that choice, and finding the right place for your loved one.

Within a matter of days of admission to the hospital, you will receive a clear message that the hospital wants the patient out as soon as he or she is medically stable. The family must make important decisions rapidly. Rehab? Home? Nursing facility? Whatever the eventual outcome, at this early point you should advocate for the most rehabilitation now. Scrutinize your health-insurance benefits plan and argue for the best and longest coverage possible.

Coming to Grips with Your Situation

"Why can't we just go home?"

This question often arises from the stroke sufferer, who may be confused, frustrated, frightened, and desperate for a return to life before stroke. It is an equally painful moment for family members, who are likely grappling with similar feelings of fear, confusion, and uncertainty.

Promises and guilt

You may feel bound by a promise made long ago to take care of your loved one at home if he or she ever became incapacitated. But how could you have imagined that this would mean assisting with nearly everything, including bathing, dressing, and using the toilet? Caring for someone with brain injury is a full-time job — one that would be difficult work for someone who is young and energetic and head-over-heels in love. If you are now 72 years old and have your own medical problems, it may well be a psychological and physical impossibility to take good care of your disabled spouse.

Stroke makes it even harder because in many cases the sufferer is affected in ways that only a close family member can recognize. Emotions are changed; personality is affected. Some family members say it's as if they're living with a stranger. The stroke victim may be more difficult to manage — perhaps headstrong, emotional, or depressed.

Keeping the spirit of your promise

When you promised never to put your spouse in a nursing home, what you meant was that you wouldn't just walk away in a time of need. You meant that your love would be constant and you would care for your spouse in the best way possible. Truth is, a nursing home or assisted-living facility may be essential if you are going to live up to *what you meant* when you made your promise. Any doctor can tell you about cases in which the lives of both caretaker and stroke survivor are threatened by the stress of attending to a seriously ill spouse.

Remember when your children promised they would feed the puppy every day if you would let them keep it? Or how much more difficult having a new baby in your lives turned out to be than you even suspected — that half the stress was simply dealing with a being who couldn't listen to reason or follow your schedule? Now, imagine that your baby is as big as you and will be with you for the rest of your life. If you're dealing with a spouse with brain injury, you don't have to imagine.

Nursing home: Often the most loving decision

If the stroke victim is severely *aphasic* (language problems), has difficulty getting out of bed, and suffers from incontinence, poor memory, or dementia, the safest, most loving place may be a care facility with experienced staff. Similarly, the amenities of assisted living can maximize the independence of some people who have less severe disabilities. Nursing homes are expensive because caring for a disabled stroke patient takes a lot of psychological and physical effort — beyond the capability of many adults. It concerns me that too many stroke sufferers are cared for at home because the cost of nursing home care is so high.

Getting Your Game Plan Together

As I write this book, I try to put myself in the places of the stroke victim *and* family members. I keep running into a lot of emotional and philosophical hurdles. The resources available for stroke care are limited compared to the need. A couple's life savings can be consumed in a few months. The strain placed on a relationship can be almost unbearable. Adult children find their lives turned upside down as they confront a new relationship with a parent who needs their care.

I have struggled with these challenges in my own family. I wonder if I could be doing better as I balance the needs of my own life, my children's interests, and a parent in a nursing home. And like many in this situation, I wrestle with "if onlys." If only the illness hadn't happened. If only there was a cure. If only I had known this would happen.

Eventually, though, you and I have to put aside all thoughts about how things *could* be or *should* be and deal with how things *are*. So for the rest of this

Hiring a care manager

If you feel incapable of assessing your loved one's needs, analyzing your resources, and deciding on a care facility, then consider hiring a care manager to help you navigate the process. A care manager can research your options, determine what you can afford, help find financial aid if that's necessary, and facilitate communication among family members.

A good care manager looks for resources and works with the family to reach a consensus on what can be done. Care managers are not just for the wealthy, as they often offer advice that optimizes limited resources. They can be paid by the hour and will work with hospital social workers to find the best options for each family. A good care manager knows where the system is flexible and helps you get the most for your dollar. This is like hiring someone to do your taxes for you — the service may well pay for itself. Care managers are not regulated, so be sure to get one who has good references.

chapter I will assume that you have realized you can't change the medical care system fast enough to meet your needs. You can't go back and buy insurance you don't have now or save money you haven't saved. Just accept where you are right now and deal with that. To survive these overwhelming challenges — and you will survive them — it's critical to get your game plan together. Because each situation is so unique, I can't map out that plan for you in all its detail. I can only give you some tips and suggest some general strategies.

Deciding to put a loved one in a nursing home is no small problem. Especially on top of the overwhelming trauma you've just experienced. It is an effort that you may have to manage on your own — and you *can* do it.

With a severe disability you have a *big* problem. The best way to solve a big problem is to break it down into small problems and solve them in turn. Here's how I suggest approaching the problem of where to live after a severe stroke:

✔ Define your care needs.

✔ Determine your resources.

✔ Choose the facility that best meets your needs *and* resources.

Defining Your Care Needs

Does your loved one need nursing-home care? Evaluations from hospital staff are helpful in determining this. You want to get a clear understanding about the brain injury suffered and the likelihood of rehabilitation. After you understand the expectations for the stroke patient, then ask the hard questions: Does this mean my husband can't bathe himself? Will I have to feed my wife? Will my spouse need close attention while I'm at work every day?

Incontinence and inability to eat, walk, or get up from a bed or a chair are just some of the physical limitations you might anticipate. Depression, anger, and frustration are behavior problems that predict things won't go well at home. Stroke can make a person impossible to manage because of angry outbursts, refusal to cooperate, or overwhelming despondency.

Once you understand the limitations your family member is likely to experience, then you want to anticipate which situations you can handle — and which you can't. Are you capable of getting your husband in and out of the shower? Will you be able to prepare meals and feed your wife three times a day? Are you prepared to attend to the most intimate and personal needs of your parent?

Sometimes a nursing home is a temporary or transitional alternative before a return home. Some stroke sufferers need a little more time to regain their strength or benefit from additional therapy. A short-term nursing-home stay may also allow the family to prepare the home for the patient's return.

It helps to list these situations and rank them in order of your comfort level with attending to them. You might have a few rankings, ranging from "No assistance needed" to "Impossible even with my help." Table 15-1 is one example of a helpful list and ranking system.

Table 15-1		Worksheet for Determining Care Needs				
Type of Activity	Needs No Help	I Can Help	Difficult	Impossible	Home	Care Facility
Get out of bed			X			X
Move to bathroom		X			X	
Urinate		X			X	
Bowel move- ment				X		X
Wash, shave, comb	X				X	

(continued)

Table 15-1 *(continued)*

Type of Activity	Needs No Help	I Can Help	Difficult	Impossible	Home	Care Facility
Take shower or bath			X			X
Get dressed			X		X	
Move to eating area	X				X	
Prepare food	X				X	
Feed self	X				X	
Use telephone	X				X	
Move to car				X		X
Get in/ out of car				X		X
Get to doctor's office				X		X
Range of motion exercise	X				X	

Go over the list of situations in Table 15-1 and consider the four scenarios offered in the first four columns: First, the stroke patient is capable of this activity and doesn't need help. Second, the patient may need help, but you feel comfortable helping. Third, you know you'd have to help, but would be very taxing on you. Fourth, you know you *couldn't* manage this.

Fill in these boxes with checks, then move to the final two columns and put an X under "Home" or "Care Facility." For each row, if you put an X in the "No Help Needed" or "I Can Help" categories, then place an X under "Home." If you checked "Difficult" or "Impossible," you probably want to put an X under "Care Facility."

Tally up the results when you're done — and you will have a pretty good idea whether your loved one will be better off in a care facility. A single X in the last column might be enough to make the decision for you. If you have three or four Xs under "Care Facility," there may really be no choice for anyone.

In some situations, the choice may not be that clear. There may be financial issues (which I address in the next section). The caretaker may also need money or retirement benefits to survive. Here are some other considerations.

Plan for today's needs

Don't make inadequate plans hoping the stroke patient will get significantly better. Plan for things staying the way they are. Accept the prognosis from your doctors, nurses, and therapists regarding your loved one's limitations. They may be wrong, but they have more experience than you do.

They are not likely to be overstating the problem. Doctors, particularly, may be overly optimistic. Perhaps this is because they don't want you to give up and refuse treatments that will help.

Allow for changing needs

Avoid long-range commitments at first. Stroke disabilities *do* usually improve somewhat over time, but stroke patients also suffer brain injuries that may not become apparent until the patient is out of the hospital. Serious problems with thinking and controlling emotions can be overlooked or attributed to being away from home. Patients often have other medical problems that may get worse after a stroke. Most changes occur in the first months after leaving the hospital. Year-long commitments to a particular residence or program may not be flexible enough to meet your changing needs.

Include caregiver priorities

The patient isn't the only one disabled by the stroke. The primary caretaker and the whole family may find their time and energies diverted into coping with the stroke. It's like waking up one day and the grocery store is gone. Either you hire someone who knows how to raise a garden, or you have to grow your own food — even if no one ever taught you how. Of course, other family members may want to help, but the primary caregiver may have other priorities that mustn't be neglected. This could be raising children who are still home, for example, or maintaining your employment. Caregiver priorities also belong on the list of considerations — and quite high up.

Determining Your Resources

Nursing and assisted-living facilities cost money, ringing up somewhere between $54,000 and $90,000 a year. And that's not including medications and treatments. Don't waste time pondering choices you don't have. *Wanting* to do something is a lot different then *being able* to do it. You've identified the critical services you need, and now your goal is to determine your available resources. This boils down to what you can afford using insurance, disability, savings, Social Security benefits, Medicare, or other income.

The person who has always managed the family finances may be the person in the hospital bed. That means *you* have to go through unfamiliar files and bank records at home to find all the possible resources. It also means that you may have to take control of something you have never dealt with before.

Make a list of assets

To the list of care needs you made, add another sheet of paper to your clipboard and start listing all the financial resources that could fund the patient's care. Get it all down — from your insurance benefits to retirement funds to savings accounts.

The hospital social worker is a valuable source of information regarding financial possibilities you may not be aware of (see nearby sidebar for more). A good social worker can usually size things up in a few minutes by looking at the doctor's notes and seeing the condition of the patient. Take this as your starting point. Go over your clipboard's list of needs with him or her.

You may need to do some homework. Do you understand all the intricacies of your private insurance? Do you have a long-term care plan that covers nursing home care? If so, does it cover all costs or only a percentage? Does it stipulate a minimum- or maximum-length stay? Are there other limitations and criteria? If Medicare is on your list, are you sure you are eligible? Do you understand what it covers and what you are expected to pay for?

Medicare is a government program that provides health care for individuals 65 and older, as well as for individuals with certain disabilities. But it doesn't cover all types of medical services, nor does it cover qualified services at

---

Social workers are valuable resources

The role of the hospital social worker is to help families navigate through the complex medical care system — from assessing what insurance will cover to finding workable solutions to finance shortfalls. A good social worker is intimately familiar with the resources available — from rehab centers to nursing home facilities — and the best ways to access them.

Hospital social workers are overworked these days, so you want to maximize the few minutes you may have with them. Have as much of your homework done ahead of time — gather all the information about your loved one's needs and the resources you have and provide it for them. Prepare questions. Take notes. Then go over your notes at the bedside while your loved one is asleep or off getting a test. Prepare more questions. The more answers you can gather from your social worker *before* you leave the hospital, the better. If your social worker is inexperienced or unhelpful, ask for another one. Most hospitals employ more than one.

---

100 percent cost. As of this writing, Medicare covers nursing home costs for 20 days, once you pay the deductible (in 2005, the deductible is $912) and if your case meets certain criteria. For the next 80 days of nursing home stay, Medicare covers a percentage, but you pay a coinsurance fee. According to www.medicare.gov, coinsurance is $114 a day in 2005.

When you can't afford the care you need

If you're fortunate, your research will reveal that you and your spouse have the resources to fund the needed care. Perhaps you wisely purchased a long-term disability policy that offers maximum coverage for nursing-home care. Maybe you have a very healthy retirement plan that will support your current lifestyle and care for your spouse as well.

You're lucky. More often than not, a severe stroke and its outcome can quickly and easily deplete any and all resources. When you finish evaluating your financial status, you may find that although you have some resources, you can't afford the level of care that you've determined is necessary — for as long as you're likely to need it. Should you give up, then? Assume you'll have to handle the care in your home? Not necessarily. You just have to be more resourceful.

Managing on your own

The fewer resources you have, the more you must do on your own. If you can't afford to hire a care manager (be sure to look into it because with all their advice they can pay for themselves sometimes), you or someone in the family will learn how to wade through all the Social Security claims, insurance programs, and medical bills. You'll become adept at cajoling, demanding, and reading a lot of fine print. On your own means a lot of research, connecting with other patients, spending hours on the telephone, and making countless trips to different institutions.

On your own may also mean reducing your expectations from "would likes" to "must haves." Where is the *best* place to invest your limited resources? Maybe instead of placing your loved one in the nursing home permanently, you arrange for a few months in the facility until you learn how to take care of your spouse at home or arrange to have another relative come to help you.

Medicaid is a government program for low-income people. It pays for some health services, including long-term nursing home care. Medicaid eligibility and coverage is state-based and varies from state to state. To be eligible for Medicaid, you basically have to be depleted of all your assets. I hope you don't have to consider this sort of help, but be aware that it exists. For more information about Medicaid, visit the Web site at www.cms.hhs.gov.

Asking for and accepting help

Accept help from anywhere and anyone. I'm not just talking about financial help, but informational and emotional support as well. You may get financial advice from a neighbor who is an accountant. Or an adult child has a healthier investment portfolio than you'd imagined. Overcome the tendency to keep the stroke private. Spread the news about the problems you are dealing with. You will get more help than you expect.

Stroke support groups

Find out about stroke support groups. Going to meetings is good, but even a phone call can connect you with other stroke caretakers who have faced similar challenges. You can get advice about nursing homes, special programs in your city or state, and tips about what to do and how not to waste time or money. Social workers or nurse care managers can connect you to stroke support groups.

An inadequate system

The realities of chronic long-term care for the disabled are grim indeed. Medical insurance and social-welfare programs do not provide enough resources to care for all those whose brains are injured by stroke. The programs cannot always accommodate those with unusually severe financial or medical problems.

To complicate matters further, many eligibility standards for such programs emphasize the physical impairments of mobility and employability. In stroke, a major portion of the disability involves the patient's inability to communicate, think, and control emotions. Many stroke patients develop a form of *dementia* (see Chapter 7). These "mental" changes often do not qualify for coverage or care in a nursing home or assisted living facility.

Making the best of a bad situation

Here's the bottom line: The medical care system struggles to spread a few resources among a huge number of people with needs far beyond its capability. The last thing you as family members want to do is blame each other for the inadequacies of the system. That only adds to the difficulties. It's not you — it's the system. You have to look out for yourselves. My best advice is to do all you can to understand the system in all its complexity so that you can take advantage of every possible bit of help.

And having learned first-hand of this really difficult situation that many if not most of us will face in our lifetime, you might ask, "Isn't it our responsibility to demand that our society do a better, fairer job of addressing this problem in the future?" I think you might be right. Getting involved in healthcare reform can help you feel good that you are helping better things for everyone.

Considering Nursing-Home Care

A skilled nursing facility offers complete care. Such places are set up to handle patients who are bedridden and require 24-hour assistance. Skilled nursing facilities are carefully regulated by the states. Many are certified for Medicare and Medicaid.

Whether you're anticipating a short stay or a permanent placement in a nursing home, the search for the best facility is important. The care and well-being of a loved one is at stake, and there are many factors to consider — from location to cost to quality of the professionals who work there.

Visit any nursing home you are considering. For an apples-to-apples comparison, it's important to gather the same information about each nursing home. I like lists (can't you tell?). Make a list of the factors you are comparing: cost, staffing, food, location, and the like. Take your list with you. And ask lots of questions of the staff persons you meet. Don't be shy — they're not going to volunteer their shortcomings.

Investigating costs

The cost of nursing-home care runs about $150 to $250 dollars a day. That's $4,500 to $7,500 per month. That doesn't include the cost of medications, which are added to the bill. There are different cost levels depending on the work required for the nurses and aides. Check whether you're locked into a minimum stay. Also, verify whether the facilities are Medicare or Medicaid certified if that's important to your needs.

Location, location, location

Choosing a nursing home that is accessible to family is important. For the stroke patient who's lived alone and far from family, it may mean moving to another city or state to be near children who can visit regularly. For others, it may mean selecting a facility that is within a short drive of a spouse for daily visits.

Also, keep in mind that the stroke patient may be back in the hospital or emergency room more than once or twice a year. In that case, you'll also want to consider the distance between the nursing home and a preferred hospital. And if you plan to retain a particular stroke specialist and anticipate the need for frequent office visits, then proximity to the doctor's office is a consideration. (See if your specialist works with a particular nursing home, possibly even making "house calls" to that facility.)

Meeting the medical and professional staff

Ask how often the nursing-home doctor sees the patients. Find out that physician's specialty. If you can, try to meet the doctor. Ask families of patients about the doctor. How easy is it for the family to meet with the doctor?

Nurses are also a critical consideration. You absolutely must talk to someone on the nursing staff during your exploratory process. A stroke patient is bound to have a number of medical problems. It's a given that doctor visits will be much less frequent than contact with nurses — so you want the most knowledgeable nurses possible on staff. If different nurses are on shift every day, it becomes very hard to monitor changes in a patient's condition. (For example, they may not recognize that a patient has had a second stroke if they haven't been on shift for the past week.) Are the nurses trained in the needs of stroke patients? Do they know the importance of range-of-motion exercises needed to keep paralyzed limbs flexible and braces to increase mobility and prevent muscle atrophy?

Some stroke patients require regular physical therapy. Find out if physical and occupational therapies are part of the program. Ask about additional cost. Meet with the therapists on staff if you can.

Don't overlook the nonmedical staff at the nursing homes. The aides and assistants who attend to the residents play an important role in their welfare. Staffing is a difficult problem for most facilities. The for-profit nursing homes tend to have tighter management but may hire less qualified aides or be understaffed.

Be sure to meet with or at least observe the aides and support staff as they interact with patients. Do they seem caring, compassionate, and attentive? As they walk through the halls, do they greet and talk to patients? Do they listen and show respect? Or do they seem frazzled and irritated?

Sizing up the place

Quality of care is, of course, the most important consideration when choosing the right nursing facility. But other factors carry a lot of weight, too. A thorough visit to each facility will help you size up the place. Be sure to investigate the following:

- **Food:** Institutional food is easy to complain about, but there are different levels of quality. Check that the menu offers variety — or that it at least serves choices that the stroke patient finds appetizing. Are there alternatives if the patient has dietary restrictions beyond the basic medical prescriptions? (Are there vegetarian options, for example?) Visit during mealtime and even taste the food, if you can. Remember, though, you're in a nursing home — not an upscale restaurant. Make sure your expectations are realistic.

- **Cleanliness:** Scrutinize the hallways and common rooms, the dining room, the bathrooms. Check out a private room or two. Do floors and fixtures appear to be scrubbed regularly? Does the facility *smell* clean? Do you see maintenance staff emptying trash cans before they overflow?

- **Rules:** Find out the rules and times for visiting. Can you visit any time, day or night? Flexibility and a liberal visitation policy may be important to family members who work or live some distance away. Limited visiting hours could prove unworkable. Ask about regulations on patient activity, as well. Excessively restrictive policies, such as curfews, bedtimes, dining hours, and more could prove frustrating to a resident with greater abilities and independence.

- **Care-planning meetings:** Find out how often care-planning meetings are held and whether your family members can arrange to attend.

- **Complaints:** How are problems resolved? Most nursing homes must list formal complaints and make them available for review.

- **The social scene:** If the stroke patient's thinking is fine — and even if it isn't — chances are that the social climate will have some importance in a successful transition to nursing-home life. Are there other stroke patients at the facility? Are there opportunities that bring residents together for some social activity — whether simply watching a movie or gathering for a celebration?

Getting a second opinion

Before signing on the dotted line, check with your area's regional support center of the government Administration on Aging (visit www.aoa.gov to find how to contact your support center). This agency has an ombudsman office where you can get help and advice about nursing homes in the area. Call to find out if there are any specific complaints registered against the facility.

You can also talk to other residents and their families. Ask questions of the other families you see visiting patients. Often they will sit in a lounge or outside in the sun with their family member. Approach them about problems, the friendliness of the staff, what they would change, and anything else that seems important to you.

Evaluating Assisted-Living Facilities

Assisted-living facilities go by a number of different names: *personal-care homes, adult homes, retirement residences,* and *group homes,* to name a few. Such places are for those who can't live independently but who don't require daily *nursing* care. These facilities may offer help with bathing, dressing, meals, and housekeeping. They also offer a safe environment for individuals who are beginning to lose their memory.

Assisted-living centers may offer more than nursing homes in the way of a social life for their residents, though they still provide nursing care and staff to help with medication and monitor conditions such as stroke and diabetes. They may not be as tightly regulated as nursing homes, so there may be greater disparity in quality of services and facility. A careful inspection is equally important when considering an assisted-living facility — to be sure your needs match with their services.

Just as with a nursing home, you want to devote the same careful attention to the quality of the medical services and the experience of the staff. Compare feedback from residents and families about their experiences. Examine the facility for cleanliness. Chat with the staff and observe how they interact with residents. Visit the dining room. (See previous section on nursing homes for what to check for.) There are differences.

Cost is still significant

Assisted living is a lot like renting an apartment. The rent varies based on location and convenience, as well as on the quality of the services. You might pay $2,500 to $5,000 per month, depending on what you get. It is important to keep your focus on your prioritized list of needs. One place can cost a lot more because it has good staff with low turnover and good credentials.

Another may cost more because of the fine-quality furniture and gourmet food. Medications, medical services, special group outings, and activities may add to costs. Be sure you understand what is included in the basic fees.

Transportation to appointments

Unlike a nursing home, an assisted-living facility doesn't provide around-the-clock medical attention and a 24-hour professional staff. Residents likely have medical appointments and therapy sessions offsite. A stroke patient will certainly need to visit doctors and physical therapists regularly. Find out whether the facility offers a driving service to get residents to appointments or arranges for therapy sessions on site. Ask about costs for these services — if not, be sure it's realistic for a family member to serve as chauffeur.

A community as well as a home

More so than nursing homes, assisted-living facilities promote themselves as *communities*. This aspect is more critical to the well-being or recovery of a stroke patient than the colors of the curtains and the furniture in the lobby. A major problem with stroke is depression and withdrawal. An attractive social program may get the patient to interact with others.

Ask about eating arrangements — they can vary widely. Some facilities provide small cooking areas where residents can prepare one or more meals per day. Most provide three meals per day in a dining room — another opportunity for social interaction.

Check out the rules, which can be surprising for those not used to communal living. In a small community, everyone has to agree to rules of behavior.

Dealing with the bad stuff

Because assisted-living facilities are not closely regulated, it is harder to discover problems, and resolving them is not as easy. You should at least ask about the process for resolving complaints and working out ways to meet special needs that aren't currently anticipated. This is one thing you should definitely talk to others at the facility and their family members about.

Life in a New "Home"

Adjusting to life in a nursing home or even an assisted-living facility is a challenge. For the stroke survivor, it may mean withdrawal and a dip into depression. For the spouse waking up to an empty house every morning, it may mean feelings of guilt and the burden of daily visits.

It is crucial to make progress toward recovery from stroke during the early days. It is the rare stroke survivor who actively seeks out treatment and strives to do more each day. The family member can also play an important role, serving as advocate for the resident on a daily basis. Try to visit once a day for at least the first two weeks of your loved one's stay.

Getting to know the nursing staff

You can assume most good nurses are thinking about quitting. These facilities demand a lot. The nurses are often overworked. The few times you may see them at the station, they may be catching up on paperwork. When you visit, find out who is on duty — it may not be the person at the station, but the individual down the hall.

Understanding the pressures of the nursing staff helps you utilize their skills and expertise to your loved one's advantage. Nurses cannot wait hand and foot on you and your family. They give medications, monitor vital signs, and test blood glucose in diabetics. They check for bed sores and make sure patients are eating and drinking. Too many patients and family members assume that the staff is there to resolve the patient's dissatisfaction with the dinner entrée or fix the television reception.

Make it your goal to get to know all of the staff by name — especially the evening and night staff. For stroke patients, most bad things happen at night or early in the morning. You want to do everything possible to be sure that the staff gets to know your loved one so that any changes can be noted.

I recommend taking pictures of the staff with your digital camera. Print them and tape them on the wall in the patient's room, writing the staff names on each. This way you get to know the staff, and it lets them know you think they are important. While you're at it, put up pictures of you, the patient, and family members, too. The staff can use these as conversation starters for an otherwise withdrawn or uncooperative stroke patient.

Keep two phone numbers with you at all times: the numbers of the nursing station and the stroke patient's room. They can save a life. I suggest calling both of the phones from your cell phone while you are visiting in the nursing home. That way, you can hear the phones ring, see who answers, and have a picture in your mind of what is happening when you call from your home or office. You don't want the office number that rings in the manager's suite. You want the number for the nurse who is on duty during the day and night.

Don't abuse the nursing station number, though. Until you establish a degree of comfort with the staff, use it only when you have important medical concerns.

When problems arise

Your loved one reports that the nurse didn't bring medication on time. Maybe it's something more personal — perhaps the patient had an accident because no one was available to assist with getting to the bathroom. You're upset, of course, and you head for the nurses' station to find out what's going on.

Take a deep breath. If you're angry, wait until you are calm. You don't need two strokes in the family. *Then* try to talk with that staff member before you complain to a supervisor. Listen to the person. I have seen that stroke survivors can easily get mixed up or perceive the situation in the entirely wrong way. Even if the complaint is legitimate, you're unlikely to do your loved one any service if you scream, yell, and threaten the nurse in question. Conveying that you are a reasonable and understanding individual who is proactively looking out for your loved one will go a lot further in establishing the best care.

Advocating for the stroke patient

It takes a lot of time and energy to visit a nursing home. Your visit can produce a number of benefits, though. First, it brightens your loved one's day. Second, it can help you to evaluate and improve the care your stroke survivor is receiving.

Asking the stroke patient what is going on in the nursing home is not the best approach, however. By communicating that you are expecting problems, you may create them. Instead, do your "checking up" with the staff. That doesn't mean you shouldn't keep your ears open to any new or unusual problems. But listen to complaints about the food and the slow response of the staff patiently, as you would listen to complaints about the weather — something you really have no control over.

Watch out for bed sores and bruises

You do need to check the patient's physical condition to be sure there are no bed sores or serious scrapes or bruises. Look for indications of falls or other injuries. Ask about anything that seems unusual. However, you have to use some judgment. Someone who is disabled is naturally more prone to bumps and falls that can't always be prevented. And many stroke patients are on aspirin and therefore bruise more easily.

You may be uncomfortable checking out your loved one's backside, but insist and do it regularly. This is especially important in cases of weakness or numbness on one side. A patient may be left sitting in the same position for hours. With a stroke-numbed side, the individual may not feel the discomfort of pressure and fail to move or adjust. Pressure sores are the dangerous result.

Keep tabs on medications and changes

Find out what medications are being given and when. Double-check this with the information you received at the hospital and confirmed with your physician. Almost all stroke patients should receive treatment to lower blood pressure. Patients who suffered a white type of stroke (see Chapter 3) should be on aspirin or an equivalent drug to reduce the risk of blood clots. Blood lipids should be controlled with medication in many patients.

The nursing-home doctor may have a different approach to stroke prevention or managing other diseases. This difference may be an improvement in care. However, you should understand why any changes are made.

If you have medical power of attorney, you can arrange to be notified whenever any medical care or medication change is advised.

Vary your visiting time

Time your visits so you can get to know *all* the staff. If you have a predictable time to come, the staff will help your stroke survivor get ready. However, an unexpected visit in the morning or later in the evening may give you more insight into what is really going on. Also, visiting at different hours keeps the staff on their toes.

As you get to know the staff, ask them about any problems or things that are needed. This gives you important information and will keep them alert and observing, wanting to have something to say the next time you see them.

Monitor therapy

Be *sure* therapy is being given. Therapists may come in the door, try to interact with the patient, and be rebuffed. Your gentle stroke survivor may be belligerent and refuse treatment when you are not around. Ask the nurse to read the notes or call the therapists to be sure they are getting the cooperation they need. You can see for yourself if lack of therapy is a concern. Check out weak or paralyzed arms and legs — can you move the joints through their full range? Do this every time you see the patient. If the muscles tighten up, serious and painful deformities can develop in a very short time.

Chapter 16

Challenges During Recovery

. . . .

In This Chapter

▶ Understanding muscle spasticity

▶ Handling depression and psychological changes

▶ Adapting to driving limitations

▶ Dealing with incontinence

▶ Managing swallowing difficulties

. . . .

*P*aralysis. Speech and language impairment (aphasia). Difficulty walking. Loss of memory. As if the major insults caused by stroke weren't enough, it often results in related challenges for the victim. Challenges that make the recovery and adjustment processes all the more frustrating.

Take driving, for example. You may have diligently adhered to your physical therapy and recovered some use of your affected arm and leg. You may now be able to walk and move unattended — yet when it comes to getting behind the wheel, you still can't quite drive safely.

In this chapter, I focus on some of the issues that make recovery or adjustment to life with stroke just a little more of a challenge: painful muscle spasms and contractures, driving limitations, depression and other psychological conditions, swallowing difficulties, and incontinence.

Taken together, the problems from a stroke can be frustrating and at times overwhelming. If you can find the emotional strength to confront them one by one — the divide and conquer approach — you will discover that they are indeed conquerable. You can take steps to make a difference and find community resources for help with even the most difficult challenges.

Muscle Spasticity

Perhaps you've seen stroke victims with an arm bent at the elbow, the wrist pulled in and the fingers forming a clenched fist. Even several months after a stroke, this may be the normal resting position of the hand. Maybe *you* are the survivor of the stroke and you've experienced this, or you've noticed your leg bouncing up and down with absolutely no input from you.

Sometimes stroke survivors develop a condition known as muscle *spasticity*. It typically kicks in several months after the stroke and affects approximately 20 percent of stroke patients. What happens is this: Muscles that are weak become tense and contract abnormally, resulting in severe and painful spasms. Spasticity does not seem to be related to severity of stroke.

With stroke and muscles, you are likely to think more of paralysis than of overactive muscles. But overactivity is exactly what is happening with spasticity. Here's what's going on: Say you're at the doctor, and she taps your knee tendon with her hammer. Nerves from the tendon carry electrical signals to the spinal cord. A normal brain receives these signals and reduces the speed and strength of the built-in rate of the electrical activity transferred back to the muscles. So, when you feel the hammer's tap on your knee (at a certain location on your tendon), your muscles move your leg in a slow and smooth manner. With an injury to the brain, your spinal cord is in charge. Instead of a smooth and controlled kick of your leg, the leg jerks rapidly and can swing widely. This isn't a good excuse for kicking your neurologist. You are likely to become hyper-reflexic in your weak arm and leg.

Injured brain and uncontrolled muscles

If a brain has been damaged by stroke, it may not be communicating correctly with the muscles. Muscles are still wired into the spinal cord, so there are still reflexes, but they are not *controlled* — as before — by the brain. Instead, signals are immediately transferred to the nerves near the muscles, and they react vigorously, out of control. In other words, spasticity occurs when your reflexes get out of control.

It doesn't take a doctor's reflex hammer to cause a spastic reaction — the touch of a hand, a brush against furniture, constant contact with clothing, even an ingrown toenail or bladder infection can be enough to stimulate the muscles and cause spasms. The result is increased tension in all muscles, which inevitably can interfere with walking, hand movement, even talking.

It may surprise you to hear that spasticity is a condition of *increased* muscle tone. Now, increased muscle tone — as those of you who work out with weights appreciate — isn't bad, even for the stroke survivor. Tight muscles may keep an injured leg straight and help someone walk.

But the tight muscles associated with spasticity can be painful and disabling. The sensation of spasticity is not unlike those "charlie horse" spasms that have sent many of us into painful hopping antics as we try to stretch and relax the muscle. With spasticity, these painful spasms are more frequent and harder to control.

An arm that has spasticity will be hard to bend back and forth. Because of increased muscle tone, the muscles resist any movement. Usually either the set of muscles that retract a limb or extend it win out over the opposite set, and without stretching and exercise, the arms, for example, may be pulled into a flexed, curled-up position. The legs tend to extend straight.

Contractures: When muscles "freeze"

Serious problems can develop when muscles become frozen in position and can't be straightened out. These rigid muscles are called *contractures.* Unless a person *diligently* stretches out these tight muscles, sometimes against a lot of resistance, they may become frozen in unusual postures. A paralyzed hand tightened into a ball and an elbow and shoulder pulled against the body make proper hygiene a challenge. The crevices and spaces created by the deformed postures are difficult to keep clean, leading possibly to infection and injury to skin and bones. And, obviously, it can be painful.

Recognizing and treating spasticity

Spasticity — uncontrolled, violent muscle movement caused by brain injury — can cause a host of symptoms for the stroke survivor:

- ✔ Stiffened, "frozen" joints that are difficult to move, making even simple tasks a chore, especially those that require fine movements

- ✔ Uncontrollable and painful muscle spasms that can interfere with sleep

- ✔ Problems with walking, legs crossing uncontrollably

- ✔ Exhaustion from extra effort to walk, move, and undertake most tasks

- ✔ Deformed limbs that can restrict movement and create hygiene challenges, leading to bed sores and serious infections

In the final assessment, spasticity can make someone more dependent. The inability to control muscles can make everyday activities difficult, from dressing to grooming, from writing to eating. This often means relying on others and further loss of independent living. Muscle spasms tend to occur at night, meaning spasticity can interfere with sleeping.

The disability from spasticity creates emotional effects as well. Because it can affect your appearance and, by constricting throat muscles, even the sound of your voice, spasticity may make you more withdrawn and less will-ing to go out into the world. And that only aggravates the depression that so often follows stroke.

Treatments for spasticity are numerous, but let me warn you, some are extreme — and permanent . . . cutting or poisoning nerves so that tense mus-cles can relax, for example. You certainly don't want to use those options until you are *sure* that the benefits outweigh the risks, and all other treat-ments have failed. Spasticity treatments work to some extent and can help free up frozen or painful joints. Perhaps the best solution is a very careful combination of several treatments designed to fit your needs exactly.

Physical therapy

Physical therapy may be the most important step you can take to overcome spasticity. It involves working with a physical therapist who knows how to work your muscles so that they stay loose and controllable. Stretching is crit-ical to keeping your muscles flexible and at their full length. Physical thera-pists also work with you to strengthen your muscles. Strength becomes important as brain function begins to return — when muscle function returns, you want to be strong enough to do some work.

Therapists teach you important exercises so that you can do them *on your own.* You're unlikely to be in a situation in which you can work with a thera-pist two or more times a day — the minimum amount of time necessary to maintain flexibility. You must do this yourself, perhaps with the assistance of a friend or family member.

Wearing braces or splints

Braces and elastic splints can keep muscle contractures from forming and help stretch out muscles. One of the most common braces is a *footdrop brace* that keeps the ankle flexible by preventing the calf muscle from overpowering the muscles that bend the ankle. Of course, you have to actually *wear* the braces regularly for them to work. Follow the instructions, and you will pre-vent deformity and pain. If you already suffer from contractures of muscles, braces can help reverse the deformity.

Controlling the reflexes that start spasms

You can avoid spasms to some extent by avoiding stimuli that set off the reflexes in the first place. Tight clothing, a bladder infection, or resting a limb on a hard edge can start a spasm.

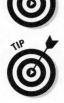

When you have a spasm, see if you can determine what stimulus caused it. If you can do that, then you can reduce the spasms by eliminating the stimulus that causes them.

If you get really good, you can *use* spasticity by setting off muscle spasms at the right time and using their force to help move yourself. Sometimes you can shorten muscle spasms by bearing down on the leg or arm that is in spasm by pushing down with your hand or foot either on the floor or on a table. Ask your physical therapist for more ideas about using such a technique in your particular case.

Controlling spasticity with drugs

Four drugs are used to reduce spasticity, each with side effects and drawbacks that you should consider before taking. Some are very addictive. All must be followed carefully without changing the dosage or stopping suddenly without a physician's guidance. You may need to get blood tests in order to ensure that you can safely take them.

Baclofen

Baclofen (Liorisal) often helps reduce painful muscle spasms by loosening muscles so they move more easily and stretch farther. Baclofen has some side effects: fatigue, drowsiness, mental confusion, and lightheadedness, and these are further aggravated if you drink alcohol while taking baclofen. With higher doses, your muscles may seem weaker and too loose and floppy. Work with your doctor to adjust the dosage so it works best for you.

Don't stop taking baclofen suddenly — or you may experience serious side effects, ranging from stiff muscles to increased and more painful spasms — even seizures.

Diazepam (Valium) and clonazepam (Rivotril)

These are both in an addictive class of drugs called benzodiazepines. They relax the muscles and they have multiple uses, from relieving anxiety to stopping epileptic seizures. If they work well for you, you may notice fewer muscle spasms and greater ability to straighten your arm or bend your knee. Your muscles may feel loose and more relaxed. As a matter of fact, you may feel pretty relaxed yourself. You may sleep more and experience lower blood pressure. You may also feel a little "hung over" and unsteady. The muscle relaxation may come at the expense of a loss of strength.

Sudden withdrawal from either drug can lead to epileptic seizures. Overdoses can stop you from breathing. And if that's not enough, they can turn off your memory. The fact that they can also upset your stomach seems like a minor problem at this point. Bottom line: Benzodiazepines are not advised for regular use and are best considered for special occasions when you may be anxious and you want your muscles to behave.

Dantrolene

Dantrolene changes the way muscles contract. It improves the range of movement of paralyzed muscles and decreases muscle tone, resulting in fewer painful spasms and looser muscles. Dantrolene also causes dizziness and drowsiness, not to mention diarrhea and possible injury to the liver. Before you start dantrolene and while you are taking it, to monitor your liver your doctor will undoubtedly recommend blood tests before and during usage.

Tizanidine

Tizanidine is the new kid on the block. This medication appears to reduce muscle spasms while not weakening the muscles. Side effects include dry mouth, drowsiness, low blood pressure, and possible liver injury. Like dantrolene, this drug requires blood testing to protect your liver in case you should be susceptible to injury. Some people have reported hallucinations with tizanidine.

Botox

Muscles contorted by spasticity can be temporarily paralyzed for a few months by injecting them with *botulinum toxin,* better known as botox. The result is a muscle that can't contract at all, and the risk is that your muscle will be weaker, leaving you more disabled. Fortunately, the effects of a botox injection are not permanent, although they can shut down a muscle for several months. During those months, the muscle can shrivel from lack of use, and once the botox wears off, you may have to rehabilitate the muscle before it is useful again. Botox is best used in one or two small muscles that cause you a lot of pain or interfere with your recovery from stroke.

Surgery: Cutting and fusing

After years of spasticity without any significant improvement, you may have to resort to surgical procedures such as cutting tendons and fusing joints. Surgical procedures are usually irreversible and may have good or bad results. You need to be confident that the good results will outweigh the bad. Different surgeons approach the problems differently. Neurosurgeons may recommend destroying nerve cells in the spinal cord that contribute to spasticity, whereas others may take aim directly at the muscles and joints. These procedures are not done that often, and there is little established proof of their effectiveness or long-term benefits.

For the treatment of a neurological problem, I highly recommend that you get a consultation with a neurologist before you go ahead with any procedure. Since there are many different ways surgeons can treat a problem, you may also want to consult with someone other than a surgeon. A neurologist can give you independent advice on whether surgery is worthwhile. I also suggest that you talk to patients who had the surgery several years before. Be careful. Surgeons have good intentions, good training, and good reason to recommend surgery as the right thing for you. But they don't have the data to prove their claims in this case, and you need to be aware of that. Have the courage to seek other opinions, especially from your neurologist.

Depression and Other Psychological Changes

After a stroke, your brain is different. And because your personality, emotions, and thoughts are wrapped up inside it, they may be different, too. The stroke may have affected who you are and the way you behave. One of the most common outcomes of stroke is increased emotionality. Sometimes it is revealed with excessive laughing, but more often negative emotions such as sadness and anger predominate.

The change in who you are may not be apparent to you, the stroke survivor. In fact, you might not even be interested in whether you have changed — you may just want to be sure breakfast is on the table when you are hungry. Lack of interest in the social aspects of life is another common outcome of stroke. Sometimes the disinterest you show can be painful to others who are used to your participation and interest in their lives.

The spark, the wit, the special characteristics that made you *you* may be gone. Others who love you may be searching for the old you, and the *new* you may not even be aware of what these people expect and hope to see. This can lead to some unhappy situations, particularly if your stroke has made it more difficult for you to control your frustration and anger.

It is useful to know that some of these changes are worse in the first few months after a stroke and that with some encouragement, old patterns of behavior may return to a limited extent. Don't give up too soon.

Personality changes and more

It's not just your personality and interest that may be affected. After a stroke, you may not do as good a job of planning and looking out for yourself. You may have trouble inhibiting some of your impulses if the cerebral cortex, the part of the brain that controls such impulses, has been partially destroyed. The impulsiveness that makes you more emotional can also make you less likely to spend the time and thought needed to make a good decision.

This is not always as bad as it sounds. I have heard wives say that they like their husbands _better_ after a stroke because they are more relaxed and easygoing. Children have reported that their mother had a better sense of humor and was warmer and more affectionate after stroke. Nevertheless, be aware that your thinking may not be as clear as you believe — you may want to seek the advice of others when making decisions more so than in the past.

And let's be completely honest here: Once you've had one stroke you may have plenty of life left, but it is still time to start planning to turn some things over to your spouse or the next generation. Maybe you have already taken care of these things. That would be great. But you may not be as sharp and insightful after a stroke as you were before, and you may not know it.

Depression: Hiding behind other emotions

The matter gets even more confused by the high incidence of depression after a stroke. You can't really tell how well you are thinking and planning and controlling your emotions after a stroke until you have taken care of any depression that may be present. Depression can make you more emotional, more impulsive, and less apt to plan well and analyze problems. Again, you may not be aware you are depressed.

I have heard people say, "Of course I'm depressed, I was just disabled by a stroke. Do you expect me to be happy?" My answer is: "Yes." After a reasonable period of adjustment, most people recover their good spirits and get on with an admittedly more limited life. If they don't, one possible reason is depression. Like all depression, it can hide beneath anger and social withdrawal. Usually someone else points out that a stroke patient seems depressed. But there's no reason that you can't just say, "I feel depressed." Once it's out in the open, depression is relatively easy to deal with. Counseling and antidepressants are two very effective treatments.

Testing for depression

How do you solve these difficult problems where you can't even see the difference in yourself or know for sure whether you are depressed? The ideal solution is to have full neuropsychological and psychiatric evaluations. These are not as expensive as MRI or CT scans and they can tell relevant information about yourself. Just like blood tests for diabetes, tests can measure depression. It may not seem as accurate as some chemical test done on your blood, but the results are very consistent and help predict how someone will progress in the future. Tests can also give a physician insight into the best possible approaches for dealing with a stroke survivor's problems.

Will you be proven mentally incompetent and taken away to a nursing home if you let someone give you a psychological test? Not unless you were already bound in that direction. It's not unusual for the results to help family members recognize that the old man isn't as bad off as they thought! With a little treatment, he might begin to show some of his old spark for life.

And you don't have to worry that the whole world will know about your mental state. Test results, as in other medical matters, are kept private. The results of the testing should be confirmed by the impressions of the neuropsychologist or psychiatrist. Otherwise, further testing or evaluation may be recommended to understand the results. Just like a cholesterol test, some preparations help ensure sound results from the evaluation. Get a good night's sleep and avoid taking the tests if there are specific and acute stressors in your life at that moment — so that you can get the most accurate assessment. Nobody thinks psychological tests are the only deciding factor. Many doctors trust their intuition more than tests and will change their clinical diagnosis only if there is clear supporting evidence.

In addition to tests for depression, I suggest some tests to pin down some of the more practical problems that come from stroke and may add to your depression. These include tests of manual dexterity, decision making, language, memory, and your ability to recognize different objects that you see. In addition, it would be helpful to have your eyesight and hearing tested. Stroke can affect your vision without any obvious difference to you. If you were hard of hearing before your stroke, it may be more difficult for your stroke-stressed brain to make the extra effort it takes to understand conversation. Hearing aids that you didn't really need before your stroke can make a significant difference after your stroke.

Treatment often leads to happy outcomes

Once you identify depression, you can take action to treat it. And the good news is, depression is one of the most treatable outcomes of stroke! If you were struggling with poor hearing or poor vision, you'd certainly take measures to correct these problems — getting a hearing aid or glasses. Likewise, depression is a medical condition that ought to be treated.

Too often, individuals self-treat depression — with alcohol, sleeping pills, withdrawal, and other means that are not only ineffective, but may worsen the problem. Many are resistant to taking antidepressants — for various reasons. But drugs like Prozac and other SSRIs have been in use for more than 20 years. They are not addictive and do not cause you to hallucinate or act silly. Millions of depressed people have taken them and gained more productive and happy lives. I hesitate to mention a specific medication because there are so many. For someone who is older or has brain injury, the general principle is to start with low doses and slowly increase dosage until there is a good response.

The bottom line is that you have a lot to gain from a psychological evaluation after a stroke. Physical and occupational therapy help you handle certain problems caused by stroke. Why not undertake therapy for the rest of your stroke-injured brain, as well? Going with your spouse or family to a psychiatrist isn't unreasonable, particularly if you have had a change of personality — even if you aren't depressed, your spouse may be.

Adapting to Driving Limitations

How would you feel about heading out into traffic knowing that someone backing out of his driveway couldn't connect the sound of your honk with its message? Or that the woman at the stoplight didn't have the spatial cognition to make a left turn from a multilane intersection? Or the man in the SUV no longer understood what an octagonal red sign stood for? If you've had a stroke, one of these drivers could be you!

Reading the signs

Whether you have doubts about your driving ability after stroke — or you're confident that you are completely competent behind the wheel, please stop to consider these warning signs that you may need to hand in the car keys:

You feel afraid while driving.

Passengers act afraid while you are driving.

You've had several near-miss accidents.

You've been finding dents and scrapes on your car and property.

You have difficulty getting on and off highway entrances and exits.

You are the object of frequent honking.

Friends or relatives avoid a ride with you.

You get lost easily.

You find yourself stopping at green lights (my personal favorite).

You drift into other lanes (very common in stroke patients).

Driving may be your means to socialize and work, a necessity for acquiring food and clothing, and a connection to your family. It's a cherished privilege for many who value the independence it affords. But if you've suffered a stroke, the damaged parts of your brain may affect your ability to drive — even if you appear to have recovered and are successfully functioning at home and work. Most seriously, you may have experienced damage that prevents you from even recognizing that you have problems driving! I hope it is obvious to you, however, that you don't want to drive unless you are undeniably capable and don't pose a risk to yourself or others by doing so.

Here's my advice about driving after you've had a stroke: Don't drive — no matter how minor your stroke — until a physician has thoroughly checked you out and determined that you still have the ability to drive safely. You can appear and behave completely normal to most people and still have disabilities that make you a danger to yourself and others on the road.

Getting evaluated for driving

Two concerns should stop you from getting behind the wheel until you've been evaluated: The first is whether you are likely to have a stroke while you are driving. If you still have transient symptoms of stroke even as little as once a day, you need to see your doctor — but you also need someone else to drive you there. You don't belong behind the wheel if another stroke is likely to occur while you're there.

The second problem is the existing brain injury caused by your stroke. Some changes are obvious. If you are paralyzed on your right side, you probably can't summon up the physical effort to drive without special equipment, and may not even be capable then. You may also have subtle but critical impairments that affect your driving. Your ability to make quick decisions, react to sudden changes, and concentrate on the driving task can all be severely limited by stroke. These limitations may not be obvious to you. Sometimes well-intentioned caretakers know there are problems with your driving but don't say anything because they don't want to discourage you.

When it comes to driving after a stroke, no laws require you to be tested or to ensure that you haven't lost important brain function necessary for the high levels of coordination needed for driving. If you are older, the system may catch you because older drivers are required to have more frequent driving tests in some states. In other cases, you may be free to drive even when it is obvious to you or others that you are a road risk.

Because no laws require stroke victims to prove their driving skills, there isn't an official test that you can take to know you're "safe." The best course is to talk to your occupational therapist who may be able to recommend a road test that will identify problems.

Following are Web sites for some potentially helpful organizations. AARP and AAA provide online driving tests, although most are directed at the older driver rather than the disabled stroke patient. Find an occupational therapist who will assess your driving skills and help with your rehabilitation as necessary.

- ✔ **AARP Driver Safety Program:** www.aarp.org/life/drive
- ✔ **Association for Driver Rehabilitation Specialists:** www.driver-ed.org
- ✔ **American Occupational Therapy Association:** www.aota.org
- ✔ **American Automobile Association:** www.aaa.com
- ✔ **National Institute on Aging:** www.nia.nih.gov
- ✔ **Insurance Institute for Highway Safety:** www.hwysafety.org
- ✔ **National Highway Traffic Safety Administration:** www.nhtsa.dot.gov
- ✔ **Your state's Department of Transportation:** (Find on a search engine such as www.google.com or www.yahoo.com)

Identifying driving alternatives

If your endeavors to assess your driving skills prove that you are not fit to sit behind the wheel, then turn in your keys and start solving your transportation problems. Of course, you may be lucky enough to have a caretaker who can drive. Otherwise, you may have to call on children, family, friends, and volunteer groups to help get you around. Some local groups may be able to help you with transportation. You will probably have the best luck if you explore the organizations you are already associated with, including your community, place of worship, or local government.

Finding yourself "grounded" can threaten your stroke recovery if you don't take action to get out in the world. If you are completely isolated and alone, consider moving to a community where an automobile is not required for everything you do. If you are in a supportive community, the increased interaction that getting yourself around requires is probably healthy and will help prevent the depression and withdrawal that often accompany stroke.

Stroke can impair your driving in ways that are not readily apparent to you or your caretaker. By being tested and trained to drive with your disability, you reduce the risk of a serious automobile accident. Occupational therapists can evaluate your driving — as well as vision, hearing, reaction time, and concentration — and provide appropriate training to increase your driving safety. In

CASE STUDY

Discovering a "blind spot" the hard way

Upon stopping at a routine fender bender, a policeman found that the 65-year-old man who apparently ran into a parked car was confused and claimed he hadn't seen the car. Another driver who saw the accident told the policeman that the man had been driving far to the right side for a block or more before hitting the car. He had not been weaving or changing lanes erratically. "It was like he just didn't see the parked car." The policeman called a tow truck and offered to drive the man home. The man didn't mention that he had had a slight stroke a month ago and this was his first time back on the road.

Because he was concerned, he had his wife drive him to an ophthalmologist appointment.

The ophthalmologist found damage to his peripheral vision on his right side — a "blind spot." The doctor explained how stroke can affect vision and that he may not be aware of the loss.

The ophthalmologist advised the man to stop driving for the time being and seek out an expert on driving for the visually impaired. The doctor said he doubted, however, that the man would ever be able to drive safely unless his vision was corrected. He asked the man to return for more testing in three months.

some cases, everyone concerned will be relieved if you just face reality and turn in your keys. Finding alternatives for transportation can actually increase your contact with other people and speed your recovery from stroke.

Dealing with Incontinence

Incontinence — fecal or urinary, occasional or frequent — is a real problem for 10 to 40 percent of stroke patients. For a number of reasons, stroke patients may lose the ability to control their bladders or bowels. Incontinence happens when you can't get the signal to your bladder or bowel to wait a bit until you get to the toilet. Or, even if you do have what would normally be adequate control, your stroke has decreased your ability to get to a toilet. In most cases it is a little bit of both — you have trouble getting to a toilet and your brain doesn't have the ability to control strong urges. Treatment of both fecal and urinary incontinence involves taking action before the signal to go gets too strong. That way you have more time to get yourself to the toilet and you don't need as much effort from your brain to keep things under control.

Incontinence is more common with severe stroke. Problems with both types of incontinence tend to clear up within three months of the stroke. But when they don't, serious, longstanding problems are often reasons for deciding to admit someone to a nursing home. Even the most dedicated caretaker cannot maintain standards of hygiene if your mobility is limited and you remain incontinent for an extended time.

Certainly, incontinence is likely to prevent you from being sent home from the hospital with a family caretaker. If you are incontinent after your stroke, there's a possibility you may have had problems with incontinence before your stroke, but could handle them yourself. The disability from your stroke may not have caused your incontinence — but it may reduce your ability to cope with the problem.

Mentioning the unmentionable: Fecal incontinence

Why not tackle the tough things first? We all dread losing control of our bowels more than our bladders. I'm sure it comes as no surprise that one of the biggest problems you're bound to face with fecal incontinence is the difficulty in talking about it and seeking help. To give in to your modesty is possibly to fail to find out some really useful information — and a solution to an embarrassing problem.

I've got some good news, though. Once you swallow your pride and disclose your condition to a professional, you'll discover that to a great extent, fecal incontinence can be reduced and controlled. But first, know that much of the fecal incontinence due to your brain injury usually clears up in a few weeks. While other stroke symptoms continue to improve, fecal incontinence can actually worsen even though it's potentially treatable. Mentioning the unmentionable is a good idea because you can learn about potential treatments and effective ways to deal with the problem.

The part of the brain associated with bladder and bowel control is your *frontal lobes,* the same area that controls your emotions. Another area associated with incontinence is in the right side of the brain above your ear. If you have brain injury here, you have trouble knowing that you are disabled. You are unaware of problems moving your left arm or left leg and tend to deny knowledge of any problem if you are asked. This failure to respond to normal stimuli may be part of incontinence.

How common is it?

Like most medical conditions, when you start talking about fecal incontinence, you find it's more common than you might have suspected. A couple of studies have indicated that fecal incontinence, either frequent or occasional, occurred in about 30 percent of stroke patients in the first seven to ten days after stroke. This improved to only 10 percent at three months to a year. There was a slight increase to 15 percent by three years. It is most common in stroke patients who have some degree of dementia.

Regaining bowel control

Although some of the steps for overcoming incontinence are fairly basic, you are likely to optimize your success if you get professional guidance. Not all methods work for all stroke patients, and it takes some experience to know what will work best for you and your situation. There are visiting nurses who specialize in this problem, national associations that have volunteers, and doctors who take the problem very seriously. And you needn't worry — none of them drive up to your house in white trucks labeled "Incontinence, Inc."

Four fundamental approaches will help you improve or regain control of your bowels:

- **Watch what you eat and drink:** Your diet may be having an effect on your incontinence issues. Your diet may make you constipated, which, as you'll read below, leads to a lot of urgency and incontinence. A low-fiber diet and dehydration tend to make you constipated. Eat plenty of fiber and drink lots of water.

- **Avoid constipation:** The link between fecal incontinence and constipation may seem surprising, but when you don't have regular bowel movements, liquid stool begins to leak out. Don't postpone going to the toilet when you need to. For the stroke patient, constipation may be caused by medication you are on that may also slow colon activity. The medical term for such drugs is *anticholinergic*. Some antidepressants, medications that prevent nausea and dizziness, and some drugs to ease anxiety and help you control your emotions might be anticholinergic. *Diuretics* used to treat heart failure and high blood pressure can also cause constipation. Take your complete list of medications to your physician to see whether any have these effects.

- **Address problems of mobility:** Poor mobility can result in fecal incontinence. It may simply be too hard to get to the bathroom or bedside commode in time. If you have trouble communicating or recognizing that you have to move your bowels, then of course you can't get the help you need to get to a toilet. A program of physical therapy may help. A refresher course for you and your caretaker may improve your mobility. In addition, some rearrangement of furniture or new equipment may be helpful.

- **Bowel training:** By taking yourself to the toilet to empty your bowels on a regular basis, you can prevent your bowels from emptying when you don't want them to. Initially, this training program has you on the toilet quite frequently. Then, as you succeed in being continent, you increase the time between trips to the toilet. Like mental weight-lifting, this gradually increases your brain's ability to control your bowel movements.

Your fecal incontinence may be aggravated by another disability caused by stroke. These disabilities can make it difficult for you to get to the toilet or to communicate your need for assistance to others. Measures outlined in the rest of the book that enhance stroke recovery may also help with fecal incontinence.

Particularly important are good nutrition to maintain strength, good vision and hearing, relief of pain by keeping muscles flexible, good communication, and treating depression and anxiety.

If you are noticing that incontinence is getting worse, it is probably a sign of a solvable problem. You may have lost some of your muscle conditioning, you may be losing ground in your mobility, or you may have a bladder infection. Consult your doctor or an expert about your particular case.

Nursing home solution

One thing is for sure, if you and your caretaker cannot handle the problem well, poor hygiene rapidly leads to other major health problems. You will likely end up back in the hospital or in a nursing home. Fecal incontinence is also a serious burden for a caretaker, greatly increasing the chances of depression and physical exhaustion. If you can't get the problem resolved fairly quickly, a temporary or permanent move to a nursing home has to be considered sooner rather than later.

Overcoming urinary incontinence

Urinary incontinence following a stroke is more common than fecal incontinence. Some researchers report that 40 percent of stroke patients have occasional or frequent urinary incontinence at seven to ten days after their stroke, 19 percent at three months, and 15 percent at two years.

The front lobes of the brain control the bladder. When they are injured by stroke, you lose awareness of your bladder function. The bladder still functions, but it operates in an automatic mode managed by your spinal cord, which doesn't care where you are or what you are doing when it empties your bladder. Urinary incontinence related to stroke-caused brain injury usually clears on its own in the first month after the stroke. If the incontinence persists, then you've got to investigate whether something else in addition to brain injury is going on.

First, check whether you have a bladder infection. Usually a urine test does the trick. Antibiotics may treat both the infection and the incontinence. If your problem isn't due to a bladder infection, you still might have other bladder problems, such as side effects from medications. An evaluation by a urologist is worthwhile at this point. Take a list of your medications. If the urologist finds that bladder function is normal, ask about medications that could be used to help you control your bladder. There are several and they may be effective for you. One may temporarily slow down your urine production so you can make it through the night. Another may increase the tone of the muscles that control your bladder.

In a bladder training program, you take yourself to the bathroom on a frequent basis, say every hour until you stop being incontinent. Then, as you gain control for a short interval, you increase the time between trips to the toilet, building bladder muscle strength and re-teaching your brain to take control. By taking control of your bladder's schedule, your brain and bladder are able to re-learn how to keep you dry.

The National Association for Continence (www.nafc.org) has some good information on its Web site. You can also check around for a local nurse specialist continence advisor. And there are products on the market, such as incontinence pads and pants, that can go a long way toward limiting the inconvenience of incontinence. Some find a laundry service to be invaluable.

For men, a catheter can work for some. Not for the long term, but it can get you through long car or plane rides. In men previously able to cope with the problems of an enlarged prostate gland, a stroke makes things more difficult. Again, a urologist's evaluation can be important here.

Sometimes a bladder catheter that has been in place for a long time can *cause* urinary incontinence. Since they don't have to work when a catheter is in place, the bladder muscles that control urination become weak. When the catheter is finally removed, the muscles can't work and you become incontinent. Bladder training works well in this case, because the solution is simply to get your bladder muscles back in good shape.

WARNING! If you can't get your urinary incontinence under control, the constant wetness and skin irritation can lead to serious problems. Repeated bladder infections, skin breakdown and ulcers, and skin infections can result. In addition, it is a great deal of physical and emotional work for your caretaker. If you have other serious disabilities, it may just be too much for you and your caretaker to handle on your own. A nursing home might be the best solution.

Swallowing Difficulties

A week after a stroke, about 10 percent of stroke patients choke when eating. Approximately 30 percent experience abnormal swallowing. This adds up to 40 percent of stroke patients with an increased rate of death, due in part to pneumonia from food that is inhaled into the lungs. Signs of trouble:

- Choking or coughing while eating
- Slow chewing and swallowing
- Food stuck in mouth
- Chest congestion
- Gurgle-like sound to the voice

If these are problems after a stroke, some of the muscles controlling your swallowing, breathing, and chewing may have been affected. If you are having swallowing difficulties, find treatments and make diet changes in order to prevent life-threatening results. It is important to act quickly if you have swallowing problems. Notify your doctor immediately.

A speech therapist can determine possible causes of the problem. Treatments include teaching throat muscle-strengthening exercises and different head and neck positions that make it easier to swallow. More serious problems may require special food preparation or even a feeding tube until the throat recovers strength. If you have problems swallowing, you may also lose weight and become dehydrated. Long-term feeding tubes occur in rare cases, usually when other problems are associated with feeding. This is a complex medical decision and requires communication between multiple doctors.

Chapter 17

Taking Care of Family

Throughout this book, I've emphasized that stroke affects everyone in your family. In this chapter, it is the key message. I devote an entire chapter to the topic because family plays such a pivotal role in the recovery and adjustment of the stroke survivor. Certainly, the relationship between the patient and the caregivers is dynamic and symbiotic. A difficult stroke patient can cause a family member to become ill, stressed, and incapacitated. And a poorly functioning caregiver can result in problems for the stroke survivor.

It is critical, in my view, to take good care of the family — so the family can take good care of the stroke patient. This chapter is meant to help the stroke survivor see "life after stroke" from the perspective of the family — whether it's a devoted spouse who has been by your side throughout the ordeal or adult children who may live far away and are now making changes in their lives to care for you.

If you are one of the lucky 35 percent of stroke patients who return home with little or no disability, you can take your stroke as a wake-up call. A time to make lifestyle changes to reduce your chances of future stroke. A time to take steps to provide for yourself and your family, in case you don't avoid another stroke. A time to get your life in order. Yes, time to think about uncomfortable subjects such as wills and power of attorney and DNR (do not resuscitate). Your family should have as little to worry about as possible.

And if you have found yourself more than a little debilitated by your stroke and are beginning your journey toward recovery and adaptation to your limitations, these things are more important than ever. This chapter helps you understand the stress and pressure that your family is experiencing as they travel this difficult road with you. I explore the importance of keeping the family healthy — both emotionally and physically. I offer suggestions on what the family can do to make everyone's life easier and to reduce stress and upheaval. And I show you ways that you — yes, *you,* the stroke survivor — can take care of your family! Read on.

Stroke Affects Every Type of Family

You can count on the fact that your stroke will have an impact on all the members of your family — no matter what sort of family you have. Although the challenges may be different, depending upon your age, marital status, and other factors, you can still expect stroke to change your life and the lives of those close to you. Just consider the following scenarios:

- ✔ **You are one half of an older couple:** You have adult children who live away. You may be surprised by the financial bind you and your spouse find yourselves in after stroke. If you are seriously disabled, and your spouse can't take care of you alone, you may have to consider getting help in the home or going into a nursing home, both of which may be more than you can afford. The caregiver may continue to shoulder the burden of all your care and risk serious emotional and health problems. Depression, guilt, shame, and other feelings can develop without active intervention.

- ✔ **You are an older person who lives alone:** Now, you need help in the home or must move to a nursing home. You are considering moving in with one of your adult children, even though very few families can provide the quality of care that is necessary for a stroke survivor. Your adult child may have to give up employment and neglect his or her own children to take care of you. An occupational therapist could evaluate the situation to determine the feasibility of home care from your family. But be prepared that these situations often don't work out.

- ✔ **You are part of a family with children at home:** You may have earned some or all of the family income. Now, your spouse may have to become the primary breadwinner — perhaps even taking a second job if you relied on two incomes before — plus take on the full responsibility of caring for the kids. Plus now there's you to take care of. Despite all your love and commitment, stroke can be a major threat to any marriage. You may have to turn to your or your spouse's parents for help.

Whatever your family situation, your stroke disability means that now you can't do everything you once did. Someone else has to do the work for you. That someone else is almost always a family member.

The physical work may be significant. But what stresses a family member the most is the *emotional* work. Even if your spouse seems to be taking on the brunt of your stroke disability, other relationships change as your increased dependence requires adjustments in the way your spouse spends time. Your caregiver may insist that he or she is managing just fine — and you may find that all your needs are met while the house stays spic-and-span and every aspect of your lives seems under control.

Checking for signs of stress

A smooth-running household and your attentive care is no guarantee that your partner isn't experiencing overwhelming stress. Check for these signs of stress in your spouse and in your household:

- ✔ Your caregiver does not act like the same person.

- ✔ Your caregiver never talks about problems and difficulties.

- ✔ No one laughs. The family has lost its sense of humor.

- ✔ Family members are defensive about whether they are "doing enough" for you.

- ✔ Family members criticize each other.

- ✔ Your caregiver has emotional outbursts that are not typical of his or her personality.

- ✔ Your caregiver doesn't talk to you as frequently or in the same manner he or she used to.

- ✔ Family members visit you less often or for shorter periods of time.

- ✔ Your caregiver has forsaken his or her former social schedule or personal routines.

Wisdom from the trenches

Because stroke is new to most families, it's not surprising that it takes a while to adjust. Over time, family members have shared amazing insights with me — and I pass them on to you. Time and again, I've heard individuals say, "If only I'd known in the beginning that. . . ."

It's easy to underestimate the impact of your stroke if you just look at the physical disabilities.

If you go home from the hospital or rehabilitation unit after a stroke, you are not prepared for how difficult your life and your caregiver's life can become.

There are completely unexpected and serious financial burdens caused by stroke disability.

Your caregiver often tries to cover up for you, understating the problems both of you are having.

If you answer yes to even a few of these situations, you can assume that your family members are experiencing stress. If you are still in the early days after your stroke, continue to monitor the family situation, taking a "pulse" every week to see if things are changing — for better or worse.

It will take some time for you and your family to realize the full implications of your stroke. Expect some emotional peaks and valleys as you all adjust to the new limitations and demands of your disabilities. In the beginning, everyone may rally and put forth a positive front. This may be followed by an emotional dip. As the weeks and months pass, and your lives *don't* return to normal, the stress may build. In some cases, family members may become depressed and physically ill.

Struggling with the "new you"

The changes you are experiencing from your stroke have an impact on your family. Some are more challenging than others. Again, the changes that often cause the most stress for your family are not your physical limitations, but the changes to your personality or emotional state.

Stroke often causes personality change

It is common for stroke to decrease executive function, which is a fancy way of saying you are no longer a responsible decision-maker. *Executive function* refers to your ability to make decisions under pressure, to concentrate for periods of time, and to hook different ideas together in order to come up with a unifying concept or decision. You may be smart and have intact memory. You just can't use your intelligence and memory in a practical way to make plans and get anything done.

If the change is obvious, doctors or nurses may mention it. Medical professionals often offer hope that you'll return to your old self in time. Sometimes that happens, but often it doesn't. If the personality change is still present after a month or two, then you probably aren't ever going to be quite your old self. And *you* are likely not even aware of the "new you." So your family has to deal with this, as well, finding you unpredictable and, in some cases, a stranger to them.

Sometimes, but not usually, your family members may enjoy the new, more carefree you. But they may now worry about leaving you alone or letting you drive. They may be uncomfortable about treating you like a child, perhaps forbidding you to drive if you're not capable or insisting that you do the exercises your physical therapist gave you. They may even hesitate to talk about your changes among themselves, feeling that they're being disloyal or disrespectful somehow.

Stroke causes depression

Though it is one of the most treatable outcomes of stroke, depression is often undiagnosed or ignored for a variety of reasons. (See Chapter 16 for more on depression.) Too many families assume that depression is just something they have to learn to live with — or they consider it a character weakness that they should have the strength to overcome. Of course, in the family dynamic, the depression of the stroke survivor has an impact on the spouse and other members of the family. And it is common for other family members to suffer from depression, too.

Stroke causes dementia

You may not have the memory and smarts that you used to have before your stroke. You may fight against showing the limitations you sense in your memory and ability to figure things out. Your family may be hesitant to mention them. If you can manage to bring the problem out in the open, there is quite a bit you can do to help with the memory problems. See Chapter 7 for more.

Stroke can make you unaware of your disabilities

Stroke damages your brain's ability to recognize the full significance of your disability. This is most obvious with strokes that injure the right brain and paralyze or weaken your left side. Your apparent lack of concern for your serious situation can be particularly difficult for your caregiver and family. They may interpret your attitude as a sign you've given up or just don't care. If they do not understand that this is something you can't help, they may express resentment or frustration toward you.

When a loved one is changed by stroke, families find themselves in foreign territory, dealing with a "stranger." Reactions may range from extreme politeness and heroic martyrdom to boiling resentment and emotional withdrawal. A concerted family effort to pull together as a team will do a lot to help create a healthier environment for them — and you. By overlooking or avoiding a problem, the opportunity to intervene and improve your recovery from stroke may be lost.

Admitting When the Family Needs Help

Self-sufficiency is a wonderful part of the human spirit and is nourished and highly valued in our culture. This same pride, though, can make you unnecessarily miserable. Your independent spirit may blind you to how badly you need help and make it difficult for you to ask for help.

Recognizing your limitations

Don't get me wrong: I'm not telling you to give up, lean back, and let others wait on you hand and foot. The greatest success comes from stroke survivors who fight the hardest to win back everything that has been taken from them. And they usually have to do it themselves. Yes, you *are* alone to a large extent. But it basically boils down to the message imparted in the Serenity Prayer: having the courage to change what you can, the humility to accept what you can't, and the wisdom to know the difference.

This is valuable advice not just for you, but for your family members, too. Just as you will benefit from recognizing that you *can* get yourself from bed to bathroom if you continue your physical therapy, but you *can't* drive responsibly, your spouse will benefit from learning those same distinctions. A 70-year-old woman may be able to help her husband dress and get to the breakfast table, but she can't lift him into the car. An adult child may be able to attend to his disabled father regularly and arrange for visiting nurses, but he can't take on the responsibilities of his father moving in with the family.

In order to deal with these situations effectively, you need an objective assessment of how you are doing. If you and your caregiver are getting along well and even improving in your function and happiness every day, then go on doing it yourself. But if an honest assessment says that overall you are doing worse, then it's time to ask for help, and the sooner the better.

Evaluating your situation

This evaluation is probably best made by someone else — perhaps a professional who is both knowledgeable and more objective. But if you have always been the independent type, then you will probably be making your own assessment. Again, I advise you that your stroke may have left you with some limitations in your self-awareness. You benefit from involving your caregiver and other family members, perhaps even friends, your doctor, and the other health professionals who are aware of your situation.

You may have to ask some hard questions of yourself and others: Are you a difficult patient? Have you been angry, emotional, demanding, or otherwise hard to be around? Are you critical of your caregiver and others in the household? Do you have unreasonable expectations? Are you following the advice of the health pros and doing your exercises and taking medications? Is your caregiver able to meet your needs consistently? Is your caregiver meeting his or her needs as well?

The answers to these questions will give you a good idea of whether you need help. If you are not getting better, then you are risking your remaining independence by continuing to try and go it alone. You can do a lot to get back on the path to recovery, but you and your family may need to ask for help.

Taking Care of the Caretaker

Caregivers run a *serious* risk of burnout. Taking care of a stroke patient can be a 24-hour job with no time off — and no benefits. Often, the task demands more than the individual can handle — lifting a larger person from a bathtub, for example. The stroke survivor may be emotionally difficult, too. Mix all this with a little financial anxiety and the social isolation that often occurs when a spouse is disabled, and you have an unhealthy situation, indeed. Caregiving can result in feelings of anger, resentment, abandonment, fear, and guilt. Caregiving can lead to depression. Caregiving can lead to susceptibility to illness.

Preventing caregiver burnout

Enough. I'm sure you've got the idea. What can be done? Plenty! When the stroke survivor and the caregiver become aware of the risks in their situation — and that the challenges are nobody's fault — they can work together to find solutions. Here are just a few recommendations:

- ✔ **Invite help from friends and family:** Arrange to have friends and family visit and spend time with the stroke patient so that the caregiver can have some free time, whether for a couple hours or an afternoon.

- ✔ **Find a daycare facility:** Yes, daycare for adults. They do exist and they're for adults with various disabilities. A primary benefit of such facilities is to offer caregivers a fallback so that when they must attend to other responsibilities or simply need a little R&R, they can feel assured that their loved one will get quality care in their absence.

- ✔ **Join a stroke support group:** In most larger communities, there are stroke clubs that provide a chance for you to meet others with similar challenges. It isn't the type of social life that you imagined for yourself before your stroke — but it gives you a chance to learn more and give your caregiver a little free time.

- ✔ **Turn to adult children:** Families often face discomfort with the role-reversal that occurs when children must assume responsibility for parents. But if your spouse-caregiver is overwhelmed with the demands of your care, it's critical to call on the kids for help. Whether it's simply a request to help spare a parent from around-the-clock care or some additional coverage so the caregiver can take a much-deserved vacation, you'll probably find that most children are eager for a way to help out.

- ✔ **Connect with other caregivers:** Check with the local stroke support group or contact the National Stroke Association (www.stroke.org) or American Stroke Association (www.strokeassociation.org) and find out if there is a representative near you who can help. Call the hospital that took care of your stroke and ask if they provide any way for your caregiver to meet others in the same situation. By connecting with others in similar situations, your caregiver may discover tips on coping and will have an opportunity to commiserate and find support among people with like experiences.

✓ **Renew friendships and activities:** Encourage your caregiver to maintain or renew connections, social activities, and personal interests. It's typical for a stroke to overwhelm the routines and rhythms of a family's lives. After weeks of upheaval, a caregiving wife may suddenly realize she's missed the weekly yoga class or book club gatherings that she once loved. An adult child may find that he's missed his son's entire soccer season because of responsibilities to his disabled mother. It's critical for the caregiver to maintain some sense of "ordinary" and pleasure in his or her life. This also helps reduce the risk of isolation.

✓ **Get caregiver training:** Arrange for a professional nurse to visit the home, train the caregiver, and reevaluate the caregiver's ability to handle all the work required. This may enlighten the caregiver to new and efficient ways to deal with some of the responsibilities.

✓ **Get a good long-distance plan:** Or whatever it takes to open up as many communication channels as possible for the caregiver. Whether it's a call from a cousin in California or daily e-mail from grandkids in Grand Rapids, contact with other loved ones keeps the caregiver from feeling isolated and alone.

✓ **Make a doctor appointment:** Insist that your caregiver get frequent medical check-ups and perhaps some type of counseling to track his or her mental health. It's important to be alert to the possibility of depression, which is a major treatable problem (see Chapter 16).

What if the caregiver needs medical care?

What will happen if your caregiver is temporarily disabled by an illness? A frank discussion opens an opportunity to anticipate difficulties and take steps to make two lives less stressful. Knowing that you have a contingency plan in case your caregiver becomes sick may give both of you peace of mind — and, in turn, reduce anxiety that can lead to illness.

Here are a couple of options that you may not want to hear about. Nursing homes can take residents on a short-term basis. If your caregiver becomes ill, you *could* stay in a nursing home for a month or two — and give your spouse a chance to regain his or her health. Another option might be assisted living. Both of you could move into an assisted-living community where you could receive the help you need without your being dependent on your spouse. Neither has to be a permanent situation.

For caregivers only

Change for the better often starts when things seem the worst. Insist on staying healthy, both mentally and physically. Insist on getting help. And take the following advice:

- ✔ Set limits and be sure and take time off.
- ✔ Take things a day at a time.
- ✔ Get some sleep.
- ✔ Keep a list of things you need done, and when others offer help, give them something on the list.
- ✔ Maintain a support system of friends and family.
- ✔ Mind your health and finances.
- ✔ You're not perfect — just do your best.
- ✔ Join a support group.

Pull Together, Not Apart

Sometimes people get the craziest ideas in their heads — such as a 75-year-old woman believing she should be able to do all the work of three full-time nurses and be pleasant and eager to start over again every day. Or a stroke survivor thinking he can resume a job without missing a day of work or having trouble dealing with the stress of the workplace.

How has your stroke affected the way others in your family feel that *they* are doing? Are they feeling that they have new expectations that they aren't living up to? Perceived criticism from you or others can make other members of your family miserable. One of the characteristics of stroke patients is that they are impatient. They can be more critical of themselves and others and can become frustrated more easily.

Rather than a lot of introspective psychological analysis, family therapy, or expensive testing for your family, I suggest a more practical approach for starters. The psychologists and counselors can step in later if you don't make any headway. I propose that the family begin by pulling together as a team and developing a game plan for managing life after stroke. Schedule a meeting. If you can't work well enough together to run your own meeting, get a nurse in the hospital or someone else to facilitate the group.

Choose a captain — most likely not you, the stroke patient, but perhaps your spouse or an adult child — to take charge, organize the huddles, and delegate responsibilities. And do these things:

- ✔ Gather all facts on your physical, cognitive, and emotional problems.
- ✔ Identify the extra work, both physical and emotional, for everyone to deal with the problems.
- ✔ Prioritize needs.
- ✔ Review your resources.

Here's a starting list of tasks that may need to be assigned to various members of your new team:

- ✔ Arrange for a nursing home or assisted living, if necessary, or make alterations in the home for the stroke patient.
- ✔ Prepare food, clean house, do laundry, help dress, bathe, and transport.
- ✔ Schedule follow-up medical care and rehabilitation consultations at home or, more likely, in a clinic. This includes special evaluations by a neuropsychologist or an occupational therapist.
- ✔ Plan for transportation.
- ✔ Manage medical insurance and pay required doctor and hospital bills.
- ✔ Purchase medications and administer medications on schedule.
- ✔ Make an overall financial plan for life after stroke, including updating a will, creating a power of attorney, and making any medical decision-making delegations. This includes managing investments, borrowing money, setting up trusts, and dealing with Social Security.
- ✔ Manage the care of the caregiver, scheduling social outings, family visits, and telephone contacts.
- ✔ Contact stroke clubs, community centers, your place of worship, and other community resources to participate or volunteer to help.
- ✔ Evaluate progress in all areas and modify plans as necessary. This can be done at regular group meetings or by telephone.

That last item is important. Success requires diligence and sticking to the plan. If you start to fall behind, get depressed or discouraged, or start to lose ground for medical reasons, someone has to take responsibility for evaluating progress and making changes in the overall plan.

Another option, if there are resources, is to hire a temporary or permanent case manager who can do many of these tasks, including making evaluations and arranging family meetings. Costs for case managers vary quite a bit, so be sure you understand who will be doing what before you sign an agreement.

Here are some facts that are important to know when a family starts to deal with your stroke:

- ✔ Stroke changes the role of everyone in the family. The bigger the stroke, the bigger the change.

- ✔ To work together, the family has to talk together. It takes someone to organize talking together.

- ✔ The best way to get the work done is to break it up into pieces and find someone or some way to accomplish each task.

- ✔ Kids, even teenagers, can help.

- ✔ Your estimate and your caregiver's estimate of what you can do are often overly optimistic. What your stroke requires should be based on an actual list of what someone has to do for you each day for a week or two.

Financial Realities

If you were the breadwinner of the family — or your income was critical to your family's budget — you may be worried about finances along with everything else. If you can't work, how are you going to pay the mortgage? Even if you plan to return to work eventually, how will your family adjust to the reduced income in the meantime? And how will you handle all the medical expenses piling up from your hospitalization?

You may be lucky — you may have a great insurance plan that will pay for all or most of your care. You may not be the primary breadwinner in your family after all. Or, best of all, your disability may be so neglible you anticipate returning to work without missing a beat.

But if you're like most stroke survivors, you'll experience at least some financial impact from your stroke. Now, I don't claim to be a financial expert — I'm a doctor, after all — but I do know that the processes of collecting insurance, dealing with employers, and settling the accounts of someone with a major disabling illness is profoundly complicated.

Ask for guidance from a pro

Your family may have to turn to a professional to help you sort out all your options. I know, I know . . . you're concerned about your limited resources, and I'm suggesting that you *pay* someone to help you? Trust me, if your family feels as if they're drowning in financial paperwork and can't make sense of the various resources, your investment will garner a great return.

Here are some materials your financial advisor may request in order to help you make some decisions:

- ✔ All recent bills, paid and unpaid
- ✔ Insurance policies
- ✔ Social Security information
- ✔ Recent income tax returns
- ✔ Paychecks/stubs
- ✔ Investment documents
- ✔ Bank account information
- ✔ Loan statements
- ✔ Mortgages and deeds

Sharing your financial picture with the family

Always a touchy subject, money can be a difficult issue to discuss with the family. But it's critically important to talk about it with family members — especially if your financial picture is changing because of the stroke. The child who was thinking they might finance a house with their inheritance from you needs to know that your money may not be available if you require a long stay in a nursing home.

Trust may become an issue for you, particularly if your stroke has made you suspicious or overly emotional. Once you are disabled by stroke, the fact is, you just won't have as much control over your life as you would like.

It's a good idea for you and your spouse or other household members to develop a new budget for your life after stroke. Sometimes the budget may seem impossible and require drastic changes. Getting a reverse mortgage, for example, essentially lets you sell your house in slow motion to pay for medical care and nursing care. However it comes about, a good realistic financial plan can help you recover from stroke. Devote the time and energy to getting a plan developed and sharing it with your whole family.

You Can't Take It with You: Wills and Wishes

What if you had *not* survived your stroke? Would your family have known where to find important papers regarding financial issues, burial matters, and property concerns? Do you have a will? Do you have medical directives in place so that others can make medical decisions for you when you can't? Have you updated the beneficiaries of your life insurance policy?

You have just survived a close call. Many strokes are fatal. Your predicted life span is shorter now. If you have any doubts, check on the price of life-insurance coverage. And your chances of another stroke are now much higher than they were before.

Now's the time to confront that uncomfortable issue no one likes to think about: your own demise. Of course, you are going to do everything in your power to reduce your odds of another stroke — and I have faith that you will succeed. But you will feel better if you help to plan for a secure future for your family — in case you are not in the picture. Unless you are an Egyptian pharoah, you can't take it with you.

Get your affairs in order

Be sure you have the following in place:

- An up-to-date will
- A living will, if you want one
- A durable power of attorney
- Assignment of healthcare decisions to a family member
- A trust, if you need one

There are experts in *elder law,* attorneys, who can help you. The more experts you get to help you, the more likely it is that you will be able to take advantage of every program you are eligible for.

Leaving a health-oriented legacy for your kids

You have wills and powers of attorney to take care of your legal and financial legacy. The only way you have to protect your *genetic* legacy is to educate the rest of your family on what they can do to avoid or postpone having a stroke or heart disease themselves. Do your kids smoke? Have they checked their blood pressure? Do they get exercise and watch their blood lipid levels? Good health could be the most valuable part of your estate. Maybe they didn't listen to you when they were teenagers. Maybe your recent stroke experience and a few years of maturity have made them better listeners.

For good advice on these matters, check out *Estate Planning For Dummies* by Jordan Simon and Brian Caverly, or *Wills, Probate, and Inheritance Tax For Dummies* by J. Knight, both publshed by Wiley Publishing.

Appreciate the power of family

I admit I've dumped some gloom and doom on you in this chapter on family matters — but let me take a moment to counter some of the negative by focusing on the *power* of family. One of your greatest assets as a stroke survivor is your family support system. Sure, it isn't infallible and of course it can be distressed by too much pressure. But your family may be instrumental in optimizing your recovery. Here are some family strengths:

- A family increases the effectiveness of problem-solving and results in a better solution for everyone.

- A family provides emotional support for each other and, as a result, the group together is happier, more productive, and has more stamina than they would were they separate.

- A family can set priorities and establish reasonable standards and allow its members to feel they are doing their parts. Unreasonable expectations and criticisms can be brought out into the open and dealt with directly.

Your stroke disability presents immense challenges to your family. Good communication, a clear delineation of responsibilities, and recognizing when you need help increase the likelihood that you and your family will successfully adapt to life after stroke. If I am successful in communicating the key message in this chapter, then it will result in better care for you.

Part VI
The Part of Tens

The 5th Wave   By Rich Tennant

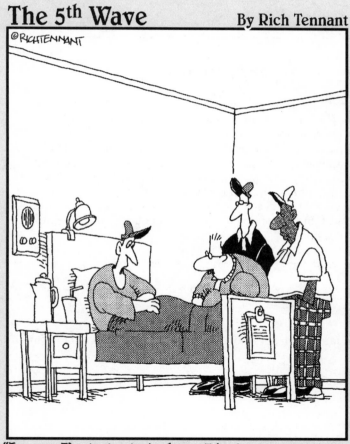

"I guess I'm lucky to be here. I had a stroke on the 18th green and then a mulligan in the ambulance."

In this part . . .

*H*ere is where I offer additional helpful information that should enhance your motivation to take care of yourself and others. From helping your community manage stroke, to inspirational stories of famous stroke victims and how they battled back. I also lay out concrete steps to improve your personal stroke care and prevent stroke. Finally, the last chapter provides a glossary of terms that serves as a helpful and quick reference to the bits of unavoidable technical jargon I have had to include in the book.

Chapter 18

Ten Ways to Help Your Community Manage Stroke

In This Chapter
▶ Encouraging your community to develop resources to combat stroke
▶ Informing others about stroke risks and opportunities to prevent stroke

After a stroke, you may be inclined to turn inward. One of the best strate-gies to energize your recovery is to turn *outward* to others in your com-munity. Not only can your community help you recover from a stroke, you can help *others* avoid stroke — by parlaying your experiences and knowledge into actions that educate friends, neighbors, and colleagues and help improve stroke treatment in your community.

Join a Group for a More Powerful Voice

Although stroke is the third-leading cause of death in the United States — not to mention a major cause of serious disability — stroke does not get the same national attention as Alzheimer's disease, Parkinson's disease, heart disease, or cancer. Add your voice to increase the volume and bring needed attention for more resources and support. Local, state, and national organizations are in place to fight stroke in the United States and Canada.

Local stroke clubs and support groups

The stroke support group or stroke club in your community offers a pathway out of the isolation that often afflicts a stroke patient. These organizations are often based in hospitals. Some are free-standing groups and others are affiliated with national organizations such as the American Heart Association (www.americanheart.org).

Involvement in a stroke support group can be critical to the caregiver, who is often struggling to juggle the demands of the stroke survivor as well as his or her own needs. The support system provides knowledge, tips, and tools for emotional survival, not to mention a network of people familiar with the stresses of caregiving. In addition to meetings, the caregiver benefits from phone contact, visits, social events, and new friendships.

Stroke clubs often sponsor stroke awareness events, arrange free risk-factor screening clinics, and work to promote better stroke care in your community. Meetings often include talks by local medical-care professionals who have a special interest in stroke.

Regional, state, and national organizations

Several organizations at the national level offer services and resources that reach down to local communities, though the availability varies by state and city. The American Stroke Association and the National Stroke Association are two voluntary organizations at the national level. You can join each of these organizations and participate in national programs to increase stroke education, promote research, and help stroke survivors and caretakers alike. The groups sponsor research and publish helpful information. Both provide extensive information for patients and professionals. You do not have to be a member to benefit from the information on their Web sites.

- American Stroke Association (www.strokeassociation.org) — closely affiliated with the American Heart Association
- National Stroke Association (www.stroke.org)

Some government organizations that offer valuable resources are

- National Institutes of Health (www.nih.gov)
- Centers for Disease Control (www.cdc.gov)
- National Institute of Neurological Disorders and Stroke (www.ninds.nih.gov)

An unusual regional organization, the Stroke Belt Consortium, exists in the southeastern United States to address the needs of this high-risk area for stroke. You will certainly find the information on its Web site, www.strokebelt.org, helpful.

Share Knowledge with Friends and Family

The only thing many of your friends and family may know about stroke is that they don't want one. You can teach them to recognize signs and symptoms of stroke and — better yet — help them prevent stroke. Through your experiences, you may persuade them to take steps to reduce their own stroke risk and learn what steps to take if someone they love is suddenly stricken with a stroke.

Think about it: As a stroke survivor, you have gained an advanced education in stroke and its prevention and care. Why not put your hard-earned knowledge to good use and teach others? From "Emergency Room 101" to graduate classes in blood pressure and cholesterol care, you have a lot to offer your friends and family.

Simply telling the story of your stroke and how it has affected you can have a profound impact. Your friends and colleagues may not pick up on the scary public service announcements in newspapers or TV — but I'll bet the story you share with them will stick and be forwarded to people they know. You can also encourage them to be aware of the need for good stroke care in your community and the importance of building community resources. Your efforts may even persuade them to volunteer to help families struggling with stroke.

Work with Local Hospitals

As the average age of the population increases, more and more people will suffer from stroke. At the same time, hospitals are cutting out every unnecessary expense in order to remain financially healthy. To make matters more complicated, stroke treatment has advanced so dramatically in the past decade that many hospitals are just now beginning to catch up.

You can, however, wield some influence over your local hospitals' budget-cut or development decisions. Community support is important to hospitals. By communicating your expectations of high-level stroke care, hospital administrators are more likely to take positive action.

Contact your hospitals to find out about special services and programs for stroke treatment. Compare their interest and commitments to providing the best care. Questions to ask each hospital include the following:

- Does the hospital have a special stroke unit with nurses trained and experienced in the care of stroke patients?

- Is the emergency room prepared to respond rapidly to stroke according to national guidelines for acute stroke centers? Which guidelines does the hospital follow?

- Is there an acute stroke-response team available on short notice to take care of stroke patients soon after they come to the emergency room?

- Is the hospital certified by the Joint Commission on Accreditation of Healthcare Organizations (JCAHO) as a Primary Stroke Center? (JCAHO is on the Internet at www.jcaho.com.)

- Does the hospital serve as a resource for patients after they are discharged following a disabling stroke? How?

Write letters to let hospitals know what you expect. Right now, hospital administrators and governing boards need to hear that you want and expect the best possible stroke care. Even if the local hospitals may have good stroke resources, they still need to hear from you in order to keep them fully staffed and up to standards. This is one area where a written letter may have more impact than a telephone call, which can be referred to a customer service representative who may not even make note of the content of your call. If your letter isn't answered, write another or call until you get a response.

Check into Emergency Medical Services

It doesn't do any good to have a great hospital for stroke if your local emergency medical service won't get you there quickly. How good is your local 911 service? The following questions will help determine how good your local 911 is for stroke:

- Are the dispatchers who answer the phones trained to recognize stroke?

- Does the service follow special stroke protocols that allow them to get a stroke patient moving more quickly to a hospital? (Sometimes this is called *scoop and run*.)

- If a stroke occurs, does the service take the patient to a special stroke center with an established record for rapid treatment of stroke?

- Are the ambulance crews trained to recognize stroke and the need for rapid transport to a stroke center? How much stroke training do they get? How frequently is it repeated?

Whom should you contact at the emergency service? I would suggest the emergency response director. However, if there is a governing board or county government agency, they may also need to receive a letter from you. Again, I'd recommend writing first. If you don't get a response, follow up with another letter or a phone call.

Educate Schoolchildren About Stroke

Several studies have indicated that what children learn in school gets passed on to their parents and the rest of their family. I've heard from many former smokers who reported that their impetus for quitting was their school-aged child who brought home the lessons learned in class. Many schools teach children the basics of heart resuscitation. Shouldn't they teach the importance of recognizing a stroke and calling 911, too? Would children knowing about the risk factors of stroke make our whole population healthier?

Many grade-school and high-school teachers welcome classroom visits from medical experts and patients on pertinent topics. Do you have children or grandchildren in the local school system? Are the kids learning about high blood pressure? Smoking? The brain? Check with the school administrators, the head of the science or health department, or the school board. Perhaps you could volunteer to speak to classes about your own struggle and recovery from stroke. Stroke is interesting from a scientific point of view because it teaches something about how the brain works.

Start Your Own Stroke Recovery Group

No stroke club or support group in your community? Why not start your own network of fellow stroke patients? You or your caregiver can serve as the hub of an effective group that deals with stroke in your own circles. Many people initially depressed and overwhelmed by stroke have found a path to sanity and a meaningful life by turning outward to help others.

How to get started? I have some ideas:

- Let the social workers and discharge planning nurses at hospitals know that you are willing to talk to any stroke patient or caregiver.

- Offer to share advice about nursing homes, adapting the home for the stroke survivor, and other recovery issues with other stroke patients.

- Let your church, synagogue, mosque, or place of worship know that you are willing to be a resource for any family with a stroke disability.

- Contact your local business clubs or other community-service organizations to find out if you might approach members who've suffered a stroke.

Suggest News Stories About Stroke Champions

People working hard to prevent or help others cope with stroke deserve some public recognition and acclaim. Collect interesting stories about stroke. Find out about doctors and nurses who've championed improvement in stroke care and are encouraging other doctors and nurses to take stroke more seriously. Gather tales of patients who've made amazing recoveries and caregivers who've supported them. Seek out news about hospitals that have recently received stroke certification or a local EMS service that has started a new stroke-education program.

These are great news stories! Let the local newspapers know if no one else has. Perhaps a local radio and television station would take an interest in stroke as a topic for a discussion panel or short news story. Maybe the newspaper might consider a feature article on "a day in the life" of a stroke patient, nurse, emergency room doctor, or caregiver.

Get Your Community to Participate in Stroke Research

Medical research is costly and slow. Yet it is critical to the advancement of treatment and prevention of stroke. Often, lack of money, conflicting priorities, and politics may mean that important research in stroke is neglected in your community.

From hospitals and nearby medical schools, you can learn whether any stroke research is being conducted in your community. None? Check the Web site for Washington University in St. Louis (www.strokecenter.org) — it lists the many ongoing clinical trials in stroke throughout the world. Stroke research evaluates new ways to prevent and treat stroke as well as enhance recovery. Not all research involves clinical trials. The goal of many important research projects is to understand or diagnose stroke better.

You can encourage hospitals and doctors to start more research. Insist that working to make things better for stroke patients is part of being a leading stroke hospital or doctor. Communicate that you want the latest treatments available in research protocols. It can't hurt. Most new treatments don't work out, but patients in clinical trials receive the best possible care. Your voice may be the one that helps a hospital board or individual doctor decide that they want to make a difference in how stroke is treated.

Volunteer for Stroke Research

You yourself can volunteer to be part of a research project. Research projects are available across the country. Numerous trials and studies seek patients who have had a stroke. Some offer a chance to receive new treatment to prevent a second stroke.

Contact doctors at stroke centers in your area and ask if there are any ongoing trials. If not, are they aware of other trials that you might be eligible for? If they are doing trials but not one that you are eligible for, ask them if they would be interested in joining a study that you are eligible for.

If you're a stroke survivor with other family members who've suffered a stroke, you may be a valuable national resource in the fight against stroke! Seek out a stroke study involving family history. This is one of our best hopes for gaining a true understanding of the causes and potential treatments for stroke.

Don't agree to participate in a trial until you have fully understood the risks and potential benefits. Doctors involved in such trials are required to explain the uncertainty and risks to you. Ask as many questions as you want and take the time to rally family support before you agree to be part of a trial. Be sure that you intend to stick with the trial before you sign up. It is important that everyone who starts a trial finishes.

Make Sense of Health Policy

How capable is your community in responding to the needs of stroke patients? Is a reasonable quality of care available to those who need it at a price they can afford to pay? Are there enough certified nursing homes in your area? Have stroke patients and their families suffered unnecessarily in your community? Are community resources sufficient to handle the demands of stroke sufferers? If not, is your community taking steps to meet these needs? Who is planning for the healthcare needs of your community?

By becoming informed on the problem of stroke as a community responsibility, you and your family can participate in forming new plans and policies.

And then run for Congress. Why not?

Chapter 19

Five Remarkable Stroke Recoveries

A president. An Academy Award winner. A writer. A musician. A beauty queen. These are just a handful of the remarkable people who've survived — and thrived — after stroke.

As you now know, stroke can have devastating consequences. But these consequences can also be overcome. There are thousands of remarkable stories from individuals who've experienced stroke and gone on to create, produce, lead, contribute, and inspire. I hope these portraits inspire you.

President Woodrow Wilson Overcomes Stroke and Leads a Country

Several strokes and evidence of *transient ischemic attack* (TIA — see Chapter 4) didn't detour Thomas Woodrow Wilson from his path toward the ultimate leadership position. Despite evidence of stroke more than 16 years earlier, Wilson persevered to become president of Princeton University, governor of New Jersey, and then was sworn in as the 28th president of the United States in 1913.

In 1896, at age 39, Wilson suffered what many believe was his first stroke while he was a professor at Princeton. The stroke weakened his right hand and arm and also decreased the sensation in his right hand. The weakness improved with time and he persisted in his career. Four years later he became president of Princeton University. It is believed that he suffered further strokes in 1904 and 1906; one further weakened his right arm, the other affected the vision in his left eye.

The symptoms from these three strokes suggest that Wilson may have had blood clots in the left carotid artery that were breaking free to injure the brain and eye on the left side. (Remember that left-sided brain problems most often cause right-sided symptoms.) It is speculated that after the 1906 episode, Wilson enjoyed a stroke-free period for a few years, although some sources indicate he complained of serious headaches during this time. This has raised speculation that he may have had severe and uncontrolled blood pressure in addition to atherosclerosis of the left carotid artery.

In 1910, he was elected governor of New Jersey. In 1912, he began campaigning for the office of President of the United States. During the campaign, Wilson had right hand and arm transient problems that suggest TIAs to many who've reviewed his medical history. He won the election, but a month after he took office he may have had his first stroke on the right side of his brain — this time, his left hand and arm were weakened.

After re-election in 1916, he continued to suffer from severe headaches — and likely had more transient strokes. At the time, the significance of transient strokes was not known, nor was high blood pressure known as a cause of stroke.

But a physician with the knowledge we have today might have predicted the devastating stroke that hit Wilson in 1919. After a series of events suggesting right-brain problems, he finally had a massive right-brain stroke that left him completely paralyzed on the left side, though still able to speak. As is often the case with left-brain strokes, he denied that he had even had a stroke.

Wilson finished his term of office without the public ever realizing his serious condition. He is thought to have become more withdrawn and depressed. He retired to private life in Washington, where he died five years later in 1924. In the meantime, his care was managed by his wife.

Although Wilson was repeatedly struck down by stroke over a period of 13 years, he fought back successfully time after time. He lived a productive life despite the problems and earned a place in American history.

Other Presidents who have had strokes include John Quincy Adams, Franklin Roosevelt, Richard Nixon, and Gerald Ford.

Miss America Jacqueline Mayer Discovers a Different Kind of Beauty

Who could have imagined that the 20-year-old college student who won the Miss America pageant in 1963 would be struck down at the age of 28 — with a massive stroke? In 1970, the young mother woke one morning to discover she couldn't move or speak. Jackie Mayer survived the near-fatal experience, and began a long, arduous seven-year journey that required relearning how to speak, walk, and even tie her shoes. Her rehabilitation was intense and even when she regained the ability to overcome almost all of her disability, her public appearances required an athletic endurance and a high level of self-discipline.

As she recovered, she turned outward and became a national spokesperson for the National Stroke Association. She shot a video, *A Different Kind of Beauty,* to increase stroke awareness, for the American Heart Association. Mayer wrote a regular column for the National Stroke Association's *Be Stroke Smart* publication. She served on the National Advisory Council of the National Institute of Neurological Disorders and Stroke in Washington and has received awards for her work in stroke. She still works as a motivational speaker. Learn more about her story at her Web site, www.jackiemayer.com.

To win the Miss America pageant and then be seriously disabled by stroke may have seemed a crushing defeat. Mayer has exhibited remarkable inner strength to undertake the physical and emotional work needed to recover from such a severe stroke. That she then devoted much of her life to helping others with stroke only adds to the greatness of her achievement.

Composer George Frideric Handel Writes "Messiah" After Stroke

George Frideric Handel enjoyed a long and fruitful career as a composer of operas and oratorios. But it wasn't until after a stroke at age 52, which left his thinking impaired and his right hand paralyzed, that he wrote his most renowned work, *Messiah.* Despite deep depression over his condition, Handel was able to recover the use of his hand. And regardless whether his thinking remained diminished by stroke, he clearly had the wherewithal to continue writing great music.

The composer was born in 1685 in Germany and exhibited a gift for music at an early age. At the age of 18, in 1703, he began his musical career as a violinist for the Hamburg Opera. His first two operas were produced before he was 20. His study and work took him to Florence, Rome, Naples, and Venice before he moved to England, where he became a royal favorite. In 1714, he was commissioned to write *Water Music,* for wind and strings. His acclaim as a composer grew.

In 1737, Handel suffered a stroke. He retreated to Aachen, Germany, where he recovered the use of his hand. He was changed by his stroke and lived a secluded life, depressed and troubled by multiple ailments. Yet in his return to England, he began writing the English choral works that eventually re-invigorated his creative life. This period culminated in his writing of the oratorio *Messiah* in 1741 in roughly three energy-charged weeks. With this success, he returned to a full life of music. He had a second stroke and then became blind in 1752, but continued to produce musical works. He died in 1759 and is buried in Westminster Abbey in London.

Writer Ken Kesey Found TPA the Drug of Choice After Stroke

American novelist Ken Elton Kesey became as well known for his Acid Test parties and Merry Pranksters cross-country antics as he was for his books *One Flew Over the Cuckoo's Nest* and *Sometimes a Great Notion.* At the height of his popularity, Kesey, born in 1935, bridged the gap between the 1950s Beat Generation and the 1960s hippie culture of California. Yet when Kesey suffered a stroke at 62, TPA — not LSD — was the drug that saved him.

In 1997, Kesey had a stroke and was treated with TPA — which had only been approved a year earlier. He responded to treatment and regained the use of his right arm, which had been paralyzed by the stroke. The stroke research community still remembers his much-publicized description of TPA as *Drano for the Brain-o.*

Thanks, most likely, to TPA, his disability from stroke was minimal. In fact, rather than slowing him down, the stroke inspired him with new energy that lead to a final burst of creativity, including a bus tour of the United Kingdom with some 30 passengers, performing a traveling version of his play *Where's Merlin?* before he died of cancer in 2001.

Actress Patricia Neal Recovers to Earn an Oscar Nomination

A year after winning an Academy Award for her role in the movie *Hud,* actress Patricia Neal experienced a stroke so devastating that it put her in a coma that lasted 21 days. Actually, she had three strokes in a single day. She was pregnant at the time. Miraculously, she survived, gave birth to a daughter six months later, and went on to star in movies — and even received another Oscar nomination. Hers is one of the better known stories of remarkable recovery and return to a full life after stroke.

Neal was 39 in 1966, when she developed a terrible headache followed by disorientation and vomiting. She had a stroke that sent her to the emergency room, where she had another and finally a third one that same day. These strokes were caused by subarachnoid hemorrhage. After surgery to clip the burst aneurysm, she fell into a coma. She wasn't expected to survive.

Three weeks later, she came out of the coma, paralyzed on her right side, unable to speak or understand conversation, and with double vision. She had to relearn to speak and walk. Her husband, writer Roald Dahl, worked closely with her to develop a rehabilitation program that kept her occupied every minute of every day. This helped her to direct her anger and frustration into the drive and determination to make her mind and body do the work necessary for recovery.

She gave birth to a daughter six months after her stroke. Her recovery continued during this time. She battled depression and setbacks, but persevered and gradually began to appear in public once again. In 1968, she starred in the movie *The Subject Was Roses* and was nominated for an Academy Award. Neal has appeared in many movies and television performances. She has also been an active spokesperson for stroke — in 1978, she helped to dedicate the Patricia Neal Rehabilitation Center, in her hometown of Knoxville, Tennessee.

Your Remarkable Stroke Recovery

Everyone who survives stroke holds within them a remarkable tale. Your life may not have been one of fame or celebrity, but the struggle you've been engaged in is no less significant than the ones mentioned here.

Take the time to consider your own experiences and write your own story. Reflect on your accomplishments — even the simplest steps forward. I'll bet when you do, you'll discover that you, too, have an inspiring story to tell.

Chapter 20

Ten Opportunities to Prevent Stroke

In This Chapter

▶ Taking steps to prevent (another) stroke

▶ Reviewing the most critical stroke risks

Medical researchers have identified a lot of valuable information that can help you prevent stroke. In this chapter I present you with a short list of these opportunities. The value of most of them is confirmed by testing in clinical trials, whereas others are based on consistent observations comparing people who have had a stroke with those who haven't. Some of it is just common sense. Because heart disease and stroke share many risk factors, there are more benefits than just preventing stroke if you choose to take advantage of one of these opportunities.

I've written most of the ten items below on the assumption that you have already had one or more strokes and want to avoid more. To a great extent, many of the recommendations, particularly those dealing with blood pressure and cholesterol, are valuable even if you are smart enough to be trying to prevent your first stroke.

The choice is yours.

Gathering Information

Any effort to reduce your chances of stroke begins with gathering data. This step may seem like a chore that forces you to face facts you wish weren't true. But it's a critical step in preventing future strokes. By having all the information about your health status and stroke history in one place, you will undoubtedly prompt more efficiency from physicians and healthcare professionals who can then propose the best treatments and maintenance plan for you.

Most of the critical data is already available in your medical records. Assembling this data may require patience, phone calls, signing forms, and waiting in line.

You need copies of the actual laboratory and X-ray reports, not just someone's summary of the report.

If you've been in the hospital recently, a copy of the discharge summary as well as all test reports is very useful. Summarizing the results on a single sheet, which includes the numerical value of the test result in addition to the date it was obtained, can be very helpful. Get it before leaving the hospital.

Having made of list of information already available and medications you are taking, you can then decide if important information is missing and track it down with the help of your doctor.

At the minimum, a recent accurate measurement of the following should be available to you if you are going to take maximum advantage of the opportunities available to you (also see the Cheat Sheet at the front of this book for a handy list you can take with you).

- Weight
- Height
- Abdominal girth (waist measurement)
- Blood pressure
- HDL and LDL cholesterol levels after eight hours of fasting
- Glucose tolerance test
- Electrocardiogram
- Chest X-ray
- Carotid ultrasound
- Hemoglobin and hematocrit
- Cardiac stress test

Treating High Blood Pressure

First, it's important to accurately measure your blood pressure at different times of day and in different circumstances. Then, some simple steps help reduce your blood pressure. These include exercising, minimizing stress, reducing caffeine, and possibly lowering the amount of salt in your diet. You can also analyze where stress comes in your routine and see if there is anything you can do about it.

Example? Commuters who drive to work are found to have higher blood pressure than those who ride with them or take public transportation.

Taking medication to reduce high blood pressure has been shown to be effective time and again for reducing stroke risk. Some medications have fewer side effects, and others are less expensive. Review Chapter 8 for more about blood pressure meds and their effects.

I'm surprised at how often people choose not to take the opportunity to treat their blood pressure. Such treatment is one of the best ways to prolong your life and increase your ability to enjoy it.

Preventing Blood Clot Formation

Numerous trials among sufferers of white stroke have shown that medication helps reduce the likelihood that more blood clots will form inside your heart and the arteries of the brain.

Aspirin is the most commonly recommended drug. Aspirin is inexpensive and generally well-tolerated in the low doses now generally recommended, either one regular (325 milligrams) or one small tablet (100 or 81 milligrams) every day. Side effects include easy bruising and stomach pain with bleeding ulcers.

You may not tolerate aspirin — or your doctor may recommend a medication found to be more effective than aspirin. Two common alternatives are clopidogrel, known by the trade name Plavix, and Aggrenox, a combination of a very small dose of aspirin with a drug called dypyridamole. Warfarin may be another medication suggested by your doctor for preventing blood clots — particularly if you have atrial fibrillation or a heart valve. But warfarin is not only more expensive, it entails some risks that require frequent blood testing.

Bottom line: It's important to take the necessary steps to prevent blood clotting if you're at risk for stroke. Medication is critical in helping with this effort. Whether your doctor recommends a low dose of aspirin or one of the other medications, be sure you understand the precautions and follow the dosage guidelines as given.

Reducing Cholesterol in Your Blood

Evidence supports this: People who exercise regularly and follow certain diets have healthier levels of cholesterol in their blood. Diet and exercise may reduce the "bad" cholesterol and increase the "good" (see Chapter 9 for a complete explanation of these fats in the bloodstream). New information is beginning to focus on the especially harmful effects of *trans* fats — processed foods such as solid margarine that have been *hydrogenated* for longer shelf life. The FDA is requiring the inclusion of data about *trans* fat on food packaging.

Diet and exercise may not result in healthy cholesterol levels for everyone. Taking statin medications has been shown to be effective in preventing stroke and heart disease in those who have high levels of LDL. Statins are expensive and may have some serious side effects. Routine testing for liver problems is critical, as is being alert to muscle pain, which may be a sign of an adverse reaction to these drugs. Repeated testing of your blood cholesterol levels should be done to determine if you are taking the correct dose for you.

Treating Atrial Fibrillation

A simple electrocardiogram (EKG) will determine whether you have an irregular heartbeat, called *atrial fibrillation*. This condition is tied to stroke risk — the uncoordinated contractions result in ineffective pumping of blood, which can lead to pooling and clotting of the blood and, subsequently, stroke.

If you do have atrial fibrillation, your doctor will likely recommend that you take the blood-thinning drug warfarin instead of an aspirin every day. Many clinical trials have demonstrated that warfarin is an effective treatment for atrial fibrillation — but there are risks.

If you take warfarin, do so with a great deal of attention to detail. Your diet, the time of day that you take the medication, and other medications can all affect the extent to which warfarin works. Taking warfarin is like driving on a road with curves. You have to pay attention or you may drive off the road — on one side or the other. With warfarin, a slight swerve (forgetting to take it or taking it too soon) can cause bleeding from blood too thin, or stroke with blood too thick.

"Steering" your warfarin dose requires strict adherence to your doctor's instructions as well as frequent blood tests. It's also critical to alert your doctor of unusual bleeding or bruising between tests. And even subtle changes to your diet — more green, leafy vegetables, for example — may have an impact. (Read Chapter 10 for more on warfarin risks.)

Checking Out Your Carotid Arteries

If you've had a stroke, be *sure* that one of your carotid arteries isn't partially blocked and about to close off completely. A carotid ultrasound test is easy to undergo, and it's a very accurate measure of whether your artery needs to be cleaned out. (You may even hear a "whoosh" sound in your head or neck — similar to when you lie down with one of your ears pressed into a pillow. This is the blood rushing past the narrow spot in the artery.)

If you do learn of a blockage, your doctor will likely recommend a *carotid endarterectomy,* a procedure that will clear the artery of blockage. Before doing so, get a second opinion. I believe the best second opinion comes for a stroke expert who is *not* a surgeon. Also, make sure your surgeon does this procedure often and has good results. Ask for numbers, not just percentages. Be especially wary if you are told your condition is too much of an emergency to get a second opinion.

Eating Right and Staying Hydrated

Ensuring that you are fueling yourself with a healthy diet and taking in plenty of fluids can have a direct impact on your risk of stroke. As discussed in Chapter 9, a diet high in certain kinds of fats (hydrogenated oils, high-fat dairy products, and, yes, those thick slabs of steak you adore) can lead to unhealthy cholesterol levels — which means greater risk of heart attack and stroke. A meal plan steeped in highly salted foods results in a sodium level that can aggravate high blood pressure. Additionally, a diet that adds pounds to your frame also adds stress to your heart. Eat moderately and watch the fats and sodium. When you are dehydrated, your kidneys don't have the water they need to function at their best, and your blood may become more concentrated. Your hydration is worst in the morning after your overnight fast. Skip the ham and eggs, but don't skip breakfast and a morning drink of water or juice.

Stopping Smoking

What more can I say about tobacco use? If you always thought lung cancer was your greatest risk from smoking, I hope you now know that far more cases of emphysema, heart attack, and stroke result from smoking. Indeed, one of the most dramatic changes you can make to improve your health is to toss the cigarettes.

You'll save money. Your clothes will smell better. Your lungs will be clearer. You'll reduce your stroke risk. Quit today.

Exercising Your Muscles and Your Brain

I don't know of any clinical trials that show that you will have fewer strokes if you exercise. I don't know if you will stay smarter longer than you would have otherwise if you exercise your brain. However, plenty of anecdotal evidence suggests that people who exercise their muscles and their brains are less likely to become demented or to have strokes.

For many, exercise is a good relief from stress and can encourage you to eat healthier food. There is no doubt that exercise helps you keep your weight down if you tend to be too heavy.

Exercise is hard to overdo, but it is possible. A regimen that's too difficult is not likely to last. If you hate to exercise and have started and failed before, I suggest trying walking. If you stay out of the way of cars, it is generally safe and results in fewer injuries than running.

A weight-training program managed by a physical therapist or experienced trainer can also be very helpful.

Writing Up a Maintenance Plan

Of course, you plan to follow some new guidelines to protect your health and prevent stroke — but such a stroke-prevention plan will work much better if you write it down and have it to refer to as you progress. It will work even better if you share your plan with your family and others who live with you. Your maintenance plan should be developed with the involvement of your stroke physician. By working together to create a written outline, you'll ensure mutual understanding of what steps must be followed to protect you from future stroke problems.

Of course, writing down the plan is only the first part of the process — you'll have to *follow* the plan diligently to enjoy the results. Consistently taking medications, getting blood tests when you need them, and having check-ups in time to catch problems early can take considerable effort. Evidence strongly supports that the effort is worthwhile.

After a stroke, you are at great risk of having another stroke, not to mention some kind of heart disease. Although you can't change your stroke history, you can proactively work to stave off future and possibly more disabling strokes. Plenty of research supports that taking certain steps — eliminating smoking from your life, lowering your blood pressure, reducing your cholesterol level, to name a few — increases your chances to prevent stroke and prolong your life. These opportunities have as much to offer you as seat belts in your car or looking both ways when you cross the street. It's your choice.

Glossary

· ·

These terms pertaining to stroke are presented in alphabetical order, so please don't get frustrated if the definition of one item refers to a term that isn't addressed until later. Not everything is covered here. If the term you seek is not here, check the index.

Acute stroke: A stroke is *acute* as it is still in the process of changing in the first hours and days after the onset of the symptoms. The acute phase of stroke, especially the first few minutes and hours, is when the injury is still not complete, and treatments have the best chance of minimizing damage.

Amyloid angiopathy: A relatively uncommon cause of intracerebral hemorrhage stroke, occurring mostly in those who are in their 70s or older, resulting from an accumulation of a protein called *amyloid* in brain arteries, which rupture and bleed.

Aneurysm: The stretching out of the rubbery wall of an artery into a balloon-like bulge. This is typically the result of damage or weakness and can lead to rupture.

Angiography: A procedure that diagnoses the presence of blood clots in blood vessels, involving the injection of a dye through the groin area, which travels up to the brain, and the X-ray photographing of the brain's blood vessels concerned.

Anticoagulant: A drug or agent whose main effect is to prevent the blood from clotting.

Aphasia: Condition that affects and causes deficits in language — including the inability to speak, understand, write, and/or read — as a result of brain damage, including damage caused by stroke.

Artery: A blood vessel that carries blood away from the heart to other parts of the body.

Atherosclerosis: A condition in which scar tissue builds up in the arteries as a result of years accumulating fat from the blood, scar tissue, and calcium. The scar tissue is called **atherosclerotic plaque** and it can block blood vessels. Because it is a rough spot on the inside of the blood vessel, blood clots may form there. These clots themselves can block the artery where they form or they can break off and travel through the bloodstream to the brain, causing damage or bleeding along the way. Atherosclerosis is also called *hardening of the arteries*.

Atherosclerotic plaque: Scar tissue in the arteries that builds up and can cause **atherosclerosis.**

Atrial fibrillation: The abnormal and uncoordinated contractions of *atria,* or upper chambers of the heart, which leads to the ineffective pumping of blood by the heart.

Berry aneurysm: An aneurysm that forms in the *subarachnoid* space underneath the brain, usually at a branch point — also referred to as a *saccular aneurysm.* When these aneurysms burst, they cause subarachnoid hemorrhage (SAH), a type of red stroke.

Blood clot: The resulting mass that occurs when blood tissue begins to collect and "harden." When this occurs inside blood vessels, it can stop blood flow and lead to heart attack and stroke.

Brain stem: The base of the brain, found at the top of the spinal cord and responsible for many of the brain's primary functions.

Carotid artery: A large artery in the neck that carries blood to the brain, often found to be involved in stroke.

Carotid endarterectomy: A surgical procedure that removes blockages such as plaque or blood clots from the carotid artery.

Cerebrospinal fluid (CSF): The clear fluid that surrounds the brain inside the skull and the spinal cord inside the spinal column.

Cholesterol: A waxy substance found in foods that come from animal sources, such as milk, meat, and eggs. It is also manufactured inside the human body. There are two types: **low-density lipoprotein (LDL)** cholesterol and **high-density lipoprotein (HDL)** cholesterol. See Chapter 9 for more.

CT scan: Also referred to as a *CAT* scan or *computerized axial tomography* scan. A diagnostic tool that takes special images of the inside of the head, as a series of 12 to 20 pictures usually printed by a computer on a single sheet of X-ray film. A CT scan can be valuable in determining whether a stroke is caused by bleeding (involved in types of **red stroke**) or blockage (**white stroke**).

Dementia: An unfortunately named condition in which damaged brain tissue results in severely impaired memory and loss of brain function, which becomes progressively worse with time.

Diabetes: A condition in which the body is incapable of producing or assimilating *insulin,* which is needed to produce energy. Diabetes can increase the possibility of cardiovascular disease.

Diastolic blood pressure: The measurement of blood pressure taken when the heart relaxes between heartbeats. The "lower number" of your blood pressure reading.

Electrocardiogram: Also called *EKG* or *ECG*. A test that measures the health of the heart.

Embolus: A piece of solid material floating in the bloodstream which travels along branching blood vessels until it gets stuck and stops blood flow. If the embolus gets stuck in a brain artery, it causes a stroke. Usually an embolus that reaches the brain is a blood clot that has formed in the heart or on a rough spot on a blood vessel.

Hemorrhage: Excessive or uncontrolled bleeding from a ruptured blood vessel. The less blood is clotting, the harder it is to stop hemorrhage.

Hemorrhagic conversion of infarction: A rare condition in which an artery injured by ischemia — or lack of blood flow (**white stroke**) — breaks and bleeds into the area of **infarction** — or dead brain tissue. Sometimes this bleeding has little impact. Other times, this bleeding can be so severe that it causes further disability and even death. Hemorrhagic conversion occurs more often in people taking drugs or having diseases that interfere with the ability of blood to clot.

High blood pressure: A condition in which the heart has to work too hard to pump enough blood through the arteries. See **Hypertension.**

High-density lipoprotein (HDL): One of the fat transporters that carries **cholesterol** and **triglycerides** in the body, often referred to as "good" cholesterol because it carries fats to the liver where they are processed and excreted from the body.

Hypertension: Also called **high blood pressure.** A chronic condition in which the pressure of the blood flowing through blood vessels is above the normal range, which is typically 140/90 or greater. Hypertension is the number-one risk factor for stroke.

Infarction: Death of cells caused by lack of blood. In the case of stroke, infarction is typically the result of blockage of blood flow in the brain because of a blood clot.

Intracerebral: One of those fancy doctor terms, in this case meaning nothing more than *within the brain.*

Intracranial: The space inside the large skull cavity occupied by the brain, as well as the leathery brain covering called the *dura mater,* the **subarachnoid space,** and the blood vessels and nerves going to and from the brain.

Intracerebral hemorrhage: Bleeding from an artery within the brain — not in the **subarachnoid space** around the brain.

Ischemia (ih SKEEM ee uh): Decreased blood flow to an area of the body, causing cells in that part of the body to starve due to lack of the oxygen and glucose the cells are supposed to be getting from the blood. Unlike much of the rest of the body's cells, the brain doesn't tolerate ischemia very well — even minutes without blood can cause brain damage or even death.

Ischemic stroke: Stroke caused by lack of blood flow (**ischemia**) — usually because a blood clot has blocked a blood vessel in the brain. (In this book, I often refer to ischemic strokes as **white strokes.**)

Lipid: A fat found in the blood.

Low-density lipoprotein (LDL): One of the fat transporters that carries lipids in the body, often called the "bad" cholesterol because it deposits fats throughout the body and causes atherosclerotic plaque, which can lead to stroke. Studies indicate that lower levels of LDL in the blood mean lower risk for atherosclerosis, heart disease, and stroke.

Magnetic resonance imaging (MRI) scan: A procedure done with a diagnostic machine that uses a magnetic field and radio waves to produce images of what's inside the body. MRI scans have been important in diagnosing types of stroke because the pictures are clear and help detect certain types of stroke earlier than other tests.

Microaneurysm: An **aneurysm** that forms in the very small arteries deep inside the substance of the brain. They are only a millimeter or so in diameter and are related to **hypertension** and **diabetes.**

Neurologist: A doctor who specializes in studying and treating problems with the brain and nervous system.

Occupational therapist: A healthcare professional trained to help individuals who suffer disabilities due to stroke or other conditions by teaching them to become independent in their daily activities, whether in the home or at work.

Physical therapist: A healthcare professional trained to help individuals who have disabilities due to stroke or other conditions by teaching them to walk again, use a wheelchair, and perform other physical functions.

Plaque: Deposits of fat and other components that build up in the blood vessels and cause damage and blood clots.

Red stroke: A term perhaps unique to this book that describes strokes caused by bleeding, referring to **intracerebral hemorrhage** and **subarachnoid hemorrhage.** I believe this helps visualize and understand what's happening with these types of strokes, but your doctor may not know what you're talking about if you say *red stroke,* so it's a good idea to also become familiar with the correct terms given in the preceding sentence.

Saturated fats: A fat that is typically solid and found mostly in animal products, such as meat and butter. Eat too much saturated fat, and you increase your risk of stroke.

Social worker: A healthcare professional trained to help individuals, including stroke patients and their families, cope with their situation and pursue helpful resources.

Sodium: A mineral found in many foods, and in high levels in table salt, that in excess can aggravate high blood pressure. **High blood pressure** is the leading risk factor for stroke.

Spasticity: A condition, linked to stroke as well as other diseases and disabilities, in which limb muscles contract uncontrollably and painfully. See Chapter 16 for more on spasticity and potential treatments for it.

Spinal tap (lumbar puncture): A fictional rock band that was the subject of a film called. . . . Okay, actually, in this book anyway, it refers to a test to determine cause of stroke that involves using a needle to extract spinal fluid from the lumbar area of the spinal column. Like most rock bands, though, its reputation is much worse than its bite. The procedure is usually no more painful than having blood drawn from your arm.

Statins or **statin drugs:** Very handy drugs that are known to simultaneously raise levels of HDL ("good" cholesterol) in the blood as they lower LDL ("bad" cholesterol).

Stroke: The sudden interruption of the blood supply to the brain caused by a blockage of a blood vessel or the rupture of a blood vessel.

Subarachnoid hemorrhage: Bleeding from a ruptured vessel in the **subarachnoid space,** which is between the skull and the brain.

Subarachnoid space: The narrow area between the skull and the brain that is filled with a clear fluid called **cerebrospinal fluid** (CSF). Nerves and blood vessels traverse this space on their way to and from the brain.

Systolic blood pressure: A measure of blood pressure when the heart is contracting — or forcing the blood in the arteries at its maximum level. The higher number in your blood pressure reading.

Tissue plasminogen activator (TPA): A clot-dissolving drug approved for treatment of **ischemic stroke** when diagnosed and implemented within three hours of the time that stroke symptoms began. TPA is proven to prevent disability, but it can cause **intracerebral hemorrhage.**

Transient ischemic attack (TIA): An **ischemic stroke** that doesn't last long enough to cause apparent permanent damage or infarction.

Triglyceride: A common type of fat found in the diet (vegetable oil, olive oil, and shortening) as well as our body. High triglyceride levels in the body indicate risk of diabetes.

Vascular dementia: A form of dementia caused by a series of small strokes.

Vein: A blood vessel that carries blood to the heart from various parts of the body.

Ventricles of the brain: The four cavities that divide the brain. Ventricles are filled with fluid that flows from one ventricle to another as well as into the **subarachnoid space** surrounding the brain. If the flow is blocked by a clot or bleeding, pressure builds up in the ventricles and can crush the brain against the inside of the skull. (It is only a coincidence that the heart has four ventricles as well, two on the right side of the heart and two on the left.)

Warfarin: A drug used to prevent blood clotting, often prescribed to survivors or others at high risk for **ischemic stroke.**

White stroke: I made this term up because I think the name **ischemic stroke** is hard to read, hard to say, and hard to remember. The brain gets whiter when its blood supply is cut off. Ischemic stroke just means that the brain isn't getting enough red blood. I thought it would help you remember the cause of ischemic stroke, so I have used this term in this book. You may not find it used anywhere else, at least not yet. The more I have used the term, the more I like it. You can thank a friend of mine, Eugene Passamani, a cardiologist who first told me strokes are like wine — either red or white.

Index

• *C* •

• S •

Notes

Notes

BUSINESS, CAREERS & PERSONAL FINANCE

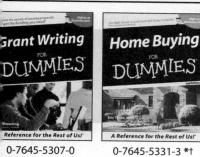

0-7645-5307-0

0-7645-5331-3 *†

Also available:
- Accounting For Dummies †
  0-7645-5314-3
- Business Plans Kit For Dummies †
  0-7645-5365-8
- Cover Letters For Dummies
  0-7645-5224-4
- Frugal Living For Dummies
  0-7645-5403-4
- Leadership For Dummies
  0-7645-5176-0
- Managing For Dummies
  0-7645-1771-6

- Marketing For Dummies
  0-7645-5600-2
- Personal Finance For Dummies *
  0-7645-2590-5
- Project Management For Dummies
  0-7645-5283-X
- Resumes For Dummies †
  0-7645-5471-9
- Selling For Dummies
  0-7645-5363-1
- Small Business Kit For Dummies *†
  0-7645-5093-4

HOME & BUSINESS COMPUTER BASICS

0-7645-4074-2

0-7645-3758-X

Also available:
- ACT! 6 For Dummies
  0-7645-2645-6
- iLife '04 All-in-One Desk Reference
  For Dummies
  0-7645-7347-0
- iPAQ For Dummies
  0-7645-6769-1
- Mac OS X Panther Timesaving
  Techniques For Dummies
  0-7645-5812-9
- Macs For Dummies
  0-7645-5656-8

- Microsoft Money 2004 For Dummies
  0-7645-4195-1
- Office 2003 All-in-One Desk Reference
  For Dummies
  0-7645-3883-7
- Outlook 2003 For Dummies
  0-7645-3759-8
- PCs For Dummies
  0-7645-4074-2
- TiVo For Dummies
  0-7645-6923-6
- Upgrading and Fixing PCs For Dummies
  0-7645-1665-5
- Windows XP Timesaving Techniques
  For Dummies
  0-7645-3748-2

FOOD, HOME, GARDEN, HOBBIES, MUSIC & PETS

0-7645-5295-3

0-7645-5232-5

Also available:
- Bass Guitar For Dummies
  0-7645-2487-9
- Diabetes Cookbook For Dummies
  0-7645-5230-9
- Gardening For Dummies *
  0-7645-5130-2
- Guitar For Dummies
  0-7645-5106-X
- Holiday Decorating For Dummies
  0-7645-2570-0
- Home Improvement All-in-One
  For Dummies
  0-7645-5680-0

- Knitting For Dummies
  0-7645-5395-X
- Piano For Dummies
  0-7645-5105-1
- Puppies For Dummies
  0-7645-5255-4
- Scrapbooking For Dummies
  0-7645-7208-3
- Senior Dogs For Dummies
  0-7645-5818-8
- Singing For Dummies
  0-7645-2475-5
- 30-Minute Meals For Dummies
  0-7645-2589-1

INTERNET & DIGITAL MEDIA

0-7645-1664-7

0-7645-6924-4

Also available:
- 2005 Online Shopping Directory
  For Dummies
  0-7645-7495-7
- CD & DVD Recording For Dummies
  0-7645-5956-7
- eBay For Dummies
  0-7645-5654-1
- Fighting Spam For Dummies
  0-7645-5965-6
- Genealogy Online For Dummies
  0-7645-5964-8
- Google For Dummies
  0-7645-4420-9

- Home Recording For Musicians
  For Dummies
  0-7645-1634-5
- The Internet For Dummies
  0-7645-4173-0
- iPod & iTunes For Dummies
  0-7645-7772-7
- Preventing Identity Theft For Dummies
  0-7645-7336-5
- Pro Tools All-in-One Desk Reference
  For Dummies
  0-7645-5714-9
- Roxio Easy Media Creator For Dummies
  0-7645-7131-1

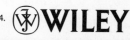

SPORTS, FITNESS, PARENTING, RELIGION & SPIRITUALITY

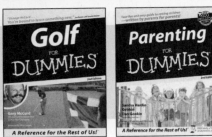

0-7645-5146-9

0-7645-5418-2

Also available:
- Adoption For Dummies
  0-7645-5488-3
- Basketball For Dummies
  0-7645-5248-1
- The Bible For Dummies
  0-7645-5296-1
- Buddhism For Dummies
  0-7645-5359-3
- Catholicism For Dummies
  0-7645-5391-7
- Hockey For Dummies
  0-7645-5228-7

- Judaism For Dummies
  0-7645-5299-6
- Martial Arts For Dummies
  0-7645-5358-5
- Pilates For Dummies
  0-7645-5397-6
- Religion For Dummies
  0-7645-5264-3
- Teaching Kids to Read For Dummies
  0-7645-4043-2
- Weight Training For Dummies
  0-7645-5168-X
- Yoga For Dummies
  0-7645-5117-5

TRAVEL

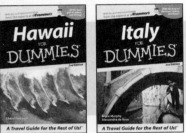

0-7645-5438-7

0-7645-5453-0

Also available:
- Alaska For Dummies
  0-7645-1761-9
- Arizona For Dummies
  0-7645-6938-4
- Cancún and the Yucatán For Dummies
  0-7645-2437-2
- Cruise Vacations For Dummies
  0-7645-6941-4
- Europe For Dummies
  0-7645-5456-5
- Ireland For Dummies
  0-7645-5455-7

- Las Vegas For Dummies
  0-7645-5448-4
- London For Dummies
  0-7645-4277-X
- New York City For Dummies
  0-7645-6945-7
- Paris For Dummies
  0-7645-5494-8
- RV Vacations For Dummies
  0-7645-5443-3
- Walt Disney World & Orlando For Dummies
  0-7645-6943-0

GRAPHICS, DESIGN & WEB DEVELOPMENT

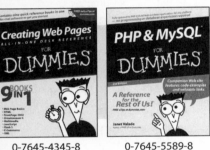

0-7645-4345-8

0-7645-5589-8

Also available:
- Adobe Acrobat 6 PDF For Dummies
  0-7645-3760-1
- Building a Web Site For Dummies
  0-7645-7144-3
- Dreamweaver MX 2004 For Dummies
  0-7645-4342-3
- FrontPage 2003 For Dummies
  0-7645-3882-9
- HTML 4 For Dummies
  0-7645-1995-6
- Illustrator CS For Dummies
  0-7645-4084-X

- Macromedia Flash MX 2004 For Dummies
  0-7645-4358-X
- Photoshop 7 All-in-One Desk Reference For Dummies
  0-7645-1667-1
- Photoshop CS Timesaving Techniques For Dummies
  0-7645-6782-9
- PHP 5 For Dummies
  0-7645-4166-8
- PowerPoint 2003 For Dummies
  0-7645-3908-6
- QuarkXPress 6 For Dummies
  0-7645-2593-X

NETWORKING, SECURITY, PROGRAMMING & DATABASES

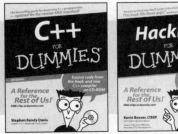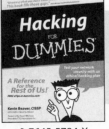

0-7645-6852-3

0-7645-5784-X

Also available:
- A+ Certification For Dummies
  0-7645-4187-0
- Access 2003 All-in-One Desk Reference For Dummies
  0-7645-3988-4
- Beginning Programming For Dummies
  0-7645-4997-9
- C For Dummies
  0-7645-7068-4
- Firewalls For Dummies
  0-7645-4048-3
- Home Networking For Dummies
  0-7645-42796

- Network Security For Dummies
  0-7645-1679-5
- Networking For Dummies
  0-7645-1677-9
- TCP/IP For Dummies
  0-7645-1760-0
- VBA For Dummies
  0-7645-3989-2
- Wireless All In-One Desk Reference For Dummies
  0-7645-7496-5
- Wireless Home Networking For Dummies
  0-7645-3910-8

ALTH & SELF-HELP

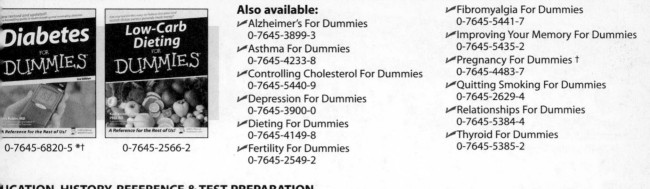

0-7645-6820-5 *†

0-7645-2566-2

Also available:
- Alzheimer's For Dummies
  0-7645-3899-3
- Asthma For Dummies
  0-7645-4233-8
- Controlling Cholesterol For Dummies
  0-7645-5440-9
- Depression For Dummies
  0-7645-3900-0
- Dieting For Dummies
  0-7645-4149-8
- Fertility For Dummies
  0-7645-2549-2

- Fibromyalgia For Dummies
  0-7645-5441-7
- Improving Your Memory For Dummies
  0-7645-5435-2
- Pregnancy For Dummies †
  0-7645-4483-7
- Quitting Smoking For Dummies
  0-7645-2629-4
- Relationships For Dummies
  0-7645-5384-4
- Thyroid For Dummies
  0-7645-5385-2

UCATION, HISTORY, REFERENCE & TEST PREPARATION

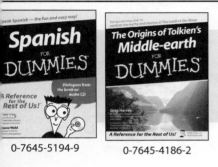

0-7645-5194-9

0-7645-4186-2

Also available:
- Algebra For Dummies
  0-7645-5325-9
- British History For Dummies
  0-7645-7021-8
- Calculus For Dummies
  0-7645-2498-4
- English Grammar For Dummies
  0-7645-5322-4
- Forensics For Dummies
  0-7645-5580-4
- The GMAT For Dummies
  0-7645-5251-1
- Inglés Para Dummies
  0-7645-5427-1

- Italian For Dummies
  0-7645-5196-5
- Latin For Dummies
  0-7645-5431-X
- Lewis & Clark For Dummies
  0-7645-2545-X
- Research Papers For Dummies
  0-7645-5426-3
- The SAT I For Dummies
  0-7645-7193-1
- Science Fair Projects For Dummies
  0-7645-5460-3
- U.S. History For Dummies
  0-7645-5249-X

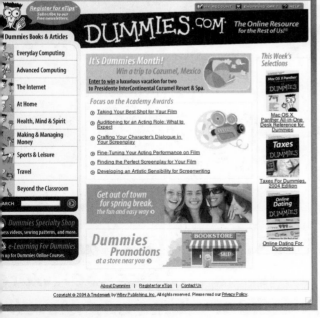

Get smart @ dummies.com®

- **Find a full list of Dummies titles**
- **Look into loads of FREE on-site articles**
- **Sign up for FREE eTips e-mailed to you weekly**
- **See what other products carry the Dummies name**
- **Shop directly from the Dummies bookstore**
- **Enter to win new prizes every month!**

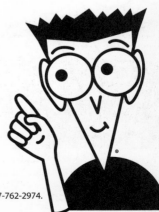

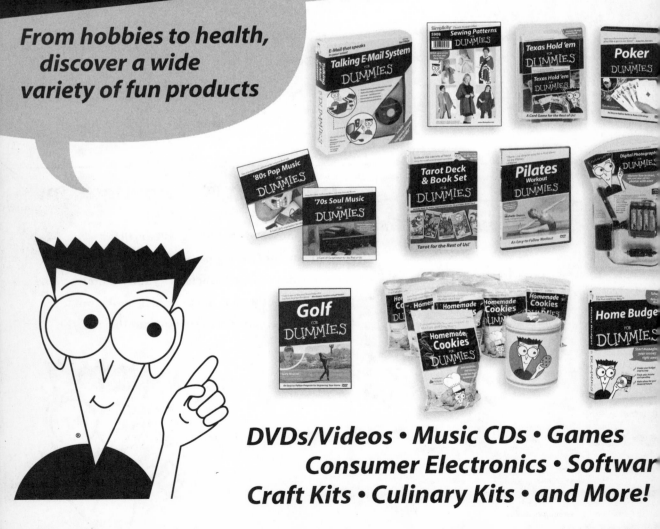
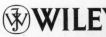